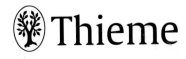

This book is dedicated to Gustav Bucky—
radiologist, inventor, teacher.
And with love to Mary and Jerry Crockett.

Getting Started in Clinical Radiology

From Image to Diagnosis

George W. Eastman, M.D.
Professor of Radiology
Virchow Campus of the Charité
Humboldt University and Free University of Berlin
Berlin, Germany

Christoph Wald, M.D., Ph.D.
Assistant Professor of Radiology
Tufts University School of Medicine
Boston, USA
Department of Radiology
Lahey Clinic
Burlington, MA, USA

Jane Crossin, M.D.
Senior Lecturer Medical Imaging
Department of Medical Imaging
Royal Brisbane Hospital
Brisbane, Australia

1035 illustrations

Thieme
Stuttgart · New York

Library of Congress Cataloging-in-Publication Data

Eastman, George W.
    Getting started in clinical radiology : from image to
diagnosis / George W. Eastman, Christoph Wald, Jane
Crossin.
        p. ; cm.
    Includes index.
    ISBN 3-13-140361-6 (GTV : alk. paper) –
    ISBN 1-58890-356-7 (TNY : alk. paper)
        1. Radiology, Medical–Outlines, syllabi, etc.
        2. Diagnostic imaging–Outlines, syllabi, etc.
    [DNLM: 1. Diagnostic Imaging–Problems and Exercises.
    2. Radiology–methods–Problems and Exercises.
    WN 18.2 E13g 2005] I. Wald, Christoph. II. Crossin, Jane.
    III. Title.
    RC78.17.E37 2005
    616.07'57–dc22
                                    2005016549

Illustrator: Andrea Schnitzler, Innsbruck, Austria

© 2006 Georg Thieme Verlag,
Rüdigerstrasse 14, 70469 Stuttgart, Germany
http://www.thieme.de
Thieme New York, 333 Seventh Avenue,
New York, NY 10001 USA
http://www.thieme.com

Typesetting by Mitterweger & Partner, Plankstadt
Printed in Germany by Grammlich, Pliezhausen

ISBN 3-13-140361-6 (GTV)
ISBN 1-58890-356-7 (TNY)

Important note: Medicine is an ever-changing science undergoing continual development. Research and clinical experience are continually expanding our knowledge, in particular our knowledge of proper treatment and drug therapy. Insofar as this book mentions any dosage or application, readers may rest assured that the authors, editors, and publishers have made every effort to ensure that such references are in accordance with **the state of knowledge at the time of production of the book.**

Nevertheless, this does not involve, imply, or express any guarantee or responsibility on the part of the publishers in respect to any dosage instructions and forms of applications stated in the book. **Every user is requested to examine carefully** the manufacturers' leaflets accompanying each drug and to check, if necessary in consultation with a physician or specialist, whether the dosage schedules mentioned therein or the contraindications stated by the manufacturers differ from the statements made in the present book. Such examination is particularly important with drugs that are either rarely used or have been newly released on the market. Every dosage schedule or every form of application used is entirely at the user's own risk and responsibility. The authors and publishers request every user to report to the publishers any discrepancies or inaccuracies noticed. If errors in this work are found after publication, errata will be posted at www.thieme.com on the product description page.

Foreword

The opening sentence says it all: "Radiology can be a lot of fun!" It summarizes what is unique about this book.

Radiology books designed for medical students have as their main purpose an introduction to the science and art of medical imaging. Behind this obvious purpose is an implicit intent also to fascinate students, and thereby to inspire some of the most susceptible and capable to choose a career in radiology. An early attempt to inspire students grew out of a classroom medical student teaching program, in which the radiologist Lucy Frank Squires was assisted by students and radiology trainees like myself. That course was wildly successful and attracted many students to a lifetime interest in radiology. What made this program unique was its light-hearted approach and the use of everyday household objects to explain radiological principles to the students, and to make them feel comfortable in the process.

This text by George W. Eastman, Chris Wald, and Jane Crossin is, in many ways, an extension of that successful humanistic formula for medical student teaching. The authors have captured our attention by introducing the subject through the eyes of fictional medical students to whom they have given form, substance, and personalities with emotions and fears. Although fictional, the characters are realistic in their foibles. What is new and different in this book is its clever use of these students to make us inquisitive about them as well as the real subject matter. This process relieves some of the inherent dryness of the topic by involving our hearts in the sharing of the uncertainties and concerns of the characters, and it captures our attention.

The thread of human connection to our fictional students weaves its way through the book. In the introduction we learn of the diverse backgrounds of the students, something of their private lives, and gain an inkling of their interactions with each other. In the chapter on chest radiology, we sympathetically experience the challenge of the subject material through their eyes.

The complexity of modern radiology is reflected in the organization and content of the book. The students' introduction to radiology starts with technical aspects of basic image acquisition and extends to the fundamentals of psychophysics in image perception, an important topic often overlooked in radiology texts. What follows includes principles of disease detection, disease diagnosis, and appropriate examination selection. As one who was a radiology trainee in the 1960s, I never cease to be amazed at how simple life was at that time. One chose between either film radiography or fluoroscopy; there was nothing else but nuclear medicine, which was then still in its infancy. Now, the wide range of imaging modalities makes it essential to learn how to choose between them to make the best use of imaging.

For this voyage of the medical student into the world of radiology, the authors have set sail toward a unique polar star that encompasses humanism as well as comprehensive imaging science. The text promises to introduce and guide a new generation of students into the fascinating world of radiological imaging.

Reginald Greene

A Word of Thanks

We would like to thank all who have so generously contributed to the development of the overall concept and final realization of this book. First of all there are the many students and residents we persuaded to act as "didactic guinea pigs" for us. Their remarks were helpful and encouraging, sometimes keenly observed: "Awkward style!" Their contributions were substantial. The same holds true for a number of residents and fellows as well as staff radiologists in our respective departments poring over parts of the book and sharing their views on particular features. To ensure that the cases provided were not only radiologically correct but also reflected the referring physicians' point of view, we asked quite a number of colleagues from other specialties to review the respective chapters. In particular we would like to thank Professor Hartmann (Ophthalmology), Dr. Schlunz (Facial and Plastic Surgery), Dr. Matthias (Ear Nose and Throat Surgery), Dr. Kandziora (Trauma Surgery), all from the Charité Hospital in Berlin; Professor Wagner (Radiology) from Marburg University; and Professor von Kummer (Neuroradiology) from Dresden University. All analogies used in Chapter 3, "Tools in Radiology", were double-checked for correctness from an engineering point of view by Dr. Anton of Siemens Medical Systems. We would also like to acknowledge the support of Thavaganeshan Vasuthevan of GE Medical Systems.

We owe special thanks to Professor Wermke of the Charité for the permission to use his ultrasound images for Chapter 9, "Gastrointestinal Radiology."

We are grateful to a long list of colleagues (see opposite) who have supported this book by supplying us with some of their best case material or in other ways.

None of this would have happened had it not been for the support of the publishers, Thieme. Special thanks go to Cliff Bergman, Juergen Luethje, and Antje Voss. They readily adopted the concept and enhanced or smoothed over parts of it where this was felt to be necessary. They accompanied the book—with patience and motivation—through the production phase.

Each one of us has—at different times in our professional lives—benefited from working with inspired radiologists who had the ability to plant the enthusiasm for practicing and teaching radiology in our heads and hearts. On G.W.E.'s side these were Drs. Jürgen Freyschmidt, Hans-Stefan Stender, Klaus Langenbruch, Reginald Greene, Dan Kopans, Ad van Voorthuizen, and Jan Vielvoye. Among others, Drs. Robert E. Wise, Frank Scholz, Alain Pollak, and Roger Jenkins from the Lahey Clinic in Boston have been an invaluable inspiration for C.W. to remain in an academic career and look beyond the obvious. J.C. thanks Drs. Gord Weisbrod, Steve Herman, and Naeem Merchant in Toronto for sharing both their enthusiasm for radiology and their encyclopedic radiological knowledge. All of us loved to learn with books by Benjamin Felson, Clyde Helms, and Lucy Frank Squire.

Our families have, of course, felt the ups and downs of this project the most. The ease and the many different ways in which our children learn about this world we live in were a great source of ideas. The critical minds of our spouses put an end to many initial little afterthoughts, that, on reflection, it would have been unwise to include in this book. Many thanks for their patience.

Finally, this book—like all of radiology—is a dynamic affair. Any comments, criticisms, and suggestions for improvement are most welcome and will be considered in its further development. All those involved in teaching who would like to contribute first-rate didactic material are also invited to do so. All contacts can be made via george.w.eastman@thieme.com.

George W. Eastman
Chris Wald
Jane Crossin

Colleagues and Co-workers Who Have Contributed Images to this Book

Contents

A Short Run through Radiological Basics

From Detection to Diagnosis and Beyond

1   Why Another Textbook of Radiology?

Can You Imagine Radiology to be Fun?

Radiology can be a lot of fun! It is this very personal experience of the authors that will accompany you throughout this book and hopefully throughout the rest of your medical life. It is also the main reason why we considered this book to be necessary. Can diagnostic imaging and the therapy of patients in need be a pleasant task? The answer is a resounding "yes." Successful management in medicine relies on keeping a certain distance from the events. Empathy and respect are essential for a trustful relationship with the patient. The optimal path to the right diagnosis and subsequent adequate therapy, however, requires primarily clear thinking. Clear thinking, in turn, greatly profits from motivation, optimism, and enjoyment of what one is doing. The enthusiasm for a "great case," which temporarily seems to ignore the often tragic personal fate of the patient, must not be taken away from the radiologist. The same is true for learning about radiology—as a student, as a young doctor: One has to enthuse the neophytes for the fascinating field of radiology!

What Is So Special about Learning (and Teaching) Radiology?

Radiology is a gigantic, continually growing specialty that gets ever more complex by the month. It is, for several reasons, not to be learned by heart. The tools of image acquisition and image analysis have to be mastered, i.e., their principles have to be understood. Understanding the principles of imaging—just like the understanding of any individual image—is primarily an intellectual challenge. It is on this foundation that specific knowledge can be accumulated, of course through reading the literature but most of all through very personal transfer of experience: "There is no substitute for a seasoned radiology teacher." In few medical fields can the exchange of knowledge between the teacher and the trainee be as intense, interactive, and multifaceted as in radiology. Radiology for that reason is a didactic specialty "par excellence." Using exemplary image material, most relevant diagnostic techniques can be taught and learned. That is the great opportunity of academic radiology—we just have to seize it.

What Makes This Textbook Different to Others?

Well . . . a lot of things. But one of the main ideas we try to convey in this book is the overriding importance of a sound indication for every radiological examination or therapy. The number of nonindicated examinations is unfortunately high; the driving forces are manifold: litigation, examinations that are "en vogue," overworked referring doctors who would rather get the scan and then examine the patient, and the practice of self-referral by nonradiologists who have a financial interest in imaging the patient in their own private practice or institution. All lead to many unnecessary diagnostic examinations with unintended consequences for our patients. Overutilization also poses a threat for the future—i.e., your professional life and our healthcare systems—as it is not economically sustainable in any of today's societies. We would like to infuse you with the right attitude and give a proper orientation of what is indicated when. The indication guidelines of the British Royal College of Radiologists under the title "Making the best use of a Department of Clinical Radiology" have thus been inserted into and adapted to this book.

How Is This Book Structured?

The first part of this book, entitled "**A Short Run Through Radiological Basics**," will describe and hopefully allow you to understand the essentials of imaging. For starters, you are going to be fed the technical principles of image acquisition. To keep this part digestible, "normal life" analogies have been recruited wherever complex technologies made this necessary and where it was felt to be didactically appropriate. Subsequently we'll take you through the phenomena and procedures that help you tackle image analysis in diagnostic imaging. We take special care to alert you to the importance of psychophysical perception: in a world filled with fantastically expensive imaging equipment it is still your visual and central nervous system that detects and categorizes disease. This fundamental truth is frequently underrepresented in other texts. Last but not least, you are going to learn about the obvious and not so obvious risks of imaging and image-guided therapy.

The second, the clinical, part of this book is entitled "**From Detection to Diagnosis and Beyond**." You will get to know not only the specific examination modalities for each organ system but also the most efficient diagnostic work-up in emergency radiology—under circumstances you will encounter in your not too distant future professional medical life when you are most likely to make crucial decisions yourself. You will be confronted with cases to solve just as if you were already engulfed in clinical routine. Every individual problem is approached by a combination of image analyses, taking into account relevant available history, and whatever clinical symptoms you might be able to verify yourself. The path to the right diagnosis is then laid out—you just have to stay on it. The differential diagnoses are described in the approximate order of likelihood, if that does not interfere with the didactic point to be made. The traditional pathologically oriented approach thus takes a step back to leave center stage to radiological morphology: it is just you and the image you have to evaluate.

Who Will Accompany You through This Book?

Five medical students will see you through this book: Giufeng, Hannah, Joey, Paul, and Ajay. All of them are bright, highly motivated kids, well prepared by their teachers and eager to solve cases on their own. It goes without saying that they eventually present their findings to "their" radiologist in charge—to get the final blessing and to learn

even more. Their first few weeks in radiology have made them inspired diagnosticians, running down interesting cases and not giving up before they find a convincing diagnosis. They are also a truly international bunch, having been attracted to this academic hospital in "down under" Sydney for a variety of reasons. (Hannah, Giufeng, Joey, Paul, and Ajay are, of course, fictitious persons. All stories relating to them are also pure fiction. We would like to thank our young colleagues and collaborators Juliane Stoll, Il-Kang Na, Ralph Patrick Chukwuedo, Ansgar Leidinger and Tino Bejach for the permission to use their pictures. Working together with them was a lot of fun. A great thanks goes to our pleasant young colleague Gero Wieners who posed as Gregory. The patients' names are also fictitious. Similarities to real persons are not intended and are pure coincidence. The cases are didactically optimized and compressed to fit the objective of this book.)

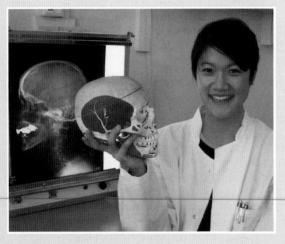

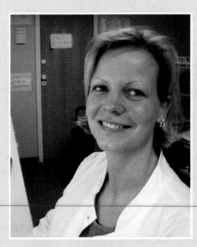

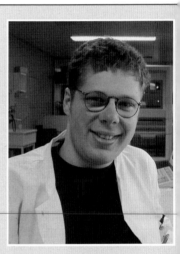

Giufeng (Chinese for "the gentle one") (Fig. 1.1) is a native of Sydney, to where her parents moved in the eighties straight from Singapore. As you can undoubtedly tell from the picture, she has developed a special interest in neuroradiology. She knows everything about the cranial nerves, their tracts and nuclei. The sensory organs are another one of her specialties. For that and other reasons, Gregory, the senior resident assigned to neuroradiology, frequently visits with her.

Hannah (Fig. 1.2) has come from Berlin for her final year in medical school. Her love of the sun, the beach, and classical music got her to the "emerald city." If she had to pick a favorite field in radiology, she would probably choose musculoskeletal radiology. She has already made up her mind to try her luck in radiology, but if that doesn't work out she will try to become an orthopod. She never loses control, however mixed-up things may be. Wiseguys get finished off by her with just a few carefully chosen words. Her private passion is—you guessed it already—surfing on Sydney's Bondi beach.

Paul (Fig. 1.3) says he sucked radiology in with his mother's milk. His father is a medical physicist, his mother a successful painter of abstract art, his brother a Melbourne investment broker almost unscathed by any bear attacks. Paul loves to dive into complex cases much like others get submerged in the latest thriller by Michael Crichton. In any case: He finds radiology a very attractive field—almost as attractive as . . . well, as far as Paul is concerned, he is getting sick and tired of this neuro guy and his interventions.

What Is There to Say about the Style of the Book?

Radiology is a thriving field with fashions, moods, fascinating personalities, and a lot of history to go around. Radiologists love to assign names to phenomena, signs, and techniques. Most of these are globally understood—radiology was a truly global thing from the very beginning. So there are a lot of Latin, German, and French terms—add a Greek cracker now and then. If they help us understand, we should use them. Some remind us of great physicians who were inventors, researchers, teachers. It does not hurt to acknowledge their accomplishments, and we support that by giving a little worthwhile or possibly useless information about them now and then in this book.

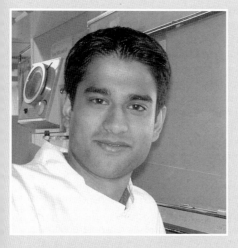

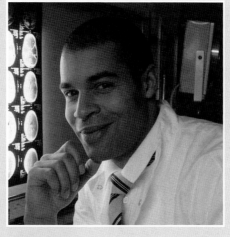

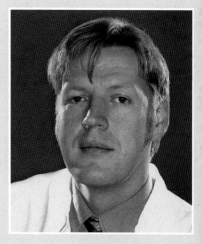

Ajay (Fig. 1.**4**) is originally from Johannesburg, South Africa, where his grandfather used to work with a certain Mahatma Ghandi. The family is rumored to be obscenely rich—car manufacturing, real estate, you name it. He is already married at the age of 25, much to the sorrow of the women around him. His wife is dashingly beautiful and three handsome kids are coming right after their father. Ajay has an untamable urge to tell delicate jokes to everyone, in one of four languages. He is interested in radiology because he loves to handle expensive hardware.

Joey (Fig. 1.**5**) has just managed to make the right histological diagnosis off just one radiograph—and seems to enjoy the experience. He will hopefully make this a habit. Joey just loves intervention. Every time he watches a difficult angiographic or drainage procedure, his fingers grab for imaginary catheters, guide wires, and needles. The interventional folks have recognized his passion for their trade and let him work with them whenever it is possible. As for his social life, he comes across as the "big loner." Apart from that he is a cheerful guy from New York who has left that city for the first time in his life to do his radiology "down under."

And then there is **Gregory** (Fig. 1.**6**), of course. As already mentioned, he is the young and enterprising senior resident with a special interest in neuroradiology. He has made it a habit to take care of the medical students—with very definite preferences and in more than one way. He is hoping for an academic career. His hormonal status is acknowledged with benevolent interest by many in the department. A nice guy at heart, he can turn into a son of a . . . at times. When you come right down to it, he is just one of us normal guys in academia.

2   Radiology's Role in Medicine

What Is So Different in Radiology as Opposed to Other Clinical Disciplines?

A radiologist primarily approaches the patients by looking at images, in a procedure quite similar to the one pathologists normally follow but quite unlike what any other clinical specialist would do. The unbiased analysis of the image is the first, and undoubtedly an abstract, intellectual step. This certainly implies that radiologists must be pretty brainy, or else they can lay down their arms right there. Thus, there should be a little Sherlock Holmes in every one of them, although county sheriffs have also been reported to survive. It is in a secondary step that we study the clinical symptoms in order to verify, improve, or—yes—dump our diagnosis and go back to square one. This procedure has many advantages, but it makes radiologists vulnerable when information is withheld or cannot be correctly evaluated.

Which Other Special Aspects Are There to Consider?

The radiology department is basically a consultative service unit for the hospital. Few other disciplines can do without it. For that reason, communication with colleagues from other fields is tremendously important and not always without glitches. At the same time it is rather transparent to the referring doctors what the radiologists do and do not do; few colleagues talk about and document their work as well as radiologists do. Patient management and the administration of reporting as well as image distribution are further cornerstones for swift and effective diagnoses and interventions.

What Else Could Improve Your Compassion for the Radiologists?

A few, admittedly cocky, statements might get you on the road. A radiologist is:

- The heroic person who presents—swiftly and accurately—hundreds of images to a bunch of hotheaded trauma surgeons in their morning round, some of whom have studied those very images with much more time and with the patient and her or his symptoms at hand. Any surgeon will tell you: There is nothing like chewing up a radiologist for breakfast before a great day in the operating room. You need a big heart and a lot of sympathy for all these colleagues whose psychological pressure at times surpasses that suffered by the radiological profession.
- The person who—on a single day—pronounces hundreds of patients to be healthy in heart and lung just on the basis of a single chest film. He or she then dares to put this down in writing, for all colleagues to see and question from then on to eternity.
- The person who—on the basis of rudimentary clinical data, if any—presents available image material at the noontime general medical radiology meeting, with listing of delicately weighted differential diagnoses for every patient, while at the same time out of the dark of the back of the room miraculously appears the hitherto unknown information that renders two-thirds of these differential diagnoses ridiculous.
- The person who has to reconsider all diagnostic and interventional procedures every half year because rapid technological and scientific developments in radiology make this absolutely necessary.
- To call it an end, the person who starts to shiver, groan, and giggle foolishly when finally coming across the splendid example of a pigmented villonodular synovitis that has been the missing link in the personal teaching file.

This has to be sufficient as justification for this book and as a peek into the soul and life of radiology.

A Short Run through Radiological Basics

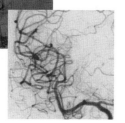

3　Tools in Radiology

3.1　Projection Radiography

Good old projection radiography remains one of the staples of radiology, although a little over 100 years old. And it is by no means obsolete even in times of multi-million-dollar high-tech imaging equipment. The bulk of all diagnostic imaging studies is still done with this technology. Mammography, a prominent representative of this group, is the only imaging study that has been proven to lower patient mortality significantly—if performed correctly and, of course, only in women. The basic technical principle of projection radiography is simple. However, the complete chain of events from generating the x-ray beam to viewing the developed image can be full of surprises to keep even the "pro" busy making sure everything is done properly and the radiograph at hand is a quality product. With insufficient knowledge or lack of experience and care, things can easily derail—there are enough catastrophic studies to prove that point.

Generation of X-Rays

A high-voltage current is built up between a cathode and an anode, all of this inside a vacuum tube (Fig. 3.1). The cathode is heated to about 2000 °C by a specific heating filament. Electrons are emitted by the cathode, accelerated by the electric field between cathode and anode, and hit the anode with considerable energy, where they induce electromagnetic radiation of the type called x-rays. These rays are richer in energy the higher the applied voltage. The area where the electrons hit the anode is called the focus. As a lot of heat is generated in the process, the anode consists of a heat-resistant disk covered with tungsten in most cases. The disk rotates quickly to disperse the heat along its circumference, thus forming a focal track. The vacuum tube is surrounded by oil inside a lead-lined housing that features only one small opening for the radiation to escape.

The generated radiation has a spectrum, or spread of energies, only a part of which can be used for imaging. Some of the so-called "soft" or very low-energy rays would be completely absorbed by the body's soft tissues and thus only increase the dose to the patient without contributing anything to the image. For that reason, they are filtered out, typically by an aluminum or copper sheet. In addition the radiation exiting the tube housing is also constrained by lead collimators that keep the beam strictly limited to the body area of interest.

Attenuation of X-Rays

X-rays are attenuated as they pass through the patient's body. Two processes play a role: absorption and scatter. With lower-energy radiation (corresponding to lower exposure voltage) **absorption** dominates. It correlates well with the atomic number of the irradiated matter. Mammography makes proper use of this characteristic and employs low-energy radiation to detect minute spots of calcium in the breast that may indicate cancer.

With high-energy radiation (corresponding to high exposure voltage) **scatter** is mainly responsible for attenuation. In this process the radiation beam loses energy and is diverted in all directions (scattered). The scattered radiation increases with irradiated body volume. It is hazardous for patients and their immediate vicinity, i.e., the angiographer standing alongside the patient to work with his or her catheters. When scatter reaches the detector, it causes an unstructured shade of gray that diminishes the contrast of the image. A scatter grid (Fig. 3.1) positioned in front of the detector reduces this "diverted" radiation.

The Guy Who Took Care of the Scatter
Gustav Bucky's name is known to radiologists all over the world for his invention of the scatter grid in 1912. After the initial presentation at a medical convention, some colleagues suggested that the images were so good it must be a hoax. Having been forced into emigration by the Nazis, he left Berlin for New York, where he continued his innovative work. With his invention of the grid that is in use in every x-ray machine to this very day he eventually earned the lump sum of $25—ingenuity is definitely not a monetary unit.

Detection of X-Rays

A variety of detectors can make x-rays visible. The simplest is **photographic film**; because of the high spatial resolution one can achieve, it is used in nondestructive testing of industrial materials such as alloy car wheels or gas pipelines. To expose film alone an incredible dose of x-rays is necessary, but that does not matter in this instance. Film is much less sensitive to x-rays than to light—any airport security x-ray scan will show you the inside of your camera without significantly damaging your valuable vacation photos, which proves the point. As light exposes film much better, in diagnostic radiology a combination is used of film and **intensifying screens** that are made of rare earth materials (gadolinium, barium, lanthanum, yttrium). These screens fluoresce when irradiated (just like

Generation of x-Rays

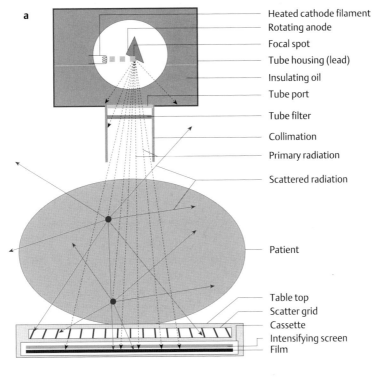

a

Heated cathode filament
Rotating anode
Focal spot
Tube housing (lead)
Insulating oil
Tube port

Tube filter

Collimation

Primary radiation

Scattered radiation

Patient

Table top
Scatter grid
Cassette
Intensifying screen
Film

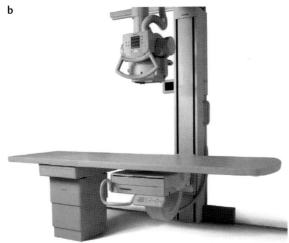

b

Fig. 3.**1 a** The figure shows the generation of x-rays, their attenuation due to scatter, and their detection.
b This is a modern digital projection radiography unit used primarily for skeletal work (by Philips Medical Systems).

the foil of "Bariumplatincyanür" that Wilhelm Conrad Roentgen used in his initial experiments) and thus expose the film. Usually the film is sandwiched between two intensifying screens inside a light-tight cassette.

❗ Film–screen combinations vary greatly in their x-ray sensitivity and spatial resolution and thus have to be selected according to the specific imaging problem to be solved. If the depiction of fine detail is important, the required dose is generally higher. If the dose must be kept as low as possible, such as in children, fine detail must often be sacrificed.

Some intensifying screens emit the main fraction of their light only after stimulation by a laser beam. These screens are called **storage phosphors.** After their exposure they are scanned in a read-out system and their information content is immediately digitized. These screens can register a larger bandwidth of radiation intensity, which is why "over- or underexposure" is widely tolerated by the digital system. The information content of the image and the dose to the patient, however, may be inadequate although the image looks normal at first glance.
Another digital detector that is currently becoming popular consists of a layer of **cesium iodide** crystals on top of

Digital Subtraction Angiography (DSA)

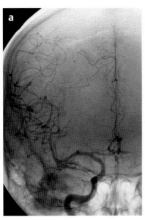 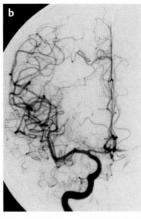

Fig. 3.**2 a**   The arterial vasculature of the brain is very complex. The bony skull is not simple either.
b If a precontrast image is subtracted from the image after contrast administration, the bony structures, especially at the skull base, disappear and the visualization of the vascular tree improves considerably.

an amorphous silicon photodiode panel. The crystals light up when hit by x-rays and their light is then converted into an electronic charge by the photodiode. This is immediately read out by special electronics.

For fluoroscopy (e.g., in small-bowel follow-through or in vascular intervention) **image intensifier systems** are used. A luminescent layer that covers a large-area cathode absorbs the x-rays. The emitted light liberates electrons in the cathode material. These electrons are focused by electronic lenses and hit a small screen that serves as anode. All this happens inside an evacuated large tube. The resulting very bright image is registered by an external television camera and shown on a viewing monitor.

Other digital detectors are used in computed tomography (see p. 9) or are being tried out for projection radiography. The resulting signal is always a digital one, permitting post-processing of images and archiving and image communication with an ease unheard of in analog systems.

Techniques of Exposure

Projection radiography: The usual radiograph is a summation image of the exposed body part. A nodule seen over the lung fields, for example, cannot generally be assigned to the lung, the anterior or posterior chest wall, or even the skin surface, because all these structures are superimposed on each other. Clinical inspection, a little brain work, a lateral projection, a fluoroscopy, or a conventional or computed tomography might help.

> ! In projection radiography, a decrease in transparency or a "shadow" (e.g., a tumor) is bright; an increase in transparency (e.g., air in the bowel) is dark.

Conventional tomography: In conventional tomography, only a single slice of the body (e.g., in the hip joint) is depicted while all others are blurred by motion. During the exposure the x-ray tube and the detector move in opposite directions parallel to the imaging plane. A steel beam connects the two and swivels around a movable axis. The

position of the axis marks the body layer that is imaged motion-free—the tomographic plane. By moving the beam axis ventrally or dorsally, other planes can be selected. Conventional tomography is a beautiful but dying art—well-equipped departments continue to use it for special, mostly skeletal, studies.

Fluoroscopy: In a considerable number of diagnostic and interventional examinations, the function and morphology of, for example, hollow organs are first evaluated in real time under fluoroscopy with image intensifier systems. Exposures of specific regions, projections, and findings are then performed separately but often with these same systems. The exposures can be viewed immediately on a monitor.

Contrast Media Examinations

To take a closer look at the **gastrointestinal tract**, it is filled with iodinated contrast solution or a barium suspension. Iodine and barium have high atomic numbers; they therefore absorb x-rays splendidly and are very visible on the radiograph. Barium suspensions can also be prepared and instilled to beautifully coat the interior wall of the air-filed or fluid-filled bowel (for example, in double contrast barium enemas).

To look at the **vascular system**, for example, in interventional procedures such as balloon dilations of the arteries, iodinated contrast solution is injected into the vessel. In angiography, subtraction is used to improve the depiction of vessels: the images before contrast are subtracted from the images after contrast administration. The resulting radiographs show only the vascular tree without the anatomical background. This is especially helpful in the abdomen and the skull base (Fig. 3.**2**).

Image Processing

Rest assured that the chemistry of traditional film processing or the post-processing of digital radiographs is all but trivial. The effects on image quality and patient dose can

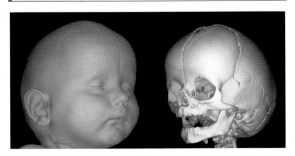

Fig. 3.**3** This complete 3D reconstruction of a child's head was performed as a special service to the plastic surgeons: They wanted a precise documentation before surgically approaching a congenital skeletal abnormality. The left part of the image shows the head with surrounding soft tissue and also the finding that worried the patient's parents. What do you make of it?

There is an accessory median suture of the frontal bone.

be tremendous. It is a regular and exciting pastime of experienced radiologists to detect and correct any mistakes that the numerous systems may come up with.

3.2 Computed Tomography

Computed tomography (CT) is currently the workhorse of radiology. Recent technical developments permit extremely fast volume scans that may serve to generate two-dimensional slices in all possible orientations as well as sophisticated three-dimensional reconstructions (Fig. 3.**3**). The radiation dose, however, remains high and continues to require a very strict indication for every intended CT.

Working Principle

In computed tomography the x-ray tube continuously rotates around the cranio-caudal axis of the patient. A beam of radiation passes through the body and hits a ring or a moving ring segment of detectors. The incoming radiation is continuously registered, the signal is digitized and fed into a data matrix taking into account the varying beam angulations (Fig. 3.**4**). The data matrix can then be transformed into an output image. In today's modern CT machines the tube rotation continues as the patient is fed through the ringlike CT gantry, thus generating not single slice scans but **spiral volume scans** of larger body

Table 3.1 **Attenuation of different body components**

Body component	Hounsfield units (HU)
Bone	1000 to 2000
Thrombus	60 to 100
Liver	50 to 70
Spleen	40 to 50
Kidney	25 to 45
White brain matter	20 to 35
Gray brain matter	35 to 45
Water	*–5 to 5*
Fat	–100 to –25
Lung	–1000 to –400

Working Principle of Computed Tomography

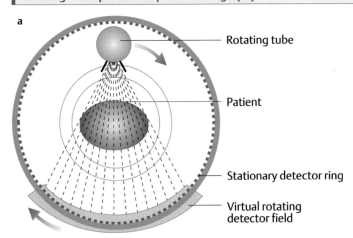

a

- Rotating tube
- Patient
- Stationary detector ring
- Virtual rotating detector field

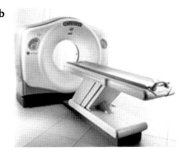

b

Fig. 3.**4 a** The x-ray tube rotates continuously around the longitudinal axis of the patient. A rotating curved detector field opposite to the tube registers the attenuated fan beam after it has passed through the patient. Taking into account the tube position at each time point of measurement, the resulting attenuation values are fed into a data matrix and further computed to create an image. **b** This is a modern volume CT scanner (by GE Medical Systems).

segments. For each picture element (pixel) the attenuation of the radiation is calculated and expressed as Hounsfield units (HU) (Table 3.**1**). Water has, by definition, a Hounsfield unit value of 0.

Contrast Media

Contrast media are used in CT to visualize vessels and the vascularization of different organ systems. They attenuate radiation because of their high atomic number (e.g., iodine and barium). Contrast media containing gadolinium (which also has a high atomic number) normally intended for use in magnetic resonance tomography could theoretically also be used in CT if the administration of iodine is contraindicated. They are, however, incredibly expensive and not registered for this use yet. To better appreciate the inside of hollow viscera, iodine or barium contrast media are also given orally or instilled into the rectum.

> **!** Fat and air are always black in CT; bone cortex and high-atomic-number contrast media are always white.

3.3   Ultrasonography

Ultrasonography ("ultrasound") is the cheapest and most "harmless" technology in radiology. For these reasons many physicians outside radiology also use the modality. Wherever ultrasound provides sufficient information and wherever radiation dose must be minimized at any cost (pediatrics and obstetrics), it is the primary imaging modality of choice. For the examination of vessels and blood flow, color-coded Doppler ultrasound may be used.

Working Principle

Ultrasound technology is simple—any bat knows how to do it. In medical ultrasonography the sound waves are generated artificially by means of **piezoelectric crystals**. These crystals are magic gadgets: when connected to an alternating current of a certain frequency, they will vibrate and thus emit a sound wave of the same frequency. If, on the other hand, they are exposed to sound waves of a certain frequency, they will produce an alternating current of that frequency.

> **!** For medical purposes sound waves of 1–15 MHz frequency are used—inaudible ultrasound waves.

If, by way of ultrasound gel, the crystal is brought into direct contact with the body, the emitted **ultrasound waves** spread through the tissue. The tissue absorbs, scatters, or reflects them.

Absorption and spatial resolution increase with higher frequencies. For that reason the maximum penetration of ultrasound waves and the depiction of fine image details correlate with frequency: in breast imaging high-resolution 7.5–10 MHz systems may be used, while in abdominal imaging 3.5–5 MHz systems are adequate to view also the deeper regions. Bone and calcifications absorb sound totally, which is why we see an acoustic "shadow" behind them (Fig. 3.**5**). Very little sound is absorbed in fluid-filled viscera, leading to the opposite effect: the echo-signal behind the fluid is stronger that in the tissue around it.

Only the *reflection* of sound back to the piezoelectric crystal will result in a signal as the basis for an image. Large and minute tissue interfaces reflect the sound. If it is an interface between soft tissue and air/gas, reflection is total—structures behind it cannot be imaged, also resulting in an acoustic shadow (Fig. 3.**5**). The ultrasound scanner calculates a two-dimensional image—how on earth does it do that? From the time passing between seeing a lightning discharge and hearing its resulting thunder we can estimate our distance to the thunderstorm. The ultrasound system measures, for each crystal separately, the time between each emitted sound pulse and the received echo pulses reflected by the tissue. The elapsed time defines the pixel matrix row that the signal is assigned to. The intensity of the echo pulse defines the respective gray value of the pixel. Hundreds of piezoelectric crystal elements are arranged in a row, and their combined data are fused into one two-dimensional ultrasound image.

> **!** In ultrasound, cystic structures are dark and show signal increase behind them. Bone and air are bright and cause an acoustic shadow.

Color-coded Doppler ultrasound: By listening to the sound of a passing motorcycle we can find out whether it is coming or going and estimate how fast it is. If ultrasound waves are reflected by moving interfaces (such as erythrocytes in flowing blood) at an angle of 10–60°, the same effect (the Doppler effect) comes into play: the echo undergoes a frequency shift dependent on the speed and direction of the blood flow. This information can be color coded into a normal ultrasound image. In color-coded Doppler ultrasound, color type and intensity tell us the direction and speed of the blood flow. As a convention, venous, centripetal flow is coded as blue; arterial, centrifugal flow as red. But take note: You accidentally rotate the scanner probe by 180° and the colors switch! And as your probe approaches a 90° angle relative to the vessel, your Doppler signal vanishes altogether. Special ultrasound contrast media further increase the Doppler effect.

3.4   Magnetic Resonance Tomography

Magnetic resonance tomography is the technically most complex imaging modality in radiology but it also holds the largest diagnostic potential. Many are terrified by the prospect of having to understand the basic principles of magnetic resonance (MR). All of this is completely unnecessary, of course: the thing is in essence nothing but a bicycle dynamo. But let's start at the beginning.

Working Principle of Ultrasonography

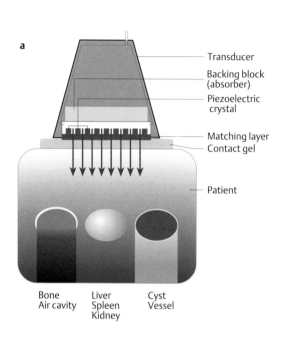

a

— Transducer
— Backing block (absorber)
— Piezoelectric crystal
— Matching layer
— Contact gel

— Patient

Bone	Liver	Cyst
Air cavity	Spleen	Vessel
	Kidney	

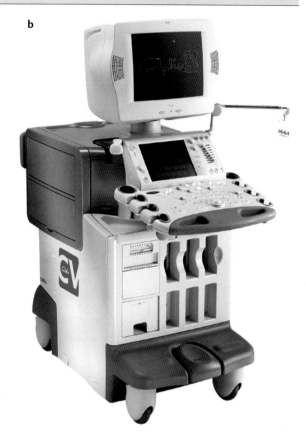

b

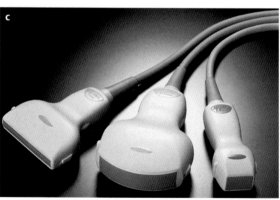

c

Fig. 3.**5 a**   If an alternating electric current is sent through a piezoelectric crystal, it vibrates with the frequency of the current, producing sound waves of that frequency. In medical ultrasound, typical frequencies vary between 1 and 15 MHz. Ultrasound gel acoustically couples the ultrasound transducer to the body, where the ultrasound waves can then spread. Inside the body the sound is absorbed, scattered, or reflected. Fluid filled (cystic) structures appear dark and show acoustic enhancement behind them. Bone and air appear bright because they absorb and reflect the sound, showing an "acoustic shadow" behind them.
b This is a modern US scanner (by Toshiba Medical Systems).
c These are transducers for different purposes.

Generation of the MR Signal

Do You Know about the Larmor Frequency?

Anyone who has sat on a swing moving legs and trunk in slow rhythm to swing ever higher, or who was the "swing pusher on duty" for a little sister or brother, daughter, or son, realizes that objects have a certain inherent frequency at which they swing (or resonate): their **resonance frequency**. If you do not know or feel this frequency or are not able to move your body accordingly (like a small child), you will never be able to swing on your own. If you are,

however, able to apply the frequency appropriately, you will go a long way with very little force. The same holds true for atoms and molecules, of course.

The nuclei of atoms spin about their axes with high frequency and some nuclei (such the hydrogen nucleus—the proton) have resultant magnetic moments. We are actually looking at small rapidly spinning "magnets." As the atoms move randomly, these "magnets" tumble about chaotically and thus neutralize each other's magnetic fields. A call to order is necessary before anything good can come out of this.

Magnetic Resonance Tomography

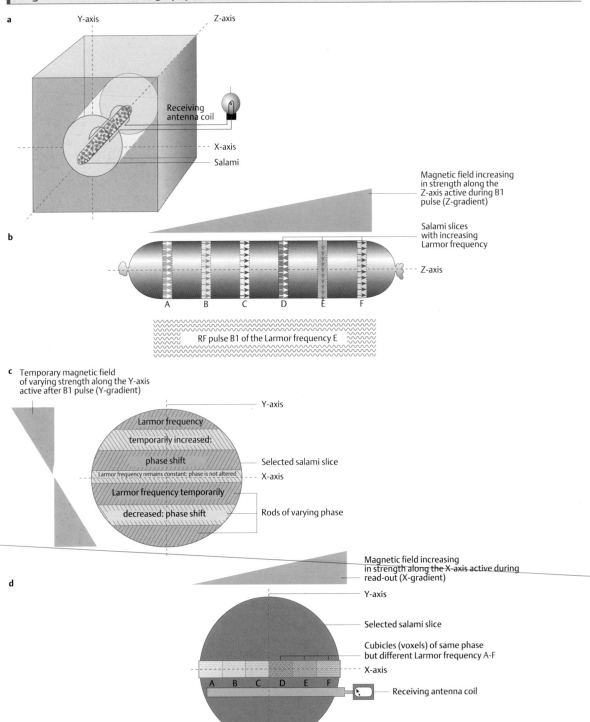

a

Y-axis

Z-axis

Receiving antenna coil

X-axis

Salami

Magnetic field increasing in strength along the Z-axis active during B1 pulse (Z-gradient)

Salami slices with increasing Larmor frequency

b

Z-axis

A   B   C   D   E   F

RF pulse B1 of the Larmor frequency E

c   Temporary magnetic field of varying strength along the Y-axis active after B1 pulse (Y-gradient)

Y-axis

Larmor frequency temporarily increased: phase shift

Larmor frequency remains constant: phase is not altered

Selected salami slice

X-axis

Larmor frequency temporarily decreased: phase shift

Rods of varying phase

Magnetic field increasing in strength along the X-axis active during read-out (X-gradient)

d

Y-axis

Selected salami slice

Cubicles (voxels) of same phase but different Larmor frequency A-F

X-axis

A   B   C   D   E   F

Receiving antenna coil

You probably remember this physics experiment from back in school: iron dust arranges itself along the lines of a magnetic field. In MR a constant external magnetic field (called B0 by the MR physicists) calls the little nuclear "magnets" to order. The protons align themselves along the axis of the magnetic field and, in addition to their spin, begin to rotate around the axis of the B0 magnetic field much like gyroscopes wobble in the Earth's gravitational field.

> **!** This rotational frequency is identical to the resonance frequency, which is also named the **Larmor frequency**. This frequency varies with the strength of the magnetic field.

The Irishman Whose Frequency We Cannot Do Without

Sir Joseph Larmor was an Irish physicist who taught in Cambridge, England, around the beginning of the last century. One of his special fields was the mathematical theory of electromagnetism. The Larmor frequency is just one of several physical phenomena

◀ Fig. 3.**6**

a The coordinate system with three axes Z, X, and Y inside the MR machine is shown. Inside of the gantry you can see the salami and the antenna alongside it in which the MR signal is induced. **b** If a gradient is superimposed on the static field along the Z-axis (Z-gradient), every slice of the salami gets its own "Larmor frequency address." An excitation pulse B1 of a frequency E will now only excite slice E. **c** Right after the B1 excitation of slice E, a temporary gradient is superimposed along the Y-axis (Y-gradient). As protons within the slice now rotate with different Larmor frequencies, the signals dephase except in the rod that keeps the original frequency. The phase shift persists until read-out. **d** During read-out, a third gradient is superimposed along the X-axis (X-gradient). Each cube in the rod now has its own "Larmor frequency address." The measured signal of that specific frequency can now be assigned to a specific voxel in the image.
e This is a modern whole-body MRI scanner (by Siemens Medical Systems). ▼

e

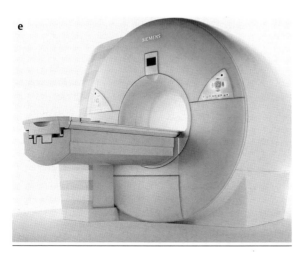

that carry his name. He was a conservative man, at times opposing most of Einstein's ideas and the introduction of baths in his college in Cambridge: "We have done without them for 400 years, why begin now?" As it turns out, he became an avid bather right after the public baths were installed.

What Is So Special about the "External" and "Internal" Magnetic Fields?

The magnets for the external applied magnetic field (B0) are large and incredibly strong (0.5, 1.0, or 1.5 tesla, the last corresponding to 30 000 times the force of the natural terrestrial magnetic field). Why do we need such a strong field? Our protons do align themselves along the field axis and wait patiently for coming sensations—they may, however, choose a parallel and an antiparallel orientation. This is where the simple magnet story comes to an end. The parallel orientation is the least energy-consuming, which is why more than half of the protons choose it. The other protons assume the antiparallel orientation. As the external magnetic field increases in power, the antiparallel orientation requires ever more energy and thus becomes less and less popular. The dominance of the parallel protons increases and thereby the magnetization of the examined body. This "internal" magnetic field initially has the same orientation as the external field B0. Its axis corresponds to the longitudinal axis of the MR gantry, also called the Z-axis (Fig. 3.**6a**). Now the stage is set: Enter a biological sample to examine—how about a nice salami?

How Do We Generate an MR Signal in a Salami?

It so happens that protons (i.e., nuclei of hydrogen atoms)—which can be beautifully studied by MR—are abundant in salamis and other organic material: in excess of 90 % of organic material consists of hydrogen. After having been moved into the B0 external magnetic field of the MR system the majority of protons inside the sausage have aligned themselves parallel to B0 and have generated an "internal" magnetic field. If we now want them to tell all, we'd better get them excited. This is done by a **radiofrequency pulse** (RF pulse), a temporary outer RF magnetic field that oscillates with the Larmor frequency of hydrogen (also called B1 by MR physicists). Remember: Hydrogen protons could not care less about RF pulses of higher or lower frequencies. The longer the B1 RF pulse is active and the stronger it is, the more the axis of the protons is tilted away from the Z-axis into the X–Y-plane. For simplicity's sake, let us consider a pulse that has the power and duration to tilt the proton axis by 90°. As this happens not only to one proton but synchronously to many protons in the salami, the "internal" magnetic field also tilts 90° and rotates with the Larmor frequency of hydrogen, much like a propeller—*or the magnet inside the bicycle dynamo* (in the X–Y plane; Fig. 3.**6a**). If you now position a wire coil along the sausage (corresponding to the receive coil or antenna of the MR machine), a measurable alternating current is induced—much like in the coils of a bicycle dynamo.

This current is the MR signal we can start our work with. Remember for later that the field signal is strongest if all protons are in phase ("listen to the same beat") which is always the case right after the B1 pulse.

After the RF pulse B1 and the resulting 90° tilt of the "internal" magnetic field, the current measured by the antenna—our signal—decreases again. The reasons are twofold: For one thing, the axis of the "internal" magnetic field moves back to the Z-axis—remember that the "external" magnetic field B0 is always present and is very strong. For another thing, the protons lose the phase synchronization they have been forced into by the RF pulse B1. As they dephase, the "internal" magnetic field power also shrinks. You will learn more about these processes later.

We now have proof that there are protons inside that salami; of course we had a hunch there would be. To look at slices of the sausage we have to assign the signals to locations in a three-dimensional coordinate system.

Spatial Allocation of the MR signal

The frequency with which I swing or push my swinging child depends, besides other things, on the terrestrial gravity. The Larmor frequency with which I can excite a proton depends on the strength of the magnetic field surrounding it. Magnetic fields can be built asymmetrically so that their strength increases along an axis. These types of fields are called gradients.

Z-gradient: If such a gradient is positioned along the longitudinal or Z-axis of the system (Z-gradient) (Fig. 3.**6a**) the magnetic field increases along the length of the salami, giving every slice of the sausage a different Larmor frequency address. If we now give the B1 pulse, it excites not the whole salami but only one slice—the one with the Larmor frequency of the B1 pulse (Fig. 3.**6b**). The bandwidth and form of the B1 pulse determine the thickness of the selected slice.

Y-gradient: After the excitation B1 pulse is over, a second gradient is positioned along the Y-axis of the system (Y-gradient). During the duration of this gradient the protons thus have different Larmor frequencies depending on their position along the Y-axis; that is, they rotate with different speeds. The subsequent phase shift persists after the Y-gradient is turned off again. The sausage slice now consists of rods of different phase (Fig. 3.**6c**). Here is the analogy to illustrate the phenomenon: If three different cars drive on a three-lane highway and adhere to a speed limit, they stay side by side. Once the speed limit is lifted, they drive with different speeds and the gap between them grows. As the speed limit is enforced again, they drive at the same speed (same Larmor frequency for the protons) and the gap between them (the phase shift) persists. This applies to law-abiding drivers only, of course. The gradient can be designed to leave the Larmor frequency unchanged in one rod that subsequently does not undergo the phase shift. Frequency and phase are thus identical to the original B1 pulse. We will now dice this rod into volume elements (voxels).

X-gradient: The last gradient is switched on during the read-out phase and is positioned along the X-axis (X-gradient). It divides the rod into cubes, assigning a Larmor frequency address to each (Fig. 3.**6d**).

Now we have the single cubes (or voxels) that we need for a two-dimensional image: a selectively excited slice of a defined thickness, and a rod in correct phase that is subdivided into cubes of different Larmor frequencies assignable to locations in a coordinate system. To calculate the image, a separate measurement must be performed for every rod (voxel or pixel row) of the image matrix; that is, for a matrix of 256 × 256 voxels, we need to repeat the process 256 times. The rest is complex electrical engineering.

Analysis of the MR Signal

Which Phenomena Do We Need to Know?

As has been described above, the MR signal measurable directly after the RF pulse decays quickly. This is due to two phenomena that can be quantified separately:

- Longitudinal relaxation: This is the process of the "internal" magnetic field returning to the original orientation (Z-axis) along the "external " magnetic field B0. This is a pretty fast process. The corresponding parameter is the **T1 value**.
- Transversal relaxation: This is the process of signal loss due to dephasing of the protons. Starting with the same rotational frequency and phase right after the B1 pulse, different protons in different locations are influenced by the magnetic forces of their neighboring atoms and the general inhomogeneity of the field and thus lose their synchronization (they "lose their common beat"). Another analogy to illustrate the phenomenon: Imagine a string orchestra fiddling away at a musical score. It is a special orchestra—the musicians hear only their own music and see nobody but the conductor. It is the conductor who gives the sign to start (B1 pulse). If he were to leave right after the beginning, the individual musicians could continue to play their score but the orchestra's music would quickly turn disharmonic—or *dephase*. As the protons dephase, the power of the rotating "internal" magnetic field decreases. This process takes time; it is called transversal relaxation and is described by the **T2 value**.

Because the T2 value tells us about the environment of the protons it is a very important parameter. You can imagine that T2 can tell us a lot about the structure of tissues.

Just How Do We Measure the T1 and T2 Values?

If some time after the excitation pulse B1 we apply an additional 180° RF pulse, we can turn the axis of the rotating protons around and let them rotate backwards to produce a signal echo. Here is the last analogy: If several cars of different maximum speed drive away from the start with top speed, gaps between them will appear and grow over time.

If they all get a radio order to return as fast as possible, they will reach the spot they started from all at the same time. It is the same with our rotating protons: after the 180° pulse the signal increases again, climaxing in an echo (spin-echo) of the original signal. The influence of constant magnetic inhomogeneities that may be due to the external magnetic field is fortunately subtracted in this process.

> **!** The difference in signal strength between the original signal and its echo tells us something about (a) the reorientation of the internal magnetic field into the Z-axis (T1; longitudinal relaxation) and (b) the local randomly distributed magnetic field inhomogeneities that cannot be compensated by the 180° pulse (T2; transversal relaxation).

If you want a T1-weighted image, you put the 180° pulse right after the primary signal. As the longitudinal relaxation is fast, the loss of signal then represents T1. If you want a T2-weighted image, you wait a long time before you give the 180° pulse to give the dephasing (transversal relaxation) time to occur. The loss of signal then represents T2.

T1 and T2 values of water, fat, muscle, and liver are quite different to each other. This is the reason for the superb soft tissue contrast in MR imaging. If the excited hydrogen atoms leave the excited slice before read-out (such as happens in flowing blood), there is no signal to measure, which is why in most MR images the vessels are black. If there are only few hydrogen atoms (e.g., in bone cortex or in tendons), the signal remains low. A variety of MR contrast media can change the T1 and T2 values. The most popular ingredient is gadolinium.

> **!** On T1-weighted images fluid (e.g., spinal fluid, urine) is dark, while on T2-weighted images it is bright. Bone cortex gives no MR signal—it is always black.

3.5   Our Perception

The outcome of an imaging study (or an intervention) does not rely only on the indication or the quality of its technical execution. The diagnostic radiologist with all his or her knowledge and experience is the last link in the diagnostic chain. The radiologist searches for relevant image information, perceives, sorts, and evaluates it, and finally comes to a (hopefully sound) diagnosis. Search, detection, and preliminary evaluation are the dominant components of perception.

> **!** Without intact and optimized perception of the diagnostician, every imaging study, sophisticated as the technology may be, is a waste of time and money. It also increases the patient's risks.

What Do We See Best?

In diagnostic images such as mammograms, incredibly small and low-contrast structures such as microcalcifications have to be appreciated.

> **!** A structure is perceived best if it is viewed at a distance at which it subtends an angle of 5° (Fig. 3.**7a**).

We implement this physiological truth in our daily work by getting closer to an image if we look for very small details—until we hit the limits of accommodation. Accommodation is, of course, phenomenal in children (if they show you a piece of paper to read, they will hold it close to your nose). Radiologists of adequate biological age, however, need to carry a magnifying glass around to compensate for their accommodation deficit. It is interesting to note that the phenomenon also works the other way around: large, low-contrast lesions are better perceived if you view them with a minifying glass. The number of radiologists carrying these around is much smaller, however. The normal crowd just takes a step back and then another look.

How well we view small structures also depends on the brightness, or optical density as the physicists call it. As typical animals of the steppe we see contrasts best at the brightness of a summer afternoon. At this optical density our optical cones work optimally while the intraocular scatter is minimal. If it becomes darker, we turn to rod vision. The detectability decreases significantly, which is why you a have a reading lamp at your bedside.

The windows of a typical ward room are only usable as "light boxes" if main rounds take place on a summer afternoon and if clear skies dominate in the region—thus in hospitals for the upper few. Late in the evening, however, a broader public can also check the healing progress while standing in the parking lot.

As our eye adapts to the brightness of the total visual field, an image on the light box should be very well masked if you do not want to miss low-contrast lesions. Room (ambient) light must also be adapted to prevent reflections on the image, and the dilation of the pupils, which would increase intraocular scatter and activation of rod vision.

The proper examination of an image that has been generated with great care is thus far from trivial (Fig. 3.**7b**). Special computer-assisted light boxes or viewing monitors that also control room light optimize our perception (Fig. 3.**7c**).

Perception

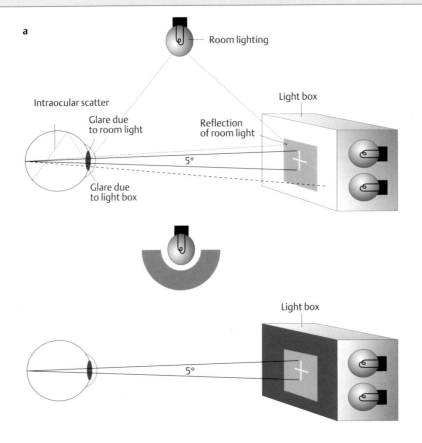

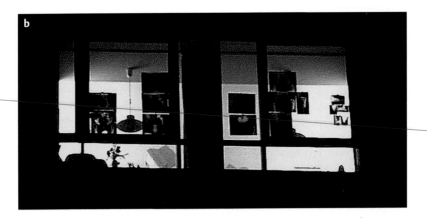

Fig. 3.**7**

a Glare and reflections in the visual field, intraocular scatter, and insufficient masking of the image on the light box are reasons for impaired perception (upper). If these mistakes are corrected and if structures are viewed so that they subtend an angle of 5° perception is optimal (lower). **b** Chief's round on the surgical ward. The films were fixed to the windows. Obviously rounds have to take place before sundown on this ward. Nice to know also that the therapeutic progress can be checked another time late at night while walking over to the parking lot. **c** This is a computer-assisted lightbox that masks the film and adapts ambient light automatically, thus optimizing perception (by Smartlight, Inc.). **d** This is a modern flat panel display used in digital mammography. In this special field the quality requirements are extremely high. The display also needs to be placed in dedicated, light-adjusted surroundings (by Fuji Medical Systems). ▶

What Else Influences Our Perception?

Even if a structure is optically well discernible it must also be perceived and, eventually, be evaluated and classified. Is the structure pathological, normal, or just a variant of the normal? The image is scanned optically and compared to an internalized standard, the "gestalt" of, for example, a chest radiograph. The more complex the normal image, i.e., the radiological anatomy, the more difficult is the detection of pathology. A given nodule is readily perceived in the periphery of the lung but is easily missed when it is close to the lung hilum, because the large vessels can look like or camouflage the nodule. The negative influence of complex anatomy on the detectability of pathology is also called **"anatomical noise"** (see p. 21).

After you have detected a definitely pathological structure, your attention may fade, especially if you are still inexperienced. This **"satisfaction of search"** effect (see p. 25) hinders the careful examination of the rest of the image. Make it a point to take the time for a second thorough pass over the image!

The independent review of an examination by another colleague (**"double reading"**) can increase its diagnostic value significantly (see p. 32)—four eyes do see more than two!

> **!** Images are generated with extremely expensive and sophisticated equipment, sometimes with substantial risk to the patient. They must be studied with great care and under optimal conditions.

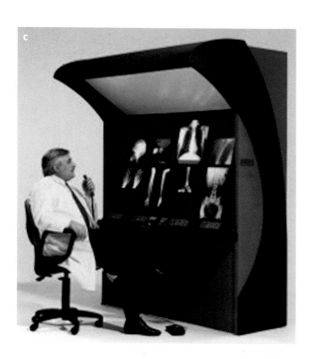

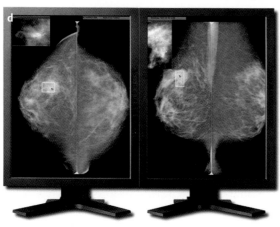

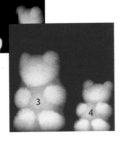

4 Phenomena in Imaging and Perception

The knowledge of some basic procedures and rules of projectional and sectional imaging is essential for the understanding of the creation of a given medical image. Other phenomena are very helpful in the interpretation of such radiological images. Some of them can be applied to every aspect of imaging, others are crucial only for subspecialties in radiology. What holds true in real life is also true here: If you know the basics and a bunch of little tricks on top of that, your fame will spread quickly.

4.1 What Do I Need to Know for Image Analysis?

Is the Quality of the Study Technically Adequate?

Checklist: Determining Study Quality

- Has the best method/modality been chosen in the given clinical context?
- Have the right body parts been imaged and completely so?
- Was the study performed properly or was imaging compromised owing to the patient's state or the situation during the examination?

Every experienced radiologist first eyes the "quality of the study" before starting a thorough image analysis. The objective of a first technical check is not to discard the study or ignore a finding (although this is also necessary in a few cases) but to establish a sound basis for the perception and decision-making process. This is a precious habit that you should also stick to. Obviously first and foremost one must assure that the images at hand indeed belong to the patient in question.

To determine the **quality of a study** we ask the following questions:
- Was the right kind of diagnostic or interventional method selected considering the clinical indication at hand? The indication lists in this book will give you an orientation on what studies are done for what problem based on science and clinical experience.
- Was the right body region imaged and is it completely represented? This is a crucial question. As an example, check Figure 4.**1a–c** for confirmatory evidence. In addition, for example, a true second projection is an absolute must in skeletal radiography (Fig. 4.**2**).

- Was the study performed properly or was imaging compromised owing to the patient's state or the situation during the examination? This includes not only study technique (e.g., exposure voltage; the use of a scatter grid in projection radiography; choice of window and filter settings in CT or frequency and probe type in ultrasonography; adequate selection of coil, sequence, and projection in MR imaging [MRI]), but also positioning (Did the patient stand upright?) and the degree of cooperation of the patient (Could the patient keep still [Fig. 4.**3**]? Did he hold his breath? Did he inhale deeply?). Having finished reading this book you should be able to answer the first two questions in 95% of all cases. If the study is of satisfactory quality, you're on your way to the correct diagnosis.

How Do I Analyze an Image?

If you track the eye movements of an experienced radiologist, you will find that they appear to be rather unsystematic or even chaotic. Their perception of findings actually takes place in the sub-second range. The neophyte, however, has to adhere to a rigid sequence to accommodate the need for longer average observation time, which conflicts with the individual's momentary attention span. You will find suggestions for such sequences in the individual chapters.

Tissue Characteristics on Radiographic Images

Speaking in terms of characteristic density on plain radiography, the human body consists of different basic components, specifically fat, water, soft tissue, and bone. These four basic densities are recognizable when a structure contains an overwhelming amount of one particular kind of tissue. Obviously that is not always the case, and, to make matters worse, since conventional radiographs are projectional images we often look at a composite shadow made up of the density of several characteristic tissues. Some additional components such as calcifications or metal are introduced by disease or by external events. Body functions can also be observed with imaging modalities; for example, the flow in blood vessels or the cerebrospinal fluid spaces or the uptake of contrast media into a specific types of tissue.

Every imaging modality has its specific characteristics, strengths, and weaknesses with respect to the depiction of these components and functions. Some modalities

Attention, This Is Your Wake-up Call!

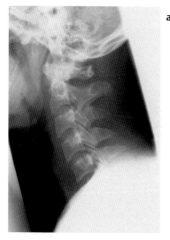 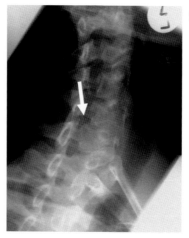 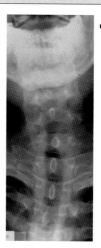

Fig. 4.1 a   Have a good look at the lateral cervical spine of this patient who fell off his bicycle. Can the stiff neck collar be taken off safely?

Only five cervical vertebral bodies are visible—this lateral view is not sufficient.

b   The additional oblique view (two sturdy trauma surgeons pulled the shoulders caudally) shows the dislocation of C6 with respect to C7 (arrow). c The anterior–posterior radiograph proves the distortion in the C6/7 segment. Had the collar been taken off without further stabilization, a spinal cord contusion could have resulted.

Diagnosis at Second Glance

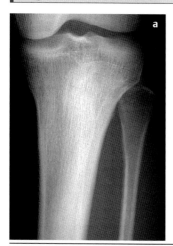 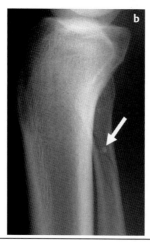

Fig. 4.2 a   The anterior–posterior radiograph shows no obvious abnormality.
b   Only the lateral projection demonstrates the fibular fracture (arrow).

No, Doctor

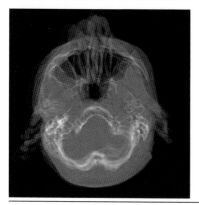

Fig. 4.3   After having been asked whether he could please hold still for just one more scan, this patient only shook his head. Not everything is possible.

What Looks How with What Modality?

a Imaging of body components

A	O	W	L	M	C	M	
							Eye
							XR (28kVp)
							XR (100kVp)
							CT
							US (in water)
							T1
							T2
							Flair
							T1 fs
							HASTE
							T2 fs
							T1 GRE

A: air; O: oil; W: water; L: liver; M: muscle; C: calcium; M: metal

b Test yourself!

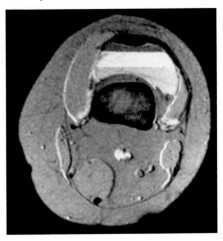

b You see a part of a study of a patient who has suffered an injury. Try to classify the study as precisely as possible and then come up with the clinical diagnosis. Use Fig. 4.**4a**, a little anatomy, and your gray matter in the process.

Fig. 4.**4 a**   Here you see the most important body components as they are depicted by the different imaging modalities. The samples are surrounded by air. Gas, fluids, and tissues are contained in rubber glove fingers. For the ultrasound, the samples were dipped in freshly drawn tap water—the little bubbles are caused by gas in that water. The calcium tablet, of course, could not be dropped into water without dissolving immediately and producing gas, so my own (G.W.E.) radius had to take its place. By the way, which metal did we choose? Copper, lead, or iron? And why?

Of course it is lead. Copper would have penetrated much better at 100 kV; iron would have flown right into the gantry of the MR machine and would have damaged the system (and what's worse, our department's slush fund).

This is an axial sectional study of the knee just cranial to the patella. You can see the complete contour of the limb—an ultrasound is thus impossible. The bony cortex and the tendons are black—that proves it is an MR image. The cancellous bone and the subcutaneous fat are comparatively dark—fat saturation would explain that. Three layers within the suprapatellar bursa are appreciated with two fluid–fluid interfaces. The middle layer is bright—compatible with serous joint fluid on T2-weighted images. The lower, dependent, layer has an intermediate signal that would go well with blood. The top layer with low signal is fat again—remember the fat saturation. The whole picture is diagnostic of a joint involving fracture of the knee, most likely a tibial head fracture. The fat is released into the joint from the bone marrow by way of the fracture line. G.W.E. likes to call this the "**Dutch flag**" sign.

"Anatomical Noise"

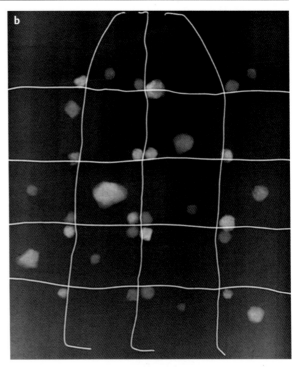

Fig. 4.**5 a**   Analyze the chest radiograph of this volunteer, who has an arrangement of wax spheres fixed to his back: large spheres are overlooked in the hilar region. **b** Compare the radiograph of the wax spheres alone: How many did you miss?

may have excellent spatial resolution (such as high-frequency ultrasound) but poor tissue depth penetration. Some have good spatial resolution (the ability to discern two small objects/points in space) but inferior soft tissue contrast resolution (the ability to discern two different types of soft tissue, such as gray and white matter of the brain). Such an example is the choice between CT of the brain versus MRI. In addition there are, in the individual modalities, special ways to enhance one aspect or another. For the beginner it is difficult—if not impossible—to get a comprehensive overview. Figure 4.**4a** is intended to help you a little. It shows the relevant components and how they are depicted by the pertinent imaging modalities. Figure 4.**4b** puts your new knowledge to the test. Please keep in mind that in projection radiography it is not only the density (Fig. 4.**4**) but also the thickness of an exposed object that determines the signal intensity (that is, the radiation attenuation in this case).

What Is a Normal, What Is a Pathological Finding?

The objective of imaging is the detection and localization of relevant disease or the exclusion of significant findings. What we consider to be pathological depends a great deal on the patient, on the societal context, and sometimes even on the immediate political or socioeconomic situation (a period of clinical depression following a catastro-

phe like 11 September 2001 in New York may be considered a normal reaction rather than disease). Calcifications in the wall of the abdominal aorta or a vertebral disk herniation without symptoms are not pathological in a 90-year-old unless their shape suggests a large aneurysm but would certainly lead to additional diagnostic work-up and possibly therapy in a young adult. Incidental findings like a closure defect of the vertebral arch of S1, a pulmonary azygos vein lobe, or a circumaortic renal vein are anatomical variants that have no relevance at all except under extraordinary circumstances: for instance, when surgery to the region is planned, e.g., laparoscopic resection of a left kidney from a healthy living donor.

As has been mentioned in the previous chapter, the normal anatomy can be so confusing that detection, localization, and classification of findings can be extremely difficult. The vascular tree of the lung, for example, with its intertwined veins and pulmonary and bronchial arteries, is so complicated that large nodules can be completely concealed (Fig. 4.**5**). This interference of the normal anatomy with the detection of pathological findings is also called "**anatomical noise**" (analogous to the bothersome noise you hear in your Dad's old stereo system).

Where is the Pathology?

To assign a lesion to a certain location we need **three dimensions**, just like in stereoscopic viewing. In sectional

Let Me Have Another Slice!?

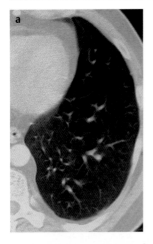

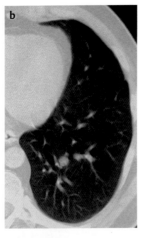

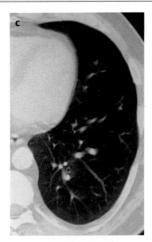

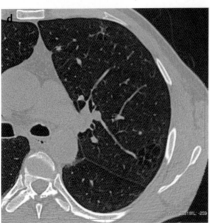

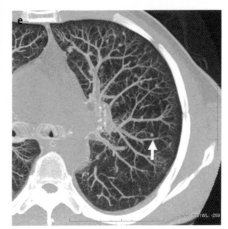

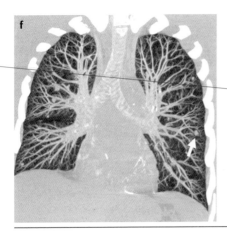

Fig. 4.**6**   The magnified view of a chest CT shows a number of little round structures (**b**). Only the review of the next cranial (**a**) and the next caudal slice (**c**) indicates that the central spot in **b** represents a nodule while the other structures are tubular and thus represent pulmonary vessels. If a thick slab reconstruction is used, things become easier: In **d** a single CT slice shows a few round suspect lesions. It is the axial (**e**) and the horizontal (**f**) thick slabs that differentiate clearly between the tubular vessels and the metastatic nodule (arrow).

imaging it is the *neighboring slices*, reconstructions or so-called *thick slab reconstructions*, that convey the third dimension. Interactive review of thin CT images on an electronic viewing system such as a workstation or PACS system is becoming increasingly popular; scrolling through stacks of contiguous images allows the interpreting radiologist to form a 3D impression in his or her head. Looking at the third dimension and the neighborhood is the only way to differentiate between a sphere (such as a lung no-

dule) and a cylinder (such as a vessel section in a chest CT) (Fig. 4.6). In projection radiography, especially of the skeleton, it is the obligatory second oblique or perpendicular projection that gives us this information in conjunction with the initial radiograph (Fig. 4.7)—*if* we see the abnormality on the other projections, which is by no means always the case. However, a simple single projection performed with a sagittal x-ray beam can also give us hints as to the localization of a lesion. We use this information

A Valid Second Point of View

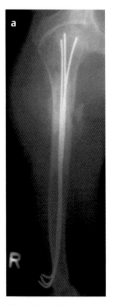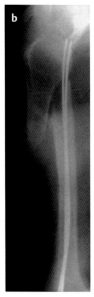

Fig. 4.**7 a**　What you see is a fracture of the humerus that has been stabilized with a number of rush pins. Looking at this projection, all looks well.
b The second projection brings a rude awakening: The rush pins lie outside of the proximal fracture fragment.

whenever a second projection is not present or does not clearly show the lesion in question.

Radiographically perceptible interfaces exist between tissues whenever their density (or signal strength) in the given imaging modality is different enough to be detected by the imaging system used (contrast resolution, see above). This is of special importance in projection radiography. The kidney contour and the border of the iliopsoas muscle, for example, are appreciated well in abdominal films because these soft tissue density structures (of kidney or muscle) are surrounded by retroperitoneal fat of much lower density (Fig. 4.**8**). If such an interface is lost or its continuity is altered, a pathological process in this region must be suspected. In the kidney the phenomenon could point to a renal carcinoma that has broken through the renal capsule; in the case of the iliopsoas muscle, retroperitoneal fibrosis or a large psoas abscess could result in the loss of its contour. When taking a closer look at the analysis of chest radiographs we will make extensive use of this phenomenon (also called "silhouette sign").

Exposure geometry also influences the image appearance and can help us to assign a finding to a specific location. For the naked eye of an observer, far objects result in a small projection and close objects in a large projection on our retina. In projection radiography it is just the other way around: looking at a radiograph we actually see through the patient at a point source of radiation, the focus. Whatever is closer to the focus, i.e., farther away from the detector, projects larger on the detector. (It is like looking at your own shadow on a wall—the closer you get to the wall the smaller the shadow gets, and the closer you get to

Radiologists Just Love Fat!

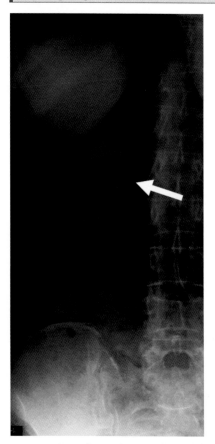

Fig. 4.**8**　The collimated view of an abdominal radiograph shows the oblique course of the iliopsoas muscle as it extends from the spine into the pelvis, made visible by its interface with the surrounding fat (arrow). The renal contour is also obvious. Sitting on top of the kidney one can, with a little imagination, appreciate the adrenal gland. The patient's breast is superimposed over it. All these retroperitoneal structures are perceptible owing to the their interface with surrounding fat, which is of different radiopacity. The dark, irregular areas represent intestinal air.

A Sharper Image, Please!

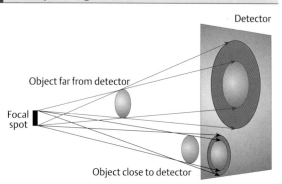

Fig. 4.**9**　The finite size of the focus causes unsharpness of the object margins that increases with growing distance to the detector.

Gummy Bears to Make You Exercise

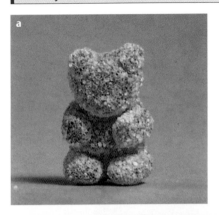

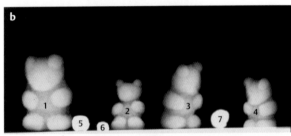

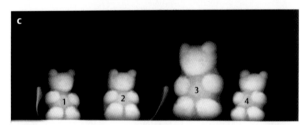

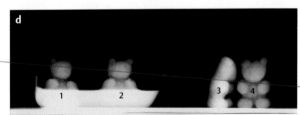

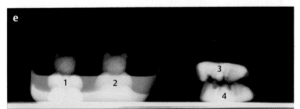

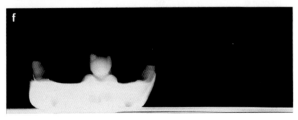

Fig. 4.**10 a**   A gummy bear made of soft-tissue-equivalent gelatin with a sugar coating. All his colleagues are of the same size and type. **b** Four gummy bears (1–4) play "lead" ball (5–7). Which bears stand close to the detector, which distant from it? Which ball is the smallest? Which ball is the largest?

Bears 2 and 4 stand close to the detector, bear 1 most distant from it. Balls 5 and 6 are of the same size and sit next to bears 1 and 2. Ball 7 is the smallest—its unsharp contour tells all: it was suspended with tape (see the faint shadow of it?) just a few centimeters from the focus.

c After the game: The gummy bears have retired into the bathroom. Bears 1 and 2 want to have a bath, bears 3 and 4 are not so sure. Which bear sits in the tub? What does it bathe in? How close to each other are bears 3 and 4? Do they have eye contact?

The tub is empty; which bear sits inside is impossible to say. Bears 3 and 4 are far away from each other; they look at each other and discuss the further course of events, but we cannot conclude this from the radiograph.

d Ten minutes later: One bear is in the tub. Which? Bear 3 has changed its position.

Bear 2 must be sitting in the tub since its contour or "silhouette" is lost—it displaces the fluid (water), which is of the same approximate density as gelatin. Bear 1 must sit outside of the tub since its shadow is added to the attenuation of the tub's water which it does not displace—its silhouette remains visible. Bears 3 and 4 have approached each other and discuss the further course of events. Both are close to the detector. Bear 3 stands at a 90° angle to bear 4. In this lateral projection it absorbs more radiation than bear 4 in the anterior–posterior position. The same is true for human beings: a lateral chest radiograph requires triple the dose of standard view! Remember this when you get a chest x-ray yourself or if you order one for a young patient.

e The evening progresses slowly. Go ahead and analyze the situation. What has happened in the tub?

There are two fluids in the tub now. Bear 2 must still be the one in the tub because its contour is still lost in the lower fluid. Its silhouette remains discernible in the upper fluid, though: The density of this fluid must be significantly lower than the gelatin's density. What wondrous fluid could that be? Of course, it is an oil bath for luxurious relaxation: The water remains at the bottom, the oil—or liquid fat—swims on top. Bear 1 still sits outside the tub in apathy. Bears 3 and 4 now both project laterally; bear 4 is now as bright as bear 3 because they absorb the same amount of radiation.

f The party is coming to an end. All bears are sitting in the tub – or has one of them left prematurely and frustrated? And what on earth is the matter with the tub?

No, nobody has left. Two bears are sitting in full harmony in the middle of the tub facing each other (do not try this in your own bathtub)—their densities add up to a higher value than the bears imaged sideways. There is another fluid in the tub now. The bears displace this fluid, showing less density than the surrounding fluid. The fluid must thus have much higher radiation attenuation than whatever these bears are made of: it is iodine contrast medium.

Summation Effect

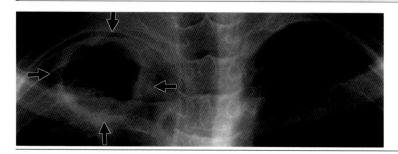

Fig. 4.**11**   You can see hyperlucent areas in both lung apices. On the patient's right side it is a real finding representing an abscess with thick walls that can be followed around the full perimeter of the lesion. The hyperlucent area on the left is bordered by the first and second ribs, the clavicle, and the spine. This is a typical summation effect—your brain tries to fool you.

the light source the larger the shadow gets). We also have to consider that the focus of the x-rays has a physical size (in plain radiography between 0.1 and 2.0 mm), and that the size predicates the inherent *unsharpness* of the image. The larger the focus or the closer an object is to the focus, the less well defined are the apparent visible margins of structures on the corresponding radiograph (Fig. 4.**9**).

You can go ahead and try out your new abilities by analyzing Figure 4.**10b–f**. Figure 4.**10a** shows a gummy bear and all the gummy bears shown have the same physical size.

What Can Go Wrong in Perception?

The fact that a lesion exists in the body of a patient does not automatically mean that it is visible. And the fact that a lesion is visible does not mean that it is always perceived by the observer. The diagnostic process is not complete, nor is it worth a penny to the patient, until the diagnosis has been communicated in writing or verbally to the responsible clinician in a timely manner and can be acted upon. During the perception of a visible lesion, a number of interesting neurophysiological and cognitive effects come into play that one should be aware of.

Like human faces, radiographic images have a "gestalt" that one can appreciate and remember after very little training. If we see the face of a good friend on the bus, we recognize them at once—we will perceive the new pimple on their face with a glance of the eye. A trained radiologist will also detect the nodule on a chest radiograph at once, in less than a second and thus without systematic search. The standardized way of generating and presenting the image supports this rapid detection. If a friend were lying on their back on the beach and you were passing behind them, you would find it much more difficult to recognize their face with certainty and even more so the pimple of course. It is the unusual orientation or "gestalt" of the otherwise well-known face that poses the problem. The same is true for other representations: Looking at fragments of an image data set (such as in multiple narrow windows of a digital image or by analyzing an image with the magnifying glass only) does not make the overall analysis of an image superfluous. Rather the combination of detailed observation and larger context of the entire image permit proper perception and interpretation. Experience and science make a strong case always

to generate, present, view, and analyze radiological images (such as chest radiographs or mammograms) in a highly standardized fashion.

Sometimes during the analysis of a radiological image we discover lesions that are not real but are conceived by our visual system as such: parts of different anatomical structures are fused into an apparent "lesion," which is a "**summation effect**." This effect can make rib crossings

"Satisfaction of Search" Effect

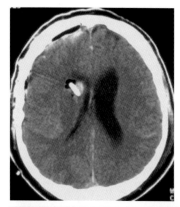

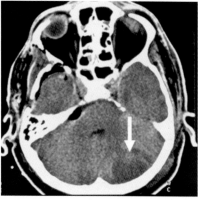

Fig. 4.**12 a**   This CT scan of the head shows a dislocated ventricle drain that led to a hemorrhage in the brain's white matter. The responsible surgeon was present. The finding was discussed animatedly, communicated, and shown to other colleagues.
b The additional infarction of the left cerebellar hemisphere (arrow) escaped attention in this setting and was diagnosed in a later review.

appear as "nodules." The lung apex is another area where the superimposition of first and second rib, the clavicle, and the spine can simulate a pseudolesion—a zone of "overinflation" in this case (Fig. 4.**11**). If we assume such a phenomenon, we have to trace the contours of the pseudolesion and dissect it into its individual components. But beware not to merely try to explain away all findings; do not automatically call all small apparent nodules in a smoker summation phenomena just because you know about this now—we do have other modalities to ensure that in fact there is no reason to worry. Comparison with previous radiographs, additional imaging, or follow-up examination after a few weeks may help work out what is going on.

Prior knowledge or findings can influence our subsequent analysis and distract us from relevant findings on the image. The discussion continues whether the patient history should be read before or after the initial analysis of the study. We suggest a preliminary analysis of the image without any knowledge about the patient's symptoms to get an unbiased first impression. Subsequently the patient history is read and the study is analyzed with this information in mind. The physician's focus on the patient's complaints is not always an advantage as it can divert from less straightforward findings and incidental diagnoses. The role of patient history and complaints with regard to the interpretation of findings is, of course, undisputed: relevant clinical points must be communicated to the radiologist or the diagnostic process goes awry. The final diagnosis then takes both perspectives into account and ideally consists of a list of differential diagnoses in the order of plausibility and probability.

A particularly tricky phenomenon has already been mentioned in Chapter 3—the "**satisfaction of search**" effect (see p. 17). If the (often inexperienced) observer has managed to find a first relevant lesion, further interest in the image may deteriorate quickly: additional relevant information is overlooked or ignored (Fig. 4.**12**). So while it is great for the neophyte to make a sound first finding right away, the analysis of a study should be continued with great discipline and care.

4.2   Can We Reach a Diagnosis that Approaches Histological Certainty?

If a pathological finding has been detected, it must be classified and the differential diagnoses must be contemplated. Going through the following questions in your mind may help you come up with a more concise list of potential diagnoses.

Are There Any Volume Changes?

Scars in parenchymal organs and pulmonary atelectasis are associated with volume loss; that is, neighboring elastic tissues move toward the pathological process. Abscesses, tumors, and metastases act quite differently: they tend to increase in volume and occupy space—they displace neighboring elastic structures.

What Happens to the Surrounding Anatomy?

Many radiographic findings (alone or in combination) can suggest an aggressive process: If neighboring vessels are invaded, bones are destroyed, fat planes, muscles, and organs are infiltrated. If the lesion has an irregular margin and/or enhances strongly after the administration of contrast, inflammation or malignancy need to be strongly considered. If the body has had time to form a capsule, if there is a sclerotic margin in bone, if a lesion is well circumscribed, a slowly developing, benign process is more likely.

What Is the Internal Structure Like?

The inner structure and potential contrast enhancement can be homogeneous or inhomogeneous. Fat, fluid, calcifications, ossifications, or even the presence of teeth (i.e., in a teratoma) help to narrow down the differential diagnosis. Fluid–fluid or fluid–gas interfaces in liquid-filled spaces permit conclusions about their constituents (see Fig. 4.**4b**).

What Pathology Commonly Occurs in a Particular Anatomical Region?

Every region has a number of typical pathological findings that tend to relate to the local organs or the function of the specific body part. A nice example is the differentiation of space-occupying lesions in the anterior mediastinum—the four great Ts: "**t**hymoma, **t**hyroid, **t**eratoma and … **t**errible lymphoma."

Sex, age, and the acute and/or general patient history further narrow down the number of differential diagnoses. At the end of it all one takes a deep breath and calls the list of "surviving" diagnoses. Depending on your individual frame of mind and your sense of suspense and drama, you call the most probable diagnosis first or last. The satisfaction achieved by reaching a relevant, complex diagnosis through crystalline logic, comprehensive knowledge, and good familiarity with the literature is difficult to surpass by any other experience—well, except one, maybe.

> **!** Please never forget: Rare things are rare and common things are common.

The sound of horse hoofs in the developed world does tend to indicate the arrival of a horse, not a zebra, although those may be more interesting to look at. More than one "zebra-diagnosis" per week should be highly suspicious, even in teaching hospitals.

5   Risks, Risk Minimization, and Prophylactic Measures

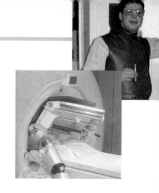

Every diagnostic and interventional procedure harbors potential risks to the patient. Risks can be very real and immediate, that is, they can directly harm the patient's health, or they can be indirect, resulting in other risky studies to prove or disprove a preliminary suspicious finding. Counterbalancing the risk of a study is, of course, the potential benefit it brings to the patient: an invasive procedure may yield a comprehensive diagnosis allowing for immediate therapy such as in angiography followed by balloon dilation.

> ! The physician's careful explanation of risks and benefits of a planned study or procedure aims to enable the patient to make an informed decision whether or not to proceed with the study.

The starting point is different for every patient. Because of the radiation dose incurred, computed tomography of the abdomen in a young woman three months pregnant will only be performed in a life-threatening emergency, for example, after severe trauma to the abdomen. In an elderly cancer patient scheduled for radiation therapy, on the other hand, the radiation dose administered during an abdominal CT is without clinical relevance. The cancellation of a study naturally also carries risks: a tumor may go undetected or an inadequate or wrong therapy might be chosen. Thus there are many reasons to take the time for a comprehensive and personal conversation with the patient and to remind yourself of the risks and relevance of your own actions.

> ! In most countries, obtaining signed informed consent of the patient or his/her legal representative (e.g., for children) is an obligatory prerequisite prior to performing procedures that carry a higher risk (administration of contrast media, interventional measures). A preparatory conversation between the patient and the physician needs to take place leaving the patient with sufficient time to ponder the options prior to the study.

Consent should be obtained from the patient prior to entering the procedure room if the administration of contrast is intended. If elective angiography or balloon dilation is planned, consent should be obtained at least 24 hours prior to the intervention. Asking patients to consent while they are already on the procedure table is legally nonbinding except in a life-threatening emergency. A countersignature of the physician is usually necessary. One should make it a habit to jot down explanatory drawings and handwritten notes on the consent form because they prove the very per-

sonal quality of the conversation. If a fully conscious patient rejects the suggested procedure—for whatever reasons—this must be accepted; that is, the patient must have the possibility to decline without further interference. A study or procedure performed in spite of the patient's refusal amounts to inflicting bodily harm, with associated potential legal consequences. If a patient loses his or her legal decision-making capacity in the further course of events—becomes unconscious, develops a psychosis, etc.—the case must be reconsidered in the best interest of the patient.

5.1   The Nonindicated Study

A study is not indicated if in a given clinical setting no information can be expected from it that could in any way alter further management. That may sound trivial. The execution of any nonindicated procedure, however, may lead to the delay or prevention of necessary, indicated diagnostic or interventional measures. As a matter of fact, it may sometime prove fatal for the patient:

Patient Paellé: Brazil Paellé (56) fell out of the bus that carried him and his friends back home from an out-of-town victory of "his" soccer team. He is not exactly sober and has suffered a bleeding skull laceration. Like all his friends who have brought him to the emergency department, he is in a splendid mood and fully oriented as to the latest league results. A radiograph of the skull is performed to exclude a fracture and turns out to be normal. After his wound has been sutured and dressed by the young doctor on call, Paellé's friends bring him to his luxurious bachelor apartment to rest. That night he becomes disoriented and helpless, and finally becomes unconscious to meet his ultimate "referee" and creator early in the morning. His body is examined by the forensic medicine department. The colleague there discovers a lethal intracranial epidural/extradural hematoma (see p. 236). The public prosecutor confiscates the patient documents. Just what went wrong?

For starters, nobody with a significant head injury should be permitted to remain without close supervision for the next 24 hours—friends or spouses can also monitor the level of consciousness in less severe cases. Secondly, the unremarkable skull radiograph lulled the on-call doctor into falsely believing that no significant injury had occurred. This was a fatal misconception since it is not the potential skull fracture that determines the course of events but the intracranial, space-occupying, and poten-

Primum Nihil Nocere

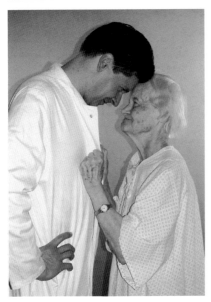

Fig. 5.**1** "Primum nihil nocere" ("First do no harm") Hippocrates and/or Galen used to say. In Greek, however. It was then as it is today: Patients undergoing treatment of any kind need to trust us with their lives and they should have every reason to do so.

tially lethal hemorrhage that may develop slowly. A radiograph cannot exclude intracranial hematoma or other significant abnormality and is therefore irrelevant. If any disturbances of consciousness develop after head injury, if a skull fracture is likely, or if the presence of a laceration or the mechanism of an accident suggest the possibility of significant intracranial injury, a head CT is indicated.

Much more frequently, however, studies are performed that burden the patient and cost time and money without improving the patient's health or quality of life at all. It is the same here as everywhere in life: an experienced professional may know very well when further investigation may not be warranted. Patients entrust themselves to us and those who cannot or do not want to question our actions must not be disappointed by too cavalier an approach of their physicians (Fig. 5.**1**).

Now, how can you quickly scrutinize the indication of a scheduled study or find the right procedure for your patient if you are not really experienced? The indication list of the British Royal College of Radiologists "Making the best use of a Department of Clinical Radiology" provides some orientation and has been integrated into this book. An adapted specific excerpt precedes each of the clinical chapters.

! Diagnostic imaging, however expensive and impressive it may be, does not replace a careful physical examination or well-thought-out therapy. In emergencies, clear indications help expedite the diagnostic process; the appropriate choice of modality depends on its power to comprehensively examine the clinical problem at hand.

5.2   The Ill-Prepared Study

Any examination can lead you astray or cause erroneous findings if it is poorly executed. Reasons may be the lack of experience of the examining physician, especially when dealing with less frequent clinical problems, or when performing a study that requires considerable technical skill but has not been performed by that particular physician in a while. When considering the choice of a radiographic modality, its particular operator dependence also needs to be taken into account. If your least-talented ultrasound technologist is on duty and is unwell because of a long night on the town the previous evening, you may need to consider doing the examination yourself or choosing a more objective method such as CT.

! Insufficient preparation of the patient, however, is by far the most frequent cause of failed studies.

The responsibility for patient preparation lies mainly with the referring physician. If the patient is restless and unable to cooperate, sedation must be considered. Special preparatory measures have to be communicated and explained to the patient with sufficient care, making sure that the information is understood. A lady undergoing an ultrasound of the abdomen, for example, should preferably be fasting because an air-filled stomach hinders optimal visualization of the pancreas. A nervous older gentleman who is scheduled for an upper gastrointestinal study with barium and air followed by a small-bowel follow-through should also be fasting to allow for a good contrast coating of the gastric mucosa. Fasting in this context means: no breakfast, no coffee, no smoking, no toothbrushing and, of course, no alcohol. For obvious reasons, the study should be scheduled in the morning hours and diabetic patients should be examined first and perhaps need to consider reducing their morning dose of insulin if applicable. Referring physician and radiologist have to cooperate well in these cases; mistakes and failures are more than irritating for the patient:

Patient Maggie Snatcher: Mrs. Maggie Snatcher (78) has been complaining about irregular bowel movements for some time. The rectal examination is normal but occult blood has been detected in her stool. You send your patient to radiology to get an air contrast barium enema (see p. 193), to exclude large-bowel pathology. You have, however, forgotten to properly inform and prepare Mrs. Snatcher. She has not been told to take a laxative the day before; she has eaten dairy products until the evening before instead of having only clear liquids and soups for two days prior to the examination. Radiologist Smith does not cancel the examination when he learns about her lack of preparation. He fights hard to make the best of it to spare the patient (and you) having to schedule another appointment. The examination takes three times longer than normal because every piece of fecal residue has to be differentiated from intraluminal tumor. Finally Smith surrenders, stating that no tumor can be found.

Four weeks later the examination is repeated after a textbook preparation and a plum-sized malignant polyp is diagnosed by Smith's special friend, Assistant Professor Newman. You should not be counting on any favors from Smith for a few months to come. And your credit rating with Mrs. Snatcher has also gone down the drain.

> ! A badly prepared study may cost you dearly in terms of time, nerves, and friends at the very least. It will certainly ruin your day.

5.3 Studies with Contrast Media

Contrast-enhancing substances are commonly used in plain radiography, CT, MRI, and sometimes even in ultrasound. They serve to improve the visualization of hollow organs, vessels, and parenchymal organs, and to document the perfusion or metabolism of tissues. Contrast media can result in a higher or lower signal intensity of structures of interest relative to the immediate anatomical surrounding—in radiography and CT the radiation attenuation is increased or decreased.

Contrast Media in Radiography and CT

Iodinated Intravascular Contrast Media

→ **Definition:** Iodinated contrast media (CMs), whether administered intravascularly or elsewhere, are currently the most frequently used type of contrast media. For the most part they are nonionic substances of low osmolality. Because of their rather high viscosity they are usually warmed before administration. The use of ionic CMs has declined in recent years because they are associated with a higher rate of allergic reactions. They are also more neurotoxic and nephrotoxic than nonionic CMs.

→ **Dosage:** Intravascular administration: 1 g iodine/kg body weight in adults and 0.6 g iodine/kg body weight in children should not be exceeded. As CMs are eliminated via the kidneys, the patient must be adequately hydrated, that is, he or she should drink a lot or should be given an additional infusion.

> ! Hydration is of paramount importance in contrast administration. Infusion therapy may be necessary in some patients.

Heart disease, hematological disease, or oncological disease: Patients with severe cardiac insufficiency (NYHA III and IV) and arrhythmias can decompensate after contrast administration. The same is true for patients with multiple myeloma, polycythemia vera, or sickle cell anemia.

Metabolic diseases: Diabetic patients should discontinue metformin medication for two days after the CM study because of the risk of lactic acidosis. If serum creatinine remains stable after contrast administration (48 hours), metformin medication can be restarted. A low dose of contrast should be used in patients with homocysteinuria.

Renal disease: In patients with latent or manifest renal insufficiency (serum creatinine in excess of 2 mg/dl), renal function can further deteriorate or cease altogether. Good hydration needs to be ensured. If needed, an infusion of saline has to be administered, the amount of CM must be minimized, and dialysis must be considered. If there is no renal function left, that is, in terminal renal insufficiency treated with regular dialysis, dosage of CM can be normal. In case of doubt, consult with the treating physician/nephrologist of the patient to determine the best course of action and renoprotective options.

> ! In renal disease, contrast media should only be given after the serum creatinine has been checked.

Thyroid disease: In patients with suspected (latent) hyperthyroidism, iodinated CM may only be given after a detailed laboratory analysis (Table 5.**1**) and in consultation with the referring physician. The sudden iodine load introduced into the patient during CM administration may lead to severe hyperthyroidism and even thyrotoxic crisis in some cases. This is a potentially lethal disease entity that requires intensive care and that can occur weeks or even months after CMs are given.

→ **Allergic reactions to contrast media:** Iodinated contrast media can cause severe adverse and allergic reactions. Slight adverse reactions are seen in about 1 % of patients, a life-threatening anaphylactic reaction in approximately 1 out of 1000 patients. It is thus essential to be familiar with the treatment of these reactions and to have the appropriate drugs and other tools available where contrast is administered. Teamwork is extremely important in severe CM incidents, which is why group training including technologists and physicians should be performed on a regular basis.

> ! A large, safely taped venous access line is required in examinations with intravascular iodinated CM. A resuscitation cart well equipped for cardiopulmonary resuscitation is also essential, together with the telephone or beeper number of the resuscitation team clearly visible on the wall.

Table 5.1 Normal thyroid hormone levels (may vary from one laboratory to another)

TSH: 0.23–4.0 mcU/ml	
TT$_3$: 0.8–1.8 ng/ml	TT$_4$: 45–115 ng/ml
FT$_3$: 3.5–6.0 pg/ml	FT$_4$: 8.0–20.0 pg/ml

F, free; T, total.

Patients with a history of asthma, atopic dermatitis, and allergies (e.g., hay fever) or reactions to contrast media in previous examinations need particular attention. Reactions to CMs that date back more than 15 years are not as worrisome as those on more recent occasions: the reason is the change of CMs from the ionic to the better-tolerated nonionic type during the course of the 1990s. Always have the patient describe the precise circumstances of a previous CM reaction so as to gauge the significance and severity of the earlier reaction—a period of intensive care after the incident is a big red flag. As a first step, the indication of the requested study should be critically reviewed. Does the potential increased yield of information outweigh the increased risk of CM administration? If the answer is "yes," the history of moderate CM reactions should prompt the administration of oral steroids (for example, three 50 mg doses of prednisone 13 hours, 8 hours, and 1 hour prior to the examination) and intramuscular antihistamines (for example, 50 mg of Benadryl 1 hour prior to the examination). Patients are advised that it is not safe to operate a vehicle for 8 hours after this medication has been administered because of its sedative effect and they should not be left alone. In patients with a history of severe CM reactions, studies with CM administration should only performed in the presence of an anesthesiologist or equally qualified physician ready to intervene.

Moderate adverse reactions: Heat sensation, unrest, an urge to cough, yawning, sneezing, nausea, vomiting, itching, edema of the eyelid, urticaria, as well as redness and edema of the skin or mucous membranes are signs of moderate reactions. Go and talk to the patient calmly (!), check heart rate and blood pressure, and, if deemed necessary, have the assisting personnel mix H_1- and H_2-antagonists in 50 ml of saline and give it via the venous access line over the course of about 5 minutes. In addition, corticosteroids can also be administered intravenously. The responsible physician in charge stays with the patient and conveys tranquility! This is the moment to give the patient the impression that as professionals we are taking good care of him/her even during a minor incident. After such an incident the patient must be monitored for a few hours and should not leave the premises before a physician has had a chance to reevaluate him or her.

Checklist: **Moderate Adverse Reactions**

1. Stay calm and calm down the patient!
2. Ensure functioning intravenous access.
3. Monitor the patient closely; check blood pressure and pulse.
4. Administer H_1- and H_2-antagonists in saline infusion.
5. Have corticosteroids available.

Severe adverse reactions: Sudden sweating, pallor, generalized exanthema, shivering, fear, back pain, dyspnea, bronchospasm, asthma, glottic edema, tachycardia, loss of blood pressure, loss of conscience, cramps, and lack of pulse are hallmarks of a severe reaction. The first step after recognizing a severe reaction is to declare a med-

ical emergency and to inform the hospital resuscitation team or the local emergency team if you are outside the hospital. If a large venous access is not yet present or not functioning, put one in now. An infusion is started; an ECG is initiated if available. The legs are elevated. The doctor stays with the patient! And remains calm—"It's the patient, who is sick!" Antihistamine medication is given intravenously; the dosage of corticosteroids is raised. If the patient goes into shock, the usual **ABC rules** apply:

- Free the **A**irways: Lift the chin forward and tilt the forehead back to open up the pharyngeal air passage; if necessary, secure the airway with instrumentation.
- Ensure **B**reathing: Ventilate the patient either mouth-to-mouth or mouth-to-nose if necessary or with airway protector and bag/mask if available; give oxygen (3–6 l/min); intubation is reserved for the experienced physician.
- Restore **C**irculation: In asystole try a precordial thump; if that is without effect, start cardiac massage with intermittent respiration (15 : 2 if you are doing it alone or 5 : 1 if you have assistance). The patient must be resting on a rigid support; the lower third of the sternum is depressed by 4–5 cm with a frequency of 70/min; in children the frequency is higher and depression is less deep. Cardiac massage must be performed with care and tailored force: rib fractures in resuscitation are normal but not desirable. Utilize cardiac defibrillation as indicated.

Checklist: **Severe Incompatibility Reactions**

1. Call the resuscitation team at once.
2. Secure the intravenous access, give volume (fluids), corticosteroids , antihistamines (in infusion) quickly i.v.
3. Clear the airways; oxygen 3–6 l/min; respire via mouth/nose or mask.
4. Monitor blood pressure and pulse; do ECG; use pulse oximeter.
5. In blood pressure loss, elevate legs 60° or more; give volume (fluids); epinephrine (1 : 10 000; 0.1 ml dissolved in 1 ml saline) slowly i.v.
6. In asystole do a precordial thump first; if that fails, initiate cardiac massage; epinephrine (1 : 10 000; 0.5 ml dissolved in 5 ml saline) slowly i.v.

If the risk of a major adverse reaction is deemed too great, the study is performed without CM (for example, in CT) or replaced by other modalities such as ultrasound or MRI. If only very little CM is needed, such as in i.v. line checks, some colleagues have used the extremely expensive but low-risk MR contrast medium gadolinium, which also appears opaque on plain radiography. This represents "off-label" use, however.

→ Contraindications: A history of severe prior adverse reaction to iodinated CM represents a relative contraindication for its use because of the significant potential associated morbidity and mortality. CM administration interferes with radioisotope therapy of the thyroid gland, for example, in patients with thyroid cancer or Basedow/

Graves disease with thyroid orbitopathy because the iodine uptake capacity of thyroid tissue may become exhausted for several months by administration of iodinated CM. You should consult the treating physician prior to CM administration in these cases to discuss risks and benefits as well as optimal timing of the study.

Contrast Media for Extravascular Use

→ **Definition:** Barium-containing as well as iodine-containing CMs are used preferentially for studies of the gastrointestinal tract. Frequently, barium-containing substances are administered together with air or methylcellulose to achieve a radiopaque coating of the luminal surfaces of hollow organs, which stand out nicely against adjacent air during so-called "double contrast" examinations.

→ **Dosage:** These CMs are administered orally or rectally. The exact dosage, viscosity, etc., depend on the clinical question, anatomy, and other circumstances.

→ **Contraindications:** If there is a suspicion of a rupture/perforation of a hollow viscus or fistula formation of the gastrointestinal tract to the peritoneal cavity, barium-containing CMs are generally contraindicated. This is due to the severe foreign body granulomatous reaction that they can induce in the peritoneal cavity when they leave the GI tract. They should also not be given to patients with partial or complete ileus because they tend to agglutinate and aggravate the peristaltic problems further. The same is true in immediately preoperative examinations because peristaltic disturbances are frequent anyway after abdominal surgery. In these cases an iodinated hyperosmolar water-soluble CM may be used, although its diagnostic efficacy tends to be poorer. It has a lower radiodensity and dilutes faster. Its hyperosmolarity also explains the therapeutic effect it has: as the CM is diluted it draws interstitial fluid into the intestinal lumen and thereby triggers peristalsis. For the same reason the patient must be well hydrated. If hyperosmolar CM is aspirated into the bronchial tree the same principles apply—the fluid transfer into the bronchial lumen leads to pulmonary edema. For this reason patients with swallowing disorders in danger of aspiration should be examined with a nonionic iso-osmolar CM, usually administered intravascularly to decrease the risk of pulmonary edema, or with thin barium-containing CMs, which do not irritate the bronchial tree or mediastinum at all (though they tend to hang around for a while . . .).

Contrast Media in Magnetic Resonance Tomography

Contrast media for magnetic resonance tomography tend to shorten the relaxation times of protons. The most frequently used CM type is a **gadolinium chelate**. It is administered with a dosage of 0.1–0.3 mmol/kg body weight and excreted by the kidneys. This type of CM is very well tolerated—significantly better than all iodinated CMs in radiography and CT—and induces considerably fewer allergic reactions.

Another type of MR contrast medium consists of **ferrite compounds** that accumulate in the intact reticuloendothelial system (RES), especially in the spleen and the liver. The contrast between the healthy and pathological tissue is thus enhanced. The development of specialized CMs in MR imaging continues at a dizzying pace and some surprises can be suspected in the future.

Contrast Media in Ultrasonography

Contrast media in ultrasonography consist of microscopically small galenically stabilized air bubbles. They are very well visible inside the vessels with Doppler ultrasound. They are only rarely used in current clinical routine but promise to be very useful in, for example, characterization of liver lesions or any other situation where vascularization of an organ or disease process is to be examined.

5.4   The False Finding

There are two kinds of false findings: the false-negative finding that ignores or overlooks a lesion, and the false-positive finding that indicates a lesion where there is none. Both kinds of false reports can have enormous consequences for the patient but they cannot be completely avoided in daily practice. Their number must be kept as low as possible, though, and false findings discovered in retrospect should always be reviewed to improve the diagnostic process.

False-negative finding: A tumor on a chest radiograph, for example, is diagnosed when its conspicuity exceeds the detection threshold of the observer. The level of the threshold depends on the experience and concentration of the observer as well as on objective factors such as exposure of the radiograph and viewing conditions (monitor or viewing box brightness, ambient light, etc.). If the lesion is detected, it must be evaluated. Is it a benign finding, for example, a harmless postinflammatory granuloma, or could it be a malignant process, for example, a bronchogenic carcinoma? Retrospective studies in patients with bronchogenic carcinoma have shown that in up to 30% of cases the tumor could already be detected on previous films that were reported as normal—if one had a real close look and in retrospect, of course. (This is in no way a phenomenon unique to radiologists. Up to 50% of all coronary infarctions are overlooked by internists even in teaching hospitals—when you ask the pathologist.) Even seasoned radiologists with years of experience will not be able to avoid false-negative reports altogether. In the worst-case scenario, life-saving therapy is delayed beyond salvage.

False-positive finding: The false-positive finding also bears a considerable risk for the patient. If, for example, a microcalcification in mammography is falsely felt to be suspicious for malignancy, a biopsy is performed. Even though nowadays this will most likely be done as a stereotactic needle biopsy under local anesthesia on an outpatient basis (rather than a surgical biopsy under general anesthesia), the psychological stress for the patient is still considerable and may induce further complications. Because the incidence of the potentially lethal breast cancer is very high and the distinction of benign and malignant calcifications difficult, false-positive findings are one price to pay for an overall high cancer detection rate. Currently only every fourth biopsy of a suspicious breast lesion turns out to be cancer.

One scientifically proven way to reduce false-positive as well as false-negative findings is to have experienced diagnosticians "double-read" the studies. This is a costly practice but it has been successfully incorporated in most quality-controlled large-scale breast screening programs worldwide.

5.5   Risks of Radiological Procedures

Risks of Projection Radiography and Computed Tomography

The terrifying experiences of the early x-ray pioneers, some of their patients, and the victims of Hiroshima, Nagasaki, and Chernobyl demonstrate the risks of exposure to large doses of ionizing radiation with dire clarity. However, the number of human beings who have been helped by the use of radiation in diagnosis and therapy exceeds that of the victims by several orders of magnitude. The injuries that can be induced by the normal procedures in diagnostic radiology are less frequent and less severe than those that occur in the course of other routine medical therapies (for example, drug intoxications) or other diagnostic procedures (for example, pancreatitis after ERCP). All the same, many patients continue to feel uneasy about x rays. They need to be comforted with truthful information, and we need to strive to limit the use of diagnostic ionizing radiation to proper indications.

Effect Does Not Equal Effect

Stochastic effect: *Even minimal radiation doses have an effect.* They increase the likelihood of developing malignant tumors (somatic effect) and sustaining genetic damage (genetic effect) that might otherwise also occur without interference by man-made technology though less frequently. There are therefore no real threshold values below which the administration of x-rays is totally safe. This effect is also called the stochastic effect. It is a fundamental effect associated with the use of all ionizing radiation in diagnostic radiology and the major reason for the general radiation protection efforts today.

Nonstochastic effect: *Higher radiation doses produce direct effects.* These are, for example, damage to the skin, the hematopoietic bone marrow, and the eye lens, and radiation syndrome. A clear relationship exists between the severity of the disease and dose. These nonstochastic effects occur mainly in radiation therapy. In interventional radiology and neuroradiology such as cardiovascular stenting or percutaneous treatment of complex arteriovenous malformations in the CNS, nonstochastic effects such as radiation-induced erythema, ulcerations, or hair loss have been reported anecdotally in patients undergoing complex procedures exposed to prolonged fluoroscopy, for example. Obviously this also poses a serious threat to the physicians involved. Radiation-induced lens injury has been reported in interventional radiology.

Stochastic Effect?

Wilhelm Conrad Röntgen died owing to an ileus 28 years after his discovery of x-rays. The young and famous surgeon Sauerbruch, a pioneer of intrathoracic surgery, tried to save him with a last-minute operation but was unsuccessful. A large-bowel carcinoma as one likely cause of the ileus could only be attributed to the stochastic effect. X-ray tubes were prohibitively expensive even in those early days—and they survived but a few exposures. For that reason Röntgen's total radiation exposure was probably low. Apart from that, the cautious old fox used to leave the laboratory while his experiments were running. Interestingly enough, there are no radiographs of Röntgen himself, but there exists one of the hand of—you guessed it—his wife Anna-Bertha.

Figure 5.**2** shows a typical nonstochastic effect from the early days of radiology as suffered by Max Levy-Dorn, one of the pioneers and first victims of the new technology.

Dose Does Not Equal Dose

Energy dose: The *irradiation of a lifeless object* is adequately described by the energy dose. This represents the radiation energy (J; joules) that is absorbed per unit mass (kg) and is measured in units of grays (1 Gy = 1 J/kg). Any impact the radiation may have on an organism is completely ignored by this descriptor.

Equivalence dose: The *effect of x-rays on living organisms* is described by the equivalence dose. To calculate it, the energy dose is multiplied by a correction factor that represents the biological effect of radiation. It is measured in units of sieverts (Sv). For the usual x-rays this correction factor fortunately equals 1, which is why 1 Sv = 1 Gy = 1 J/kg. The energy and equivalence dose are of course difficult to measure in any living organism let alone a human being. The patient would have to swallow dosimeters, which would have to be read out after the intestinal passage—a little impractical, to say the least.

Personal dose: To quantitate the effect of radiation on an individual, the personal dose was introduced—also measured in sieverts (Sv). It represents the equivalence dose at specific representative locations on the body surface where you can wear a dosimeter. Now dose becomes a parameter you can work with. Dose limits have been

Nonstochastic Effect

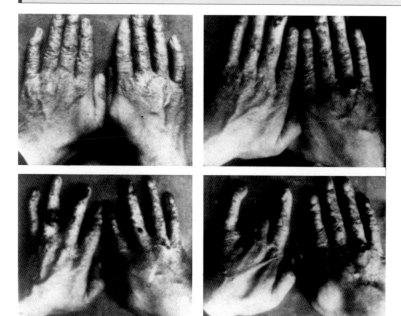

Fig. 5.**2** These historical photographs show the development of radiation injury to the hand of Max Levy-Dom, who acquired it over the duration of several years as chief of one of the first radiology departments in the world. Before starting an examination he used to test the function of the "Roentgen" tube—unfortunately using his own hand as a test object.

agreed upon (Table 5.**2**). To put these into a proper perspective, here is a comparison: The natural radiation exposure of the gonads is about 1.1 mSv/year, while radiation exposure to this area due to human activities (from medical exposures, fallout from atomic bombs, etc.) equals approximately 0.6 mSv/year.

Protection of the Patient

! The best radiation protection is to adhere to a strict indication list, reducing the number of examinations to the absolute necessary minimum, and whenever feasible to choose other imaging modalities that do not require radiation.

The technical execution of the examination by an experienced diagnostician comes next in line: fluoroscopy times are kept short, the radiated volume is kept small by careful collimation, the distance of the patient to the detector is kept short, and the examination protocols (for example in CT) are dose-optimized by experienced physicians and by clever scanner technology. Minimal dose means a dose that is just short of decreasing the diagnostic performance of the study. This is also called the **ALARA** principle: **a**s **l**ow **a**s **r**easonably **a**chievable. The choice of a dose-saving detector system, that is, a fitting film–screen combination or an optimized digital area detector, plus adequate beam filtration is essential. For the patient, the collimation of the x-ray beam is important to keep the exposure due to scattered radiation low (see Chapter 3, p. 6). Lead protectors should be used minimize the exposure of the gonads if the circumstances allow: in polytrauma, lead protection of the ovaries in women is impossible because fractures of the pelvic ring could be missed. Clever new CT scanners constantly modify the tube current and exposure according to patient thickness at each location as they proceed through an examination.

Gonadal Protection: When and Where

Radiation protection in women is more difficult than in men, for anatomical reasons. In acute polytrauma, protection is secondary in both sexes. In normal pelvic films, gonadal protection may obscure the region of interest in women. The female fertile phase ends with menopause, which makes gonadal protection less important. The law states that men need protection where appropriate. G. E.'s old chief used to put it this way: "Every man up to the age of 60 gets gonadal protection. Older men get it if they request it—but they get a piece of sweet chocolate with it."

If you translated a single-study dose into a total-body dose that would result in the same risk of acquiring genetic damage or a malignant disease, the result would be as shown in Table 5.**3**.

Table 5.**2 Legal dose limits for professional radiation exposure**

Organs/body region	Dose limit (mSv)
Gonads, uterus, red blood marrow	50
Thyroid, periosteum, skin	300
Hands, forearms and thighs, ankles	500
All other organs	150

Table 5.3 Effective total body dose in radiological examinations

Examination of organs/body regions	Typical effective total body dose (mSv)	Equivalent number of chest radiographs	Equivalent period of natural background radiation
Radiography			
Limbs and joints	0.01	0.5	1.5 days
Chest PA	0.02	1	3 days
Skull	0.1	5	2 weeks
Cervical spine	0.1	5	2 weeks
Thoracic spine	1.0	50	6 months
Lumbar spine	2.4	120	14 months
Hip	0.3	15	2 months
Pelvis	1.0	50	6 months
Abdomen	1.5	75	9 months
Barium swallow	2.0	100	1 year
Barium follow-through	5.0	250	2.5 years
Small-bowel barium enema	6.0	300	3 years
Large-bowel barium enema	9.0	450	4.5 years
Mammography	0.5	25	10 weeks
Computed tomography			
Head	2.0	100	1 year
Chest, abdomen	8.0	400	4 years
Scintigraphy			
Bone	5.0	250	2–5 years
Thyroid	1.0	50	6 months
Heart (thallium)	18	900	9 years

Protection of the Examining Physician

Most factors that serve the radiation protection of the patient also diminish the radiation exposure of the radiologist. These include the adequate experience of the examining physician, short fluoroscopy times, strict collimation of the x-ray beam, dose-minimized x-ray equipment, and a strict adherence to the indication list. One very effective protective measure is to keep the greatest possible distance (dose decreases by the square of the distance) from the primary or secondary sources of radiation (the tube and the patient). Another measure is to protect the physician with lead-lined, sometimes movable, walls, lead aprons, gloves, thyroid protectors, and awkward-looking lead-glass goggles or spectacles (Fig. 5.3).

By the way, British radiologists working between 1920 and 1945 showed the same cancer incidence as their nonradiological clinical colleagues and lived longer than the average general practitioner in the United Kingdom at that time.

X-rays Are Everywhere

A standard chest radiograph imparts a radiation dose of about 0.2 mSv; the CT study of the chest exceeds 20 mSv. A mammography takes about 2 mSv. One transatlantic flight from cool New York to old, old Europe for that cultural weekend, or vice versa, amounts to 0.1 mSv of cosmic radiation. The healthy life on an Austrian high mountain pasture increases the natural exposure to up to 10 mSv/year.

Paul Gets Real Serious

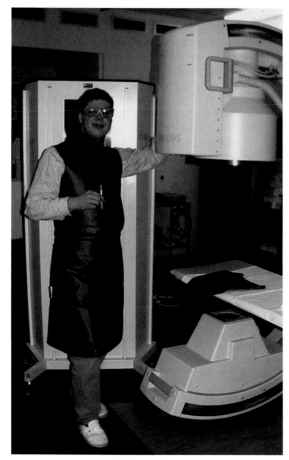

Fig. 5.**3**   Paul is well equipped for any radiological intervention, wearing a lead skirt that puts the weight on his iliac crests and not on his spine. The lead waistcoat, the thyroid protector, and the trendy lead goggles complete the outfit. In his hand he holds a quartz fiber dosimeter that is worn underneath the lead waistcoat, just like the film dosimeter, during the examination. Behind him you see a movable lead panel. Paul has thrown the clumsy lead gloves that are used in noninterventional fluoroscopy (such as barium enemas) onto the tabletop.

Risks of Ultrasound

Direct relevant risks of ultrasound techniques are not known. However, the results of an ultrasound examination depend strongly on the quality and experience of the examiner and are often difficult to document. The indirect risk to the patient due to nonultrasound procedures that follow false-positive or incorrect ultrasound findings is thus much higher than any direct hazard. There is, nonetheless, a general agreement that multiple ultrasound examinations of the unborn within the mother's womb without clinical indication ("baby-video") should not be performed because of the susceptibility of the unborn to external perils.

Risks of Magnetic Resonance Tomography

The extremely strong magnetic fields can cause malfunctions of mechanical and electronic equipment. Self trials with the inherited Rolex or the American Express card are not really recommended, but variations of the theme are reported on a regular basis. Metal buckets filled with cleaning water and carried into the MRI examination suite by inexperienced cleaning personnel off hours, which then miraculously plunge into the system gantry, emptying themselves and leaving the MRI machine unusable for weeks—it has all been heard of. Figure 5.**4** shows a particularly worrisome approach to a 1.5 tesla MRI machine that led to a total loss of the system, fortunately without any damage to human life or health. There is the story of an MRI engineer in a Great Lake City in the United States who was trying to repair something from inside the gantry of a running 1.5 tesla MRI machine propped up on a trailer truck. A fork lifter passed by the trailer; the unsecured forks were torn off the fork lifter and pierced through the trailer wall into the gantry of the machine, killing the engineer. That serves to make the point: MRI is by no means a harmless or risk-free technology. The following perils need to be considered:

- The induction of electrical currents
- The movement of metallic objects
- The noise that is generated by quickly switching gradients

Fatal Affinity

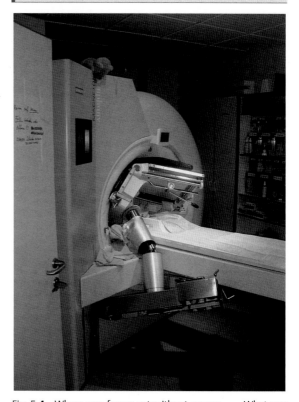

Fig. 5.**4**   Where raw forces act without reason . . . What you see in the gantry of this MR machine is a 200 kg (31.5 stones or 441 pounds) surgical table.

Induction of currents: Currents are not only induced in the MR receive coil or antenna. This occurs in all conducting structures. Flowing blood is such a conductor. The resulting current boosts the ECG curve at the time of the peak blood flow: the T-wave is raised. In cables, particularly in cable loops (cardiac pacemakers), currents are generated that can lead to overheating and even burns. Loops such as these can also be caused by faulty patient positioning: if the patient's hands or bare calves touch each other, burns can result.

> **!** Ear implants, cardiac pacemakers and defibrillators (including residual wires), neurostimulators, and implanted electronic infusion pumps prohibit any MR study.

Firmly anchored osteosynthetic material can disturb the imaging process and heat up. Metallic implants longer than 20 cm should be approached with special care. If the patient feels unwell during the examination, it should be terminated immediately. Paramagnetic materials, which are attracted little by magnetic fields, and ferromagnetic materials, which can be magnetized, can also severely compromise imaging. Tattoos may also hinder imaging and heat up depending on their ingredients. For the same reason, eye shadows (which often contain metal) and jewelry of all sorts (rings, bracelets, piercings, etc.) must be removed (Fig. 5.**5**).

Movement of metallic objects: The extraordinary danger due to metallic objects outside the body has already been mentioned. But how about metal within the body? One must ensure prior to the examination (e.g. with an orbital radiograph) that retained shrapnel or other metallic for-

eign bodies are not located in the vicinity of crucial structures such as the eye. The usual prosthetic cardiac valves do not constitute a contraindication for MR imaging. However, as a general rule, patients with loose vascular coils, stents, or filters should not be examined. At least six weeks should go by after implantation before an MR procedure is considered. MRI-induced movement of aneurysm clips on cerebral vessels are really dangerous. Lethal incidents have been reported. The type of clip—which is hopefully documented in the surgical report—and its MR compatibility should be determined with great care. Lists on the MR compatibility of almost all implanted materials are available on the Internet (see the homepage of the Food and Drug Administration, FDA: http://www.fda.gov; or that of the International Society for Magnetic Resonance in Medicine, http://www.ismrm.org).

 What Does the FDA Say?
"For a properly operating system, the hazards associated with direct interactions of these fields (static magnetic, pulsed gradient and radio frequency) and the body are negligible. It is the interaction of these fields with medical devices . . . that create[s] concerns for safety."

Noise generated in the course of gradient switching: The extremely rapid switching of gradients, particularly in modern fast and complex MR sequences, can lead to noise levels beyond 100 dB. Just to remind you: music during an exuberant disco night reaches 140 dB, a jack-hammer about 120 dB. Ear plugs or special protective headphones are thus mandatory for the patient and any other person in the same room (and for your disco visit, obviously . . .).

Further risks to human life and health due to the commonly used MR techniques are not known. Elective MR studies of women in early pregnancy (up to the third month) are nonetheless discouraged because of residual safety concerns. In vital indications in this patient group, however, MR is always preferred to CT because of the lack of definitely harmful ionizing radiation and because MR often has the same or a better diagnostic yield.

> **!** The MR room may only be entered after a thorough briefing by and in the company of the MR personnel. Any cables inside the body prohibit MR studies.

5.6   Risks of Intervention

A considerable proportion of risks in invasive imaging (such as angiography) is due to the use of contrast media, which has already been covered. Further significant risks are:
- In **angiography**, direct injury of the vessel may occur including dissection of the vascular wall, hematoma, arteriovenous fistula formation, or the development of pseudoaneurysms at the site of vascular entry. Furthermore, catheters may dislodge thromboembolic

Piercing, Yes but . . .

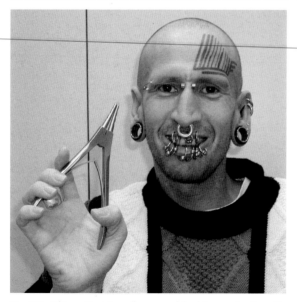

Fig. 5.**5**   This patient is well prepared for his examination. He brought a pair of pliers along to take his jewelry off. It took him about half an hour.

Table 6.1 Suggestions for diagnostic modalities in chest imaging[1]

Clinical problem	Investigation	Comment
Nonspecific chest pain	CXR	Not indicated initially. Main purpose is reassurance.
Upper respiratory tract infection	CXR	Not indicated.
Chronic obstructive airways disease or asthma; follow-up	CXR	Only if signs or symptoms have changed, asthma is life-threatening, or treatment fails.
Pneumonia	CXR	Majority of patients with community-acquired pneumonia will show radiological resolution at 4 weeks. In smokers, the elderly, and chronic airways disease, resolution may be prolonged. If patients become completely asymptomatic, no follow-up CXR is needed.
Pneumonia, adults: follow-up	CXR	If patients become completely asymptomatic, no follow-up CXR is needed in younger patients or in the absence of a significant smoking history. If symptoms persist, in the elderly and smokers, 6 weeks follow-up is advised.
Acute chest infection, children	CXR	Not indicated routinely. Initial and follow-up films are indicated in the presence of persisting clinical signs or symptoms or in the severely ill child. Children may have pneumonia without clinical signs.
Pleural effusion	CXR	Small effusion can be missed, especially on a frontal CXR.
	US	Indicated. To assess fluid consistency; to guide aspiration.
	CT	CT occasionally needed for better localization, assessment of solid components, etc.
Hemoptysis	CXR	Indicated. P-A plus lateral view. If normal and hemoptysis is significant or out of context of a concurrent chest infection, further investigations are necessary.
	CT	In conjunction with bronchoscopy. May detect malignancies not identified on CXR and bronchoscopy, but is insensitive to subtle mucosal and submucosal disease.
Occult lung disease	High-resolution CT (HRCT)	HRCT can show abnormalities not evident on CXR and may be more specific; may give valuable information about disease reversibility and prognosis.
Myocardial infarction	CXR	Assesses heart size, pulmonary edema, shows paradiagnoses tumor and pleuritis, pneumonia.
Pericarditis, pericardial effusion	US echocardiography	Assesses size of effusion, suitability for drainage, development of tamponade, concomitant pathology. Best for follow-up.
Valvular disease	CXR	For initial assessment.
	US echocardiography	Best method of sequential follow-up. TOE may be needed for prosthetic valves.
	MRI	Useful in congenital heart disease. Contraindicated in many patients after mechanical heart valve replacement.
Hypertension	CXR	Assesses cardiac size and possible associated pathology such as aortic coarctation or rib erosion from collaterals.
	US echocardiography	Most practical method for assessing LV hypertrophy.

CT, computed tomography; CXR, chest radiograph; ITU, intensive therapy (intensive care) unit; LV, left ventricular; MRI, magnetic resonance imaging; NM, nuclear medicine; P-A, posterior–anterior; PE, pulmonary embolism; PET, positron emission tomography; TB, tuberculosis; TOE, Trans esophageal echography; US, ultrasound

Table **6.1** (continued) **Suggestions for diagnostic modalities in chest imaging**[1]

Clinical problem	Investigation	Comment
Pulmonary embolism	CT	Investigation of choice; will show and exclude relevant pulmonary embolism as well as other differential diagnoses (e.g., aortic dissection); dedicated "one-stop shop" PE protocols will also demonstrate deep vein thrombosis from the knee up in the same procedure.
	CXR	To demonstrate consolidation and pleural effusion; cannot exclude pulmonary embolus.
	NM	Ventilation/perfusion (V : Q) scintigraphy can be diagnostic in patients without COPD and consolidations on CXR. Normal perfusion scintigraphy excludes significant pulmonary emboli.
Aortic dissection	CT	Investigation of choice; will show and exclude dissection as well as other diagnoses (e.g., pulmonary embolism).
	CXR	Baseline investigation to exclude other causes; rarely diagnostic.
Intensive care patient	CXR	CXR is most helpful when there has been a change in symptoms or insertion or removal of a device. The value of the routine daily CXR is increasingly being questioned. CT is a useful adjunct for problem-solving in the critically ill.
Preemployment or screening medicals	CXR	Not indicated. Justified in a few high-risk categories (e.g., at risk immigrants with no recent CXR). Some have to be done for occupational (e.g., divers) or emigration purposes (UK category 2).
Preoperative	CXR	Not indicated routinely. Exceptions before cardiopulmonary surgery, likely admission to ITU, suspected malignancy or possible TB. Anesthesiologists may also request CXRs for dyspneic patients, those with known cardiac disease and the very elderly. Many patients with cardiorespiratory disease have a recent CXR available; a repeat CXR may not be necessary under these circumstances.
Cancer patients		
Diagnosis	CXR P-A and lateral	But can be normal, particularly with central tumors. Marking of nipples may reduce number of fluoroscopies in tumor patients with suspected metastases.
	CT	Many centers proceed directly to bronchoscopy, which allows biopsy. CT is superior in identifying lesions responsible for hemoptysis.
Staging	CT chest, upper abdomen	Indicated. Despite limitations in specificity of nodal involvement, etc.
	NM	Some centers perform bone scintigraphy for possible skeletal metastases.
	MRI	Assists in estimating local invasion of chest wall, particularly for apical and peripheral lesions and mediastinal invasion. Helps distinguish adrenal adenoma from metastasis.
	PET	Specialized investigation. A single expensive investigation to identify small metastatic foci may save a lot of other investigations and inappropriate surgery.

[1]Modified after: RCR Working Party. *Making the best use of a Department of Clinical Radiology. Guidelines For Doctors*, 5th ed. London: The Royal College of Radiologists, 2003.
COPD, chronic obstructive pulmonary disease; CT, computed tomography; CXR, chest radiograph; ITU, intensive therapy (intensive care) unit; LV, left ventricular; MRI, magnetic resonance imaging; NM, nuclear medicine; P-A, posterior–anterior; PE, pulmonary embolism; PET, positron emission tomography; TB, tuberculosis; TOE, Trans oesophageal echography; US, ultrasound

Chest Radiograph Erect: Normal Findings

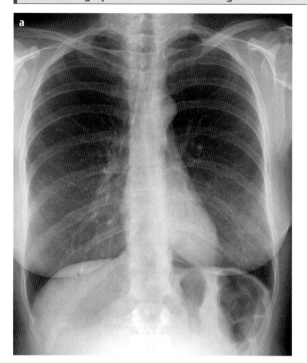

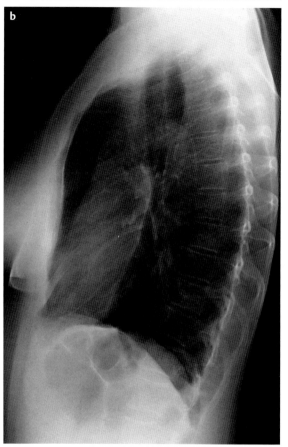

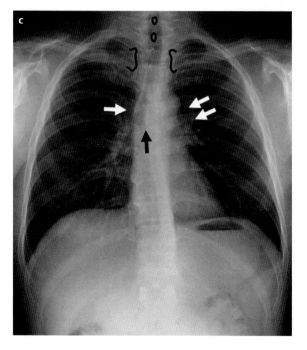

Fig. 6.1 a   This is a normal CXR of a female. Note the increased density of the lower lung due to the mammary glands. The contours of the breasts are not always visible as well as this. In a patient who has undergone mastectomy the operated side may be less radiopaque, resulting in a relative increase on the contralateral side! If one breast is missing, unintended rotation of the patient may ensue when the patient is asked to "hug" the detector or film cassette—how you control for that is outlined in **c**.

b Here you see a normal lateral view of a slim female. Once you identify left and right hemidiaphragms (silhouette sign of the heart, air in the colon and the stomach!), you can also assign the posterior costophrenic sulcus and the posterior lung margin to the proper side. Now find the aortic arch. Draw the pulmonary artery in your mind (see also Fig. 6.**2a**)

c This is a normal CXR of a male. You can appreciate the handy "spirit level" all of us carry around—the gastric bubble. The medial contours of the scapula are visible outside of the lungs. There is no doubt: this radiograph was performed with the patient erect. The spinous processes of C7 and T1 are marked as posterior point of reference, the medial borders of the clavicles as anterior point of reference. This patient is well positioned!

First follow the diaphragmatic contour: Is it well demarcated and do the costophrenic sulci show a normal depth and pointed tip? Or is there an upward-curved line (as for instance in a pleural effusion)? The right lower lobe of the lung covers the entire surface of the right hemidiaphragm;

in the left hemithorax the heart abuts the hemidiaphragm anteriorly and the left lower lobe touches the remainder of it. If the lower lobe is not aerated, the hemidiaphragmatic contour is no longer perceptible and we lose its silhouette (this is the "silhouette sign," see p. 23–24).

"Silhouette Sign"

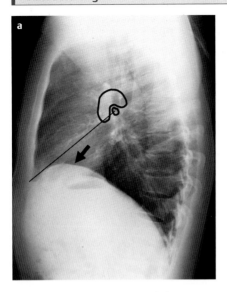

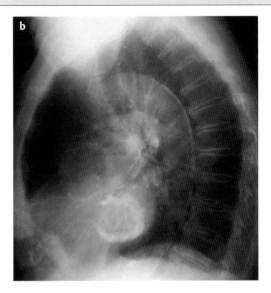

Fig. 6.**2 a**   The silhouette sign helps us to assign the hemidiaphragms to their correct side. The heart sits on the left hemidiaphragm, which is why the anterior part of the hemidiaphragmatic contour is not visible. Together with the gastric bubble, the splenic flexure of the colon is located underneath the left diaphragm. Got it all lined up? The arrow points to the right hemidiaphragm. Trace its contour back to the right posterior pleural margin and the right costophrenic sulcus. You can now assign pleural lesions such as pleural effusion to their proper side. The inverted comma is drawn for orientation—it corresponds to the left pulmonary artery. Do you recognize the "black hole" that the comma bends around? The major and minor fissures are both easily identified on properly exposed radiographs and they provide clues for orientation in the process of allocating a lesion to a specific lobe. Note how far superiorly the lower lobe extends!

b Now go ahead and use your fresh knowledge in the analysis of this image. Which heart valve is calcified in this patient?

It is the mitral valve that is most prominent, but the aortic valve is also visible.

Portable Chest Radiograph: Normal Findings

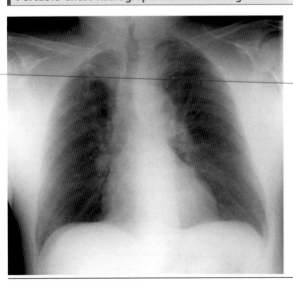

Fig. 6.**3**   This CXR was performed with the patient in bed without a scatter-reducing grid—that is why the inherent image contrast is lower. The mediastinum is compressed, the diaphragm is elevated owing to the increased abdominal pressure. The upper lobe pulmonary vessels are well filled because the hydrostatic pressure in the recumbent patient is similar in the upper lung to the pressure at the lung bases. The superior mediastinum is a little wider than usual in a bedside CXR. Do you need to worry? Have you checked the rotation of the patient?

Now trace the visible pleural border up to the lung apex: Is the pleura smooth? Is it fitted tightly to the rib cage or not—as, for example, in pleural scarring, in pleural effusion in a recumbent patient, or in a patient with a pneumothorax?

Inspect the lung parenchyma: Is the radiographic density of the lungs homogeneous and symmetric? (Asymmetry may be caused, for example, by freely mobile pleural effusions causing a more radiopaque appearance of the affected side in a supine patient.) Are there increases and/

or decreases in radiolucency (for example, regional over-inflation, opacities)? Can circumscribed opacities be seen (nodules, consolidation)? Do the vessels appear to be sharp and of normal caliber, or are they fuzzy and prominent (as, for example, in pulmonary edema)? Do they branch in a harmonic fashion or like the branches of an old apple tree (as, for example, in emphysema)? Briefly check the position of the minor fissure, the thin pleural leaf that separates the upper and middle lobes on the right side (Fig. 6.**1a**).

Have a look at the superior mediastinum: Is it of normal width? Is the trachea in midline and of normal caliber? Or is the trachea displaced and narrowed (such as in a patient with a goiter)? Does the aortic arch show a normal configuration or is it widened (as can be the case in patients with aortic aneurysm or traumatic pseudo-aneurysm)? Is its lateral contour visible ("silhouette sign," see p. 23–24)? Is the outline of the trachea immediately adjacent to the aortic arch or is there a perceptible separation between these two structures (for example, as caused by enlarged lymph nodes)? Is the azygos vein of normal caliber (approx. 1 cm; Fig. 6.**1c**), or is it enlarged (as, for example, in superior vena cava obstruction or right heart dysfunction)? Are the tracheal bifurcation and carina normally configured (Fig. 6.**1c**)? Or do they appear elevated and widened (such as in an enlarged left atrium or enlarged infracarinal lymph nodes)?

Now let us review the hila: Is the left hilum about a finger's width higher than the right (due to the left pulmonary artery crossing over the left main stem bronchus)? Or is one of the hila displaced (for example, by loss of volume or scarring in the upper lobe on that side)? Is the aorto-pulmonary window—the angle between the aortic knob and the left pulmonary artery—empty? Are the hila bilaterally enlarged (for example, in pulmonary hypertension or bilateral lymph node enlargement) or is only one hilum of irregular shape (for example, due to a tumor)?

Look at the inferior mediastinum: Is the heart contour of normal size and configuration? The width of the heart may not exceed half the maximum diameter of the chest. Do you see additional shadows projecting over the heart (for example, pericardial calcifications in constrictive pericarditis, coronary or valvular calcifications, metal valve re-placements, cardiac pacer or defibrillator electrodes)? Are the heart contours visible all around? The right heart contour is adjacent to the middle lobe, the left contour by the "lingula" of the upper lobe of the left lung (these are other potential sites for a "silhouette sign," see p. 23–24). If the lower left heart contour is rounded and extends far laterally, the left ventricle is enlarged (for example, in cardiac muscular hypertrophy due to arterial hypertension or aortic valve stenosis). If the concavity of the upper left heart contour turns convex, this may be due to pulmonary arterial enlargement in patients with valvular disease or sometimes in patients with severe pulmonary arterial hypertension.

Observe the heart shadow and the space underneath the diaphragmatic contour: About one-third of the lung is located in these areas; consequently, about one-third of the pathology also hides there. Try to trace the course of the vessels in the heart shadow and underneath the diaphragmatic domes! In perfect radiographs of perfect patients you can see the anterior and posterior margins of the costophrenic sulci.

Finish up and check the thoracic wall and soft tissues: How wide is the soft tissue mantle of the thorax; how muscular, adipose, or edematous is the patient? Is there perhaps a breast missing or are there clips in the axilla in a patient with treated breast cancer? Now analyze the cervical region: Is there any air in the soft tissue (for example, in soft tissue emphysema due to trauma or a leaky chest tube); are the vocal cords visible at the upper end of the trachea (essential to determine the correct position of an endotracheal tube!)?

Finally have a look at the thoracic skeleton: A first glance goes to the shoulders and clavicles, the second scans the spine. Then rotate the radiograph by 90° to better appreciate the ribs without your attention being distracted by the heart and lung (Fig. 6.**4**). Experienced radiologists will applaud this procedure and give you additional points in your oral exam. Now trace every single rib from the spine to its ventral end. Pay attention to discontinuities and irregularities in the rib margins and to soft tissue shadows alongside the ribs: Are variants present such as bifid ribs or do you see fractures, metastases, or destructions due to tumors such as multiple myeloma?

Checking the Ribs: Normal Findings

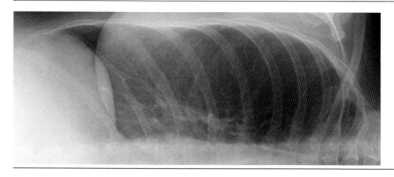

Fig. 6.**4** This is how you evaluate the thoracic skeleton best—clockwise or anticlockwise rotation (90°). Trace every single rib over its complete course. For specific bone problems, a dedicated rib series of the affected hemithorax with a different (lower) exposure voltage (approx. 80 kVp) is performed.

Now Get Additional Information from the Lateral Chest Radiograph

When looking at the lateral CXR, things only get more complicated: both lungs and hila are now superimposed. The first step is to become familiar with the appearance of normal anatomical structures so that you can recognize them on a lateral CXR like good old friends and notice when one is missing.

Begin with both hemidiaphragms: Which one is the left hemidiaphragm (see Fig. 6.**2a**)? Follow the contour of both hemidiaphragms anteriorly, starting at the bottom of the respective posterior costophrenic sulcus. Now trace the posterior pleural border toward the upper thorax. Localize both the minor and the major lobar fissures (by the way, which side was the minor fissure on?).

Analyze the hila at this time: The left pulmonary artery swings out of the pulmonary trunk up over the left main stem bronchus, assuming the configuration of an inverted comma. The left main stem bronchus is part of the "black hole" that you see on most films. On a normal CXR, essentially all visible dense structures within the lungs should show a typical vascular, branching course toward the hilum. If that is not the case, you need to explore further.

What do the heart contours tell you? The anterior heart contour corresponds to the anterior wall of the right ventricle and is seen behind the anterior thoracic wall, mainly made up of the sternum centrally, which is why this space is called the retrosternal space. If the right ventricular border reaches the mid and upper sternum, the ventricle is enlarged. The posterior heart contour on the lateral CXR corresponds to the left atrium in its upper part and to the left ventricle in its lower part. A small amount of barium swallowed by the patient prior to taking the CXR outlines the course of the esophagus and lets you better appreciate the outline of the atrium if this is of clinical importance.

Finally put everything else in order: The contour of the aortic arch is visible throughout most of its course. It runs in a wide arc over the hilum. Atherosclerosis of the aorta is easily appreciated on this projection. The "black hole" mentioned before can help us once more (see Fig. 6.**2**): If we draw a line from there to the anterior costophrenic sulcus, the aortic valve typically projects superior to the line, the mitral valve inferior to it. Pretty good trick, isn't it? Finally we take a good look at the upper retrosternal space, which should be rather radiolucent because here both lungs meet anterior to the mediastinum. In emphysema this space could be widened; if there is a tumor or goiter present, the space becomes radiopaque.

I See an Abnormality—What Do I Do Now?

You proceed as systematically as you did during the image analysis described above. First of all the diagnostic thinking needs to be pointed in the right direction!

If the abnormality concerns the **lung parenchyma**, the following questions need to be answered:

- Is it an opacity or an abnormal radiolucency?
- Is it a rather circumscribed or a diffuse process?
- Are we dealing with a solitary lesion or are multiple lesions present?
- Is the lesion homogeneous or heterogeneous?
- Does the diffuse process have a patchy (acinar) or fine linear (reticular) or diffusely nodular pattern of appearance?

If the abnormality is located in the **mediastinum**, it suffices to localize the lesion: hilar region, upper or lower, anterior or posterior mediastinum.

If the lesion is in the **thoracic wall**, any involvement of the ribs needs to be determined.

Additional studies may help to show the lesion more clearly and in more detail; for example, a quick fluoroscopy of a nodule in the central lung or an elevated hemidiaphragm, or an apical lordotic view when dealing with an abnormality in the lung apices (Fig. 6.**5**). After that the diagnostic approach starts to vary. We will see and exercise this in the respective cases. Now you should be about ready to tackle the first clinical case.

Hyperlordotic View

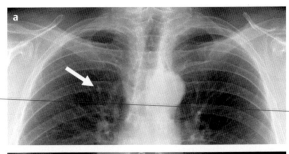

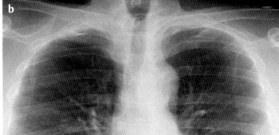

Fig. 6.**5 a**   There is a small nodule seen above the right hilum (arrow). Is it a real finding?
b The apical lordotic view shows a normal superior lung (the patient leans back during the exposure and thus elevates the clavicles up over the lung apices). In retrospect the "nodule" must have been a prominent vessel viewed end-on or "down the barrel."

6.2 Opacities in the Lung

Solitary, Circumscribed Opacity of the Lung

Checklist: Singular, Circumscribed Opacity of the Lung

- Is the radiographic appearance of the lesion homogeneous or inhomogeneous?
- Is the margin to the surrounding parenchyma sharp or unsharp?
- Is its contour smooth or irregular, straight or lobulated?
- Are any interfaces to adjacent structures (diaphragm, heart contour, aortic arch) obscured?
- Does the lesion displace its neighboring tissues or cause loss of volume with resulting shift of adjacent structures toward the lesion?

All of a sudden—a spot in the lung

Sidel Zastro (78) has come into the hospital to get his inguinal hernia repaired. Since he has not really felt well for the past months (he has not enjoyed his cigars the way he used to) and since he has got some mileage on him, a preoperative chest radiograph is performed. With a patient of this age, Paul anticipates seeing some traces of a life gone by—long, exhaustive work, war, malnutrition, diseases, smoking, surgery, and vice of any kind may leave their traces in the thorax of an individual. He expects apical (Fig. 6.**6a**) and possibly basal pleural adhesions, irregular vascular markings such as in old age emphysema, and possibly some scarring due to past pneumonias (Fig. 6.**6b**). Mr. Zastro did not, of course, bring previous films—why on earth should he have bothered? He last saw the inside of a hospital 30 years ago. Paul and Joey study the CXR (Fig. 6.**7**) together, following the analysis scheme outlined above (see p. 40, 43–46).

→ **What Is Your Diagnosis?** Paul has discovered that the right basal lung isn't as radiolucent as it should be. Or could that be a delusion? In a woman, removal of the breast on the other side could sometimes give rise to this appearance, argues Joey. How about a chest wall anomaly? The x-ray technician says the patient's chest looked normal to her. Should one consider an emphysematous overinflation of the left basal lung in a patient of this age? In that case the vessel markings should be irregular and decreased, which is not what Paul and Joey see. Both finally agree that the true abnormality is at the right lung base. They go ahead and answer all the key checklist questions one by one:

Is the internal structure of the lesion homogeneous or inhomogeneous? *Lesions with homogeneous internal structure:* In this case the parenchyma is devoid of air. A solid tumor will replace alveoli and bronchi with tumor tissue (Fig. 6.**8**). In a pleural effusion, whether mobile (Fig. 6.**9a**) or loculated (Fig. 6.**9b**), the lung is intact but displaced away from the abnormality. In endobronchial obstruction, the air distal to the point of obstruction is resorbed—a postobstructive atelectasis results (Fig. 6.**10**).

A Chest Radiograph Appropriate for Age

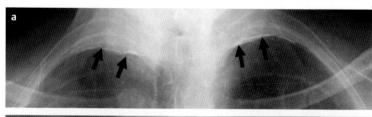

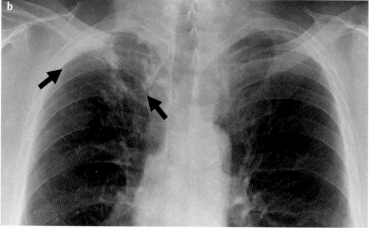

Fig. 6.**6a** During the course of the usual pulmonary infections of a long life, this patient has developed apical pleural scarring with some calcifications (arrows). No need to get exited—this finding is appropriate for age. **b** This elderly gentleman must have experienced a severe pneumonia that left a large area of scarring (arrows). Could a bronchial carcinoma hide in there? Of course! Any pulmonary scar may turn malignant ("scar cancer"). It is only the careful comparison with previous films that gives you sufficient certainty. The patient will possibly reassure you by telling you that he has had a scar in his lung for years. He may, however, not realize that there has been a change in size or appearance since the previous radiographs.

The Case of Sidel Zastro

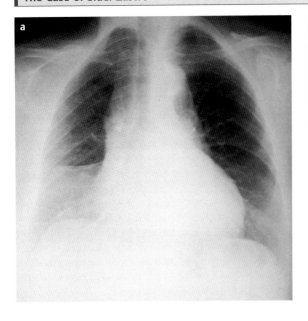

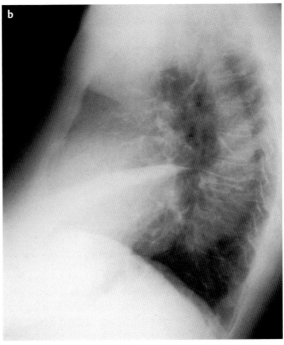

Fig. 6.**7**   Have a look at the CXRs of Sidel Zastro. Anything remarkable?

Bronchial Carcinoma

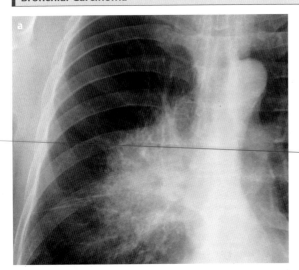

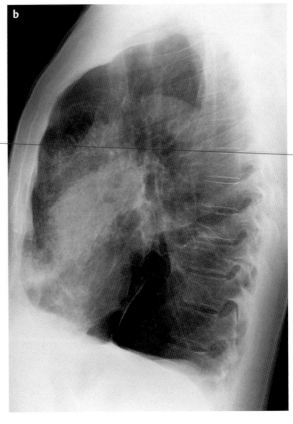

Fig. 6.**8 a**   The tumor has a relatively homogeneous internal structure because there are no aerated components. Its margins are irregular. You appreciate the pulmonary parenchyma overlying the tumor. Where is the tumor? In the lower or middle lobe? **b** On the lateral view of the patient you recognize the complete situation: the middle lobe (search for the minor and major fissure!) is homogeneously opacified and shows volume loss—the minor fissure ascends too steeply and runs too far inferiorly. This configuration is typical of atelectasis. Superiorly to the minor fissure the opacity continues, however. There it has an unsharp and irregular margin. In this patient a carcinoma developed in the middle lobe, led to atelectasis, and then continued to invade the neighboring lung tissue.

Pleural Effusion

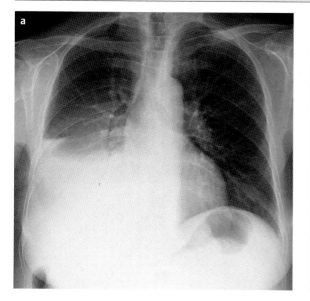

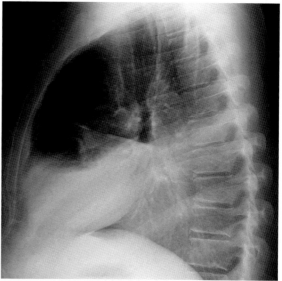

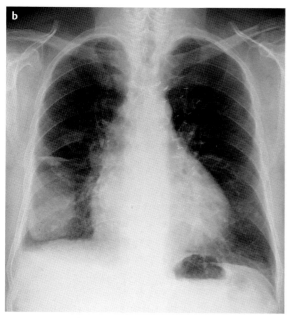

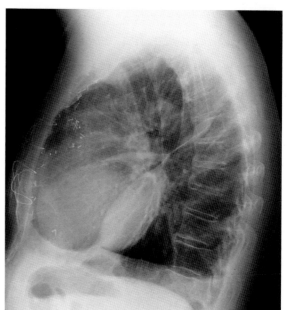

Fig. 6.9 a   Note the large right-sided pleural effusion, which obscures any internal structures (it is homogeneous). The middle lobe floats in it; the upper and middle lobes are compressed by the fluid in the pleural cavity. In the left mid-lung close to the hilum (left) you see a dark branching structure—that is the air bronchogram of the middle lobe bronchus surrounded by compressive atelectasis.

b   In this patient a previous large pleural effusion has been absorbed except for some residual fluid at the base (left) and some loculated fluid along the course of the minor fissure (right). This interlobar effusion can persist and scar down over time.

Lesions with inhomogeneous internal structure: These must be analyzed further. Do you see tubular, branching structures of radiolucency, that is, air bronchograms (Fig. 6.**11a**)? In pneumonia the alveoli fill with pus and exudate while the larger bronchi remain air-filled in the initial phase. For that reason they suddenly become visible against the backdrop of the airless surrounding alveoli (Fig. 6.**11b**). If the alveoli are filled with fluid from the interstitium, for example, in edema (Fig. 6.**12**), or with blood, for example, in a lung contusion (see Fig. 14.**6**, p. 313), the same phenomenon develops. If the lung is compressed from the outside, for example, by a large pleural effusion, the alveoli collapse while the bronchi stay open owing to the relative rigidity of their walls: compression atelectasis is the end result (Fig. 6.9a).

Postobstructive Atelectasis

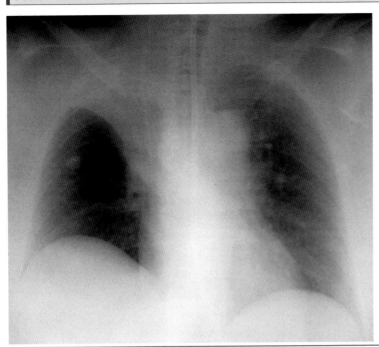

Fig. 6.**10**   The opacity of the right upper lobe has a homogeneous internal structure. The minor fissure and the hilum are displaced superiorly, which points to a volume loss. The upper lobe bronchus is obstructed and a postobstructive atelectasis has developed. The air in the alveoli and the bronchi has been absorbed.

Pneumonia

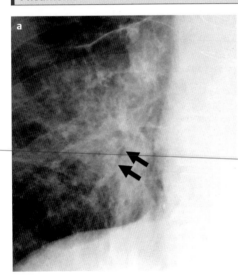

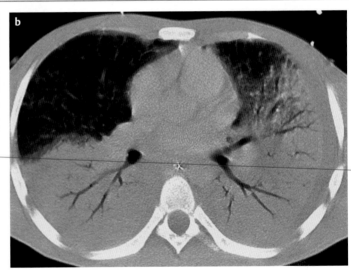

Fig. 6.**11 a**   An air bronchogram in a lower lobe pneumonia (arrows). Could a cancer look like that? Unfortunately yes! The bronchoalveolar carcinoma tends to destroy the alveoli first and leaves the bronchi open initially. The complete resolution of any "pneumonia" type infiltration must therefore be documented radiologically once treatment has been completed, especially in the elderly. **b** In this boy a severe pneumococcal pneumonia has necessitated treatment in the intensive care unit. The alveoli are filled with pus; the bronchi can be traced far into the periphery.

Space-occupying lesions of the lung can also become partially necrotic. If necrosis reaches the bronchial tree, some of the necrotic tissue may be coughed up and air may enter the ensuing cavity (Fig. 6.**13a**). The contents of a necrotic lesion can be spread along the bronchial tree (Fig. 6.**13b**). Almost all infections, especially tuberculosis, can form cavities. But malignant tumors may do the same thing (Fig. 6.**14**). If the infectious cavities heal, their wall thickness may decrease and they can turn into cysts. Naturally these dark, warm, and humid spaces provide

Alveolar Lung Edema

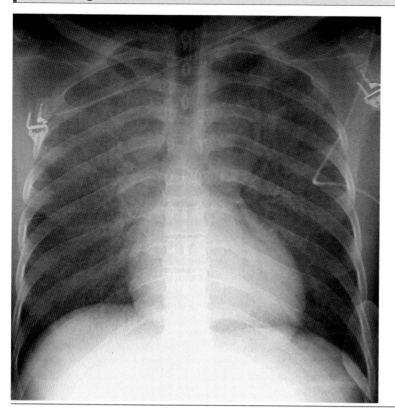

Fig. 6.**12** This is the CXR of a polytraumatized patient who received large quantities of intravenous fluid replacement within a short period of time to treat his severe blood loss. It ended up being a little too much of a good thing: The symmetrical opacification of both central lungs with air bronchograms indicates an alveolar pulmonary edema. The minor fissure is prominent, the bronchial walls are thickened, and the interlobular septae, particularly in the periphery of the right base, are well appreciated (Kerley B lines). This is an indication that there is also fluid deposition in the pulmonary interstitium. Conclusion: They'd better get the kidneys to work quickly.

Tuberculosis

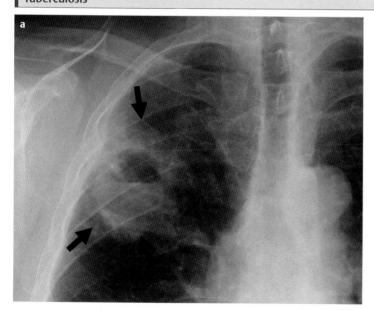

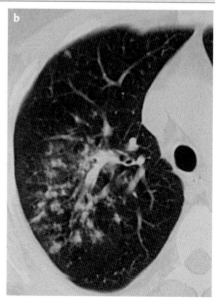

Fig. 6.**13 a** Here we see a consolidation with a central lucency (arrows), indicative of a cavity. This radiograph of a young prison inmate sent the whole chest unit team into a flurry. Before the urgently summoned Gregory had a chance to declare "Hey, mates, this is one hell of a full-blown tuberculosis," the chest unit room had already been sealed and the disinfector been called by the young tech in charge. A rather typical finding, indeed. The prison guards who accompanied the man immediately got themselves an appointment for a check-up with their own physicians.

b This CT demonstrates beautifully what else happens when the cavity erodes into the bronchial system: Infectious material is distributed all over the bronchial system and initiates satellite lesions.

Bronchial Carcinoma

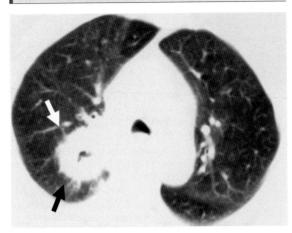

Fig. 6.**14**   This bronchial carcinoma (arrows) has turned necrotic in its center and eroded a bronchial wall vessel. The patient is coughing up blood—that was his first symptom.

perfect growing conditions for fungi (Fig. 6.**15**), which can superinfect a preexisting cavity.

Finally one has to realize that a CXR is a two-dimensional projectional image of a three-dimensional object. Several superimposed anterior and posterior pulmonary opacities can create the visual impression of a single inhomogeneous infiltrate when in fact there are multiple focal ones. This can be the case in inflammatory and neoplastic processes.

Does the lesion have a sharp or unsharp border? The margin tells us something about the localization and type of the lesion. Borders that are smooth and straight at the same time are often formed by an adjacent fissure (see Fig. 6.**10**). If you recognize the involved fissure, you know which lobe the lesion most probably occupies. If the lesion has a smooth interface with the thoracic wall, first check whether there is a pleural effusion or whether the ribs are destroyed. If the borders toward the thoracic wall and toward the lung are smooth, a pleural process such as a loculated pleural effusion or a lipoma (Fig. 6.**16**) might be present.

Is the contour regular or irregular, straight, or lobulated? A lobulated, relatively sharp contour is found in many pulmonary nodules, for example, in metastases (Fig. 6.**17**). An irregular, pointed, and jagged margin implies a disturbance of the surrounding pulmonary parenchymal architecture and is seen not only in primary pulmonary tumors, for example in bronchial carcinoma (Fig. 6.**18**), but also in infections.

Are any of the physiological air–soft tissue interfaces (diaphragm, heart border, aortic arch) obliterated? Normal interfaces between soft tissue structures like the diaphragm, the heart and the aortic arch on the one hand and the air-filled lung on the other hand disappear if the adjacent lung loses its air content at the site of contact (see p. 23–24, 44). This phenomenon, also called "silhouette sign," allows assignment of the location of underlying radiopaque lesions to certain areas of the chest:

Aspergilloma

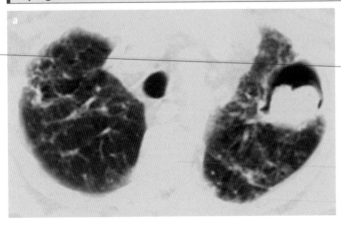
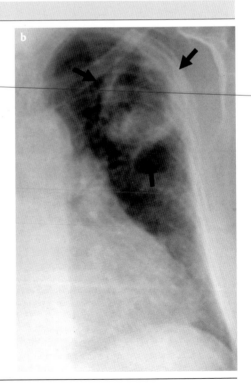

Fig. 6.**15 a**   This patient has interstitial lung disease associated with bullae due to previous asbestos exposure. One of the bullae has been colonized by *Aspergillus*.
b Under fluoroscopy the fungus ball (arrow) can be seen rolling around in the bulla! A stellar moment for any radiologist and the pathognomonic sign of an aspergilloma.

Pleural Lipoma

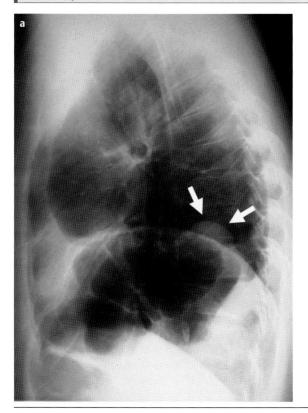

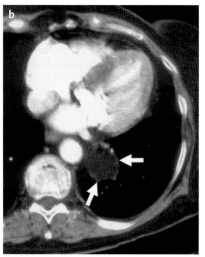

Fig. 6.**16 a** This tumor (arrows) adjacent to the diaphragm (left or right hemidiaphragm?) was found on the occasion of a preoperative chest check-up. It has a smooth margin and is not associated with a pleural effusion. It looks pretty benign.

It is the left hemidiaphragm. The air in the colon directly underneath proves this point.

b CT confirms the benign character of the lesion: The tumor (arrows) clearly exhibits fat density (compare the density of the subcutaneous fat!). It is a lipoma.

Metastases

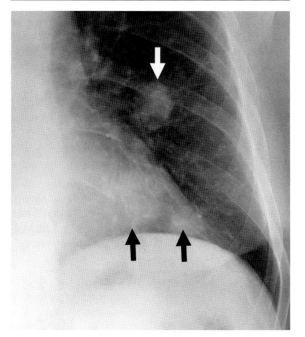

Fig. 6.**17** This is what typical metastases (arrows) look like: multiple round nodules with relatively sharp margins surrounded by pulmonary parenchyma.

Bronchial Carcinoma

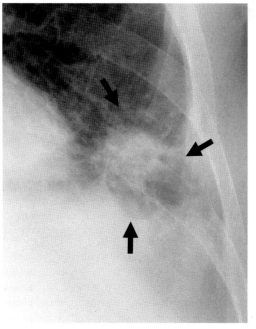

Fig. 6.**18** This bronchial carcinoma (arrows) has a spiculated border. The tumor invades and distorts the surrounding pulmonary parenchyma in the process (see also Fig. 6.**8a**).

Atelectasis

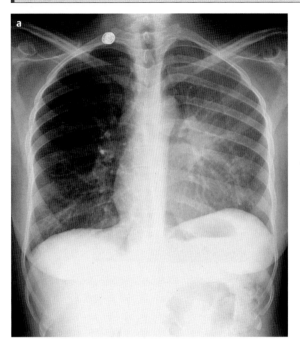

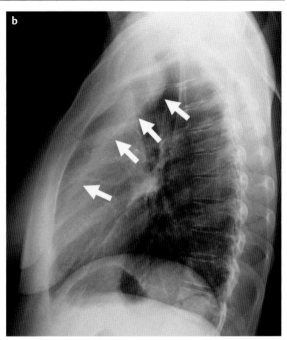

Fig. 6.**19 a**   The opacity seen on the CXR obliterates the inter-face between the left heart and the left lung—which means that it is located in the upper lobe. It demonstrates a homogeneous internal structure indicating that it is airless and it shows asso- ciated volume loss in the affected lung (the left hemidiaphragm is elevated). **b** The lateral view confirms a dense stripe retroster-nally (arrows). This is compatible with left upper lobe collapse (complete lobar atelectasis).

- Loss of the left or right lower heart border: anterior lo-cation, middle lobe (right) or lingula (left)
- Loss of definition of the aortic arch contour: mid chest, left upper lobe
- Loss of the contour of the descending aorta and/or the paravertebral soft tissue shadow: dorsal location, lower lobe.

Now you can go ahead and apply your new knowledge to Fig. 6.**19a**. Where is the pathological finding?

What is the volume effect of the lesion? The volume effect is of special relevance. The displacement of surrounding structures (for example, the fissures, the diaphragm, the mediastinum) toward the lesion implies a *loss of volume*: a loss of lung aeration (atelectasis, Fig. 6.**19**) or scarring (see Fig. 6.**6b**) causes this behavior, but a slow-growing tumor or a chronic infection may also lead to this phe-nomenon. An *increase in volume* would point toward an acute infection or a quickly growing tumor (see Fig. 6.**8a**).

→ **Diagnosis:** Paul and Joey have got it all figured out. Mr. Zastro's temperature is normal. The internal structure of the lesion is homogeneous in their opinion. The contour is sharp and straight: it is the minor fissure. The right heart contour is obliterated. The lesion seems to decrease vo-lume rather than increase it. They have made up their mind: it is obstructive atelectasis of the middle lobe. As they want to go ahead and call up Mr. Zastro's doctor, Greg, the senior resident in neuroradiology, trots by in

his search for Giufeng and stops the students: "Do you think you're done just because Mr. Zastro has an atelec-tasis? Always think of a bronchial carcinoma in this age group! Look at the hilum again and analyze it carefully, then go ahead and search the lymph node stations." Together they scrutinize the aortopulmonary window, the azygos angle, and the carina underneath the tracheal bifurcation. Nothing! Greg leaves them grumbling. A bronchoscopy will be necessary to find the cause of the obstruction and to verify it histologically.

Should a bronchial carcinoma be the cause a chest CT would be needed to stage the tumor correctly following the TNM system and to determine operability as well as the optimal chemotherapy regimen (Fig. 6.**20a, b**). Some will have this CT done even before the bronchoscopy is performed in order to give better orientation to the bro-choscopist. In any case, this CT should—as a rule—include the upper abdomen to the adrenal glands (Fig. 6.**20c**) be-cause they are a frequent and early location of metastases. Rarely a special MR study is necessary (Fig. 6.**20d**). If tumor tissue cannot be gathered at bronchoscopy, a core needle biopsy may be attempted under CT guidance (Fig. 6.**20e**).

Staging in Bronchial Carcinoma

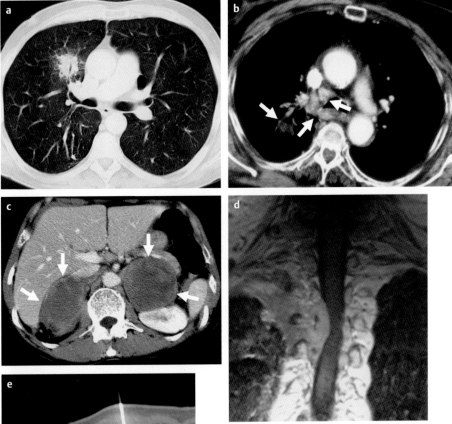

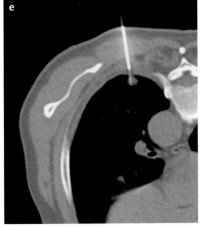

Fig. 6.**20 a**   Lung windows in this CT illustrate the spiculated contour and the size of the tumor. The cancer does not appear to infiltrate the mediastinum—thus it is not a T4 stage. **b** Soft tissue windows of a CT obtained from a different patient shows enlarged lymph nodes along the course of the azygos vein and ventral to the trachea (arrows). They correspond to an N2 stage of a right-sided bronchial carcinoma. **c** Bronchial carcinoma frequently metastasizes into the adrenal glands (arrows). **d** This MRI in a third patient depicts a bronchial carcinoma (T4 stage). This Pancoast tumor extends cranially and into the spinal canal. **e** If blood clotting tests are normal, CT-guided biopsy with a core needle is the fastest, least invasive, and for the patient perhaps the most comfortable way to obtain a tissue biopsy for histological diagnosis.

Obstructive Atelectasis in Children

Children also develop postobstructive atelectasis. Causes differ from the adult population, however: foreign bodies and mucous plugs are more common. Typical foreign bodies in toddlers are glass eyes chewed off of the favorite teddy bear or aspirated peanuts that have just the right caliber to block the trachea or a main bronchus. By the way, children in the Netherlands know just what to do to decrease this risk: As a rule of thumb, any kid who manages to reach over his or her head and insert a finger into the opposite external ear canal may eat peanuts. As you can see, Philipp may enjoy peanuts, but Paula is not ready for them yet. Her airways do not have a large enough caliber.

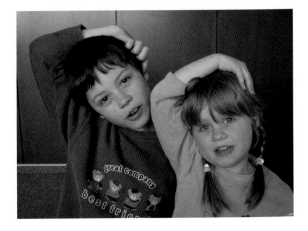

! The times of a purely "contemplative" radiology have definitely passed. The analysis of a finding is essential, but the next diagnostic or therapeutic step should always be considered. Try to reach conclusions that directly improve the patient's management in terms of time needed to diagnosis and recovery. Getting the patient back on the right track with minimally invasive diagnosis and therapy—that is the goal!

Multiple Lesions in the Lung

Checklist: Multiple Lesions in the Lung

- Do the lesions have sharp or unsharp margins?
- Are they calcified or ossified?
- Are they solid or necrotic?
- Do you know the age, history, and symptoms of the patient?

And There Are More and More Every Month

Isadora Pumpkin (65) has been feeling unwell and depressed for a few months. She has lost some weight and her primary care physician has diagnosed anemia. He has sent her for a thorough diagnostic check-up. The ultrasound of the abdomen has been unremarkable. Joey and Ajay are hanging out in the chest imaging unit and are the first to review Mrs. Pumpkin's CXR (Fig. 6.21). The finding is obvious: multiple nodules in both lungs. They discuss the relevant differential diagnoses.

→ What Is Your Diagnosis?

Metastases: The most frequent multiple lesions in the lung are, of course, metastases (Fig. 6.22). They tend to be round and sharply demarcated (see Fig. 6.17). Breast, kidney, and colon cancers as well as carcinomas of the head and neck region are the most frequent primary tumors to give rise to metastatic involvement of the lung; in young men testicular cancer takes the lead as source of pulmonary metastases. Some types of tumors show specific characteristics: osteosarcomas, for example, have a tendency to ossify, not only at the primary site but also their metastases. Multiple ossifying pulmonary nodules are therefore almost pathognomonic for this tumor in the respective—unfortunately often young—patient group (Fig. 6.23).

The Case of Isadora Pumpkin

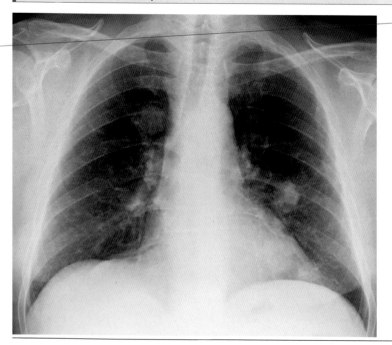

Fig. 6.21 This is the CXR of Mrs. Pumpkin. Which diagnoses do you consider?

Metastases of Testicular Carcinoma

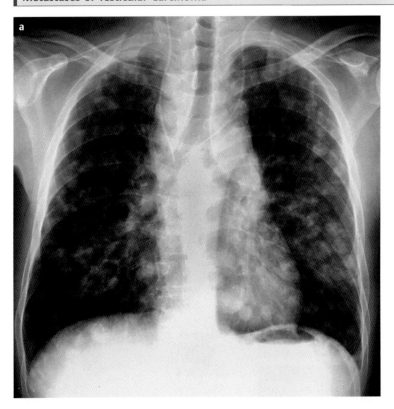

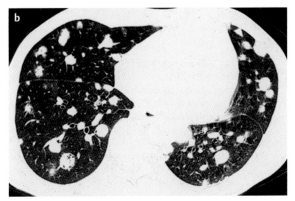

Metastases of an Osteosarcoma

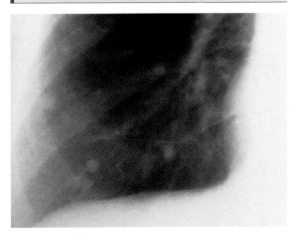

Fig. 6.**22 a**   You see the horrific findings on a CXR of a young man with a history of testicular carcinoma. Metastases of up to walnut size are observed scattered throughout the lungs. Take note of the nodules projecting over the heart shadow and underneath the diaphragmatic contour. You have to search there, too! Have you noticed the widening of the upper mediastinum? The aortopulmonary window and the azygos angle are filled with enlarged lymph nodes. The paratracheal stripe is widened considerably for the same reason (compare Fig. 6.**1**). **b** With just a little luck these masses will all but disappear with modern combination therapy and only a few scattered scars will remain.

Fig. 6.**23**   The nodules in this lung are rather dense—denser than the rib intersections! The increased density suggests ossification; in a 17-year-old an osteosarcoma is an unfortunate but likely diagnosis. Of course, calcified granulomas following an infection with tuberculosis can also be very dense. However, we tend to expect them in older patients or in patients from endemic areas.

Septic Emboli Caused by Fungal Infection

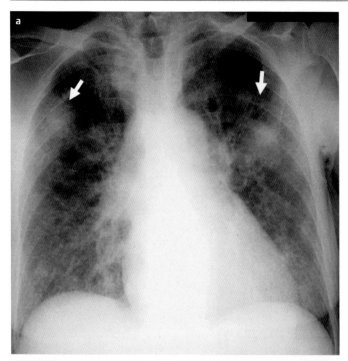

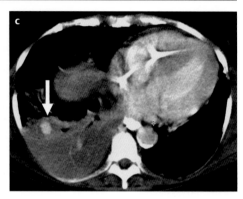

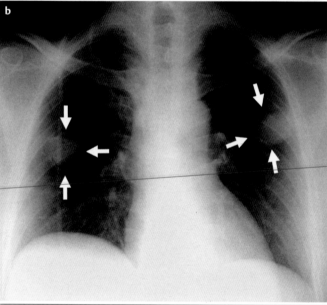

Fig. 6.**24 a** This patient has become neutropenic during the course of chemotherapy for his chronic myelogenous leukemia (CML). The aspergillus hyphae ubiquitous in his bronchial system have subsequently overwhelmed the immune system and have infiltrated through the bronchial walls into the pulmonary arterial system. Here they have become dislodged by the bloodstream into the pulmonary capillaries, where they have induced small-vessel obstruction, "fungal" infarctions. **b** The "fungal" infarctions eventually lead to necrosis of lung tissue and resulting cavitation (arrows). **c** Vessels may also be eroded. This patient developed a mycotic aneurysm (arrow) and died of a severe pulmonary hemorrhage.

Septic emboli: Septic emboli can also give rise to multiple nodules in the lungs. They tend to become necrotic centrally. If, for example, the mitral valve is colonized with bacteria in endocarditis, some of the vegetations can be dislodged into the lung vasculature and settle in the pulmonary parenchyma. In immunosuppressed patients (cancer, transplantation, long-lasting corticosteroid therapy, HIV infection), ubiquitous fungi such as *Candida albicans* and *Aspergillus* can invade the vessels and settle in the parenchymal periphery, causing life-threatening infections of the lung (Fig. 6.24). The reasons for septic emboli can be bizarre. In drug addicts the injection of contaminated material can cause multiple infections and abscess formations in the lung (Fig. 6.**25**). Whether you will see them in your life greatly depends on the type of community you work in (inner cities, etc.) and the existence of clean needle programs in that community.

Septic Emboli in Intravenous Drug Abuse

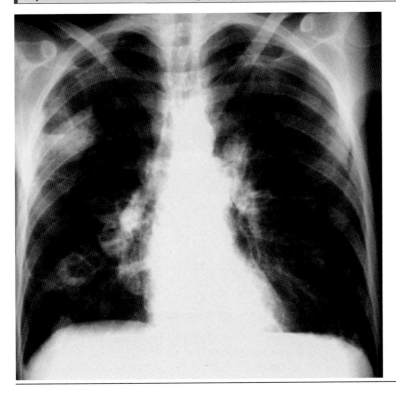

Fig. 6.**25** This young drug addict was brought into the emergency ward absolutely run-down and severely sick, straight from some abandoned harbor shack. A lot of lesions are visible in the lung, the majority of which appear centrally necrotic—septic emboli. Can metastases look like that? Yes, but infrequently. If you are looking for reasons in favor of methadone substitution therapy for intravenous drug addicts, here is one.

Wegener disease: Solitary or multiple pulmonary lesions (granulomata) can occur in Wegener disease, an autoimmune vasculitis that is frequently associated with glomerulonephritis. They tend to necrotize centrally (Fig. 6.**26**).

Wegener Disease

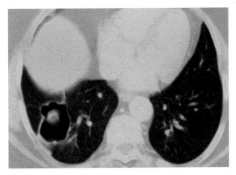

Fig. 6.**26** This pulmonary lesion is centrally necrotic. If the clinicians do not consider all of this patient's findings, diagnosis and therapy may go awry. A bright radiologist might include Wegener disease in the differential diagnosis and prompt a search for the respective clinical signs (sinus and joint problems, glomerulonephritis, and the presence of antineutrophilic cytoplasmic antibodies [c-ANCA]).

Skin tumors, nipples: As an exception, skin tumors may look like multiple lung nodules—just think of neurofibromatosis (Fig. 6.**27**). Nipples can also look suspicious. In some departments small lead markers are taped onto them to facilitate their differentiation from lung lesions. In other instances a quick fluoroscopy with a metal paper-clip taped to the areola will solve the problem.

→ **Diagnosis:** Joey and Ajay have talked to Mrs. Pumpkin. She has been pretty healthy up to now and is not the adventurous, easy-going type. For these reasons the lesions are metastases until proven otherwise. Ajay suggests an examination of the breast physically and mammographically, which would certainly be a good next step as breast cancer is a common malignancy in women of her age; someone should also take a look at her colon. If this and other tests fail to find the primary tumor, a CT-guided biopsy of one of the metastases would be the way to go (see Fig. 6.**20e**) because the appearance of the tumor cells under the microscope may provide a clue as to their origin. Bronchoscopy, perhaps with bronchial lavage, would be the next step in an immunosuppressed patient with a suspicion of a fungal infection of the lung that needs specific therapy urgently. Of course, CT-guided biopsies should only be performed if blood clotting is normal and if bronchoscopy does not provide the material with more ease.

Skin Tumors

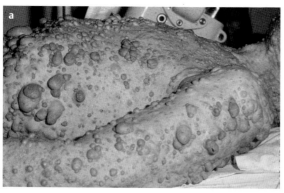

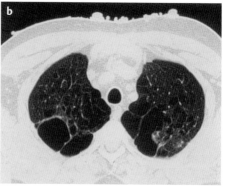

Fig. 6.**27 a** The cutaneous tumors in neurofibromatosis may certainly become visible on the CXR just as prominently as nipple shadows. A precise physical inspection and perhaps a short fluoroscopic examination after marking the nipple or any cutaneous tumors will clarify the situation.

b If the CXR becomes too complex, a CT may be necessary. In patients with neurofibromatosis it frequently also shows pulmonary emphysema.

Diffuse, Homogeneous Opacity of the Lung

Checklist: Diffuse, Homogeneous Opacity of the Lung

Unilateral
- Is the patient well positioned?
- Has the contralateral breast been resected?
- Is there any volume loss?

Bilateral
- Has the patient taken a deep breath?
- Has the film been adequately exposed?
- Is the patient exceptionally adipose?

Shortness of Breath in Search of a Cause

Jonathan Bootleg (53) has developed shortness of breath while on dialysis for his terminal renal insufficiency. The internist in charge has requested a CXR (Fig. 6.**28**). Hannah is alone this late morning in the chest unit and takes a close look at the film. She considers the list of differential diagnoses.

The Case of Jonathan Bootleg

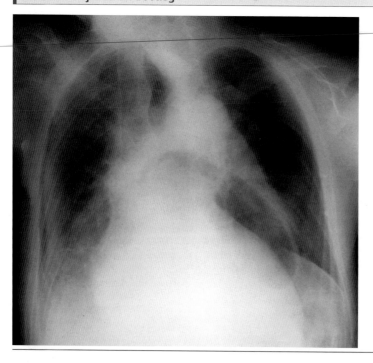

Fig. 6.**28**   Analyze the CXR of Mr. Bootleg. Does anything appear abnormal?

→ What Is Your Diagnosis?

Pleural effusion: A multitude of diseases, for example, pleural tumors (metastases, mesotheliomas) can result in a *unilateral* effusion. A homogeneous opacity of both lung fields can naturally also be caused by *bilateral* pleural effusions. The bilateral effusions may be different in quantity (Fig. 6.**29**), especially in cardiac decompensation and subsequent pulmonary venous congestion.

Do You Know Other Causes for a Diffuse Homogeneous Opacity of the Lung?
Portable CXRs are frequently performed without a scatter grid. The scattered radiation reaches the detector and uniformly increases the image density. If a grid is used it may not be properly aligned with the tube and may partially block diagnostic x-rays in one half of the chest causing an asymmetric exposure of the film. In insufficient inspiration, the density of the lung parenchyma also increases bilaterally owing to low lung volumes. Finally, any imaging technology may fail because the wrong exposure parameters have been chosen or because the patient simply was not built for imaging: patients who weigh more than 140 kg/300 pounds may need to be imaged with dedicated veterinarian equipment.

Posttraumatic loss of radiolucency: Trauma can result in a diffuse unilateral opacity of the thorax; a chest wall hematoma, possibly due to a serial rib fracture, or a hemothorax (Fig. 6.**30**) after an injury of intrathoracic vessels (intercostal arteries or the aorta) may be the cause.

Atelectasis: An atelectasis of the left upper lobe or of a total lung can increase the density of a complete hemithorax (see also Fig. 6.**19a**).

Swyer–James syndrome: Sometimes it is difficult to differentiate between an opacity on one side and an increase in radiolucency on the other. An early childhood pneumonia causes a circumscribed hypoplasia of the lung in Swyer–James syndrome. The change is characterized by a decreased vascularity and an increased aeration due to air trapping (Fig. 6.**31**).

→ **Diagnosis:** Initially Hannah was going to report a pleural effusion in Mr. Bootleg's chest, but the dark stripe along the right thoracic wall has made her hesitant: Could this also be a pneumothorax? Sitting in front of the viewbox, she scratches her head as Joey, Giufeng, and Ajay come by to pick her up for lunch. "It's a skin fold," Giufeng declares, "the density slowly increases laterally and then suddenly falls off. Above the aortic arch on the left side you can see two more of those folds." "That does not explain it all, Giufeng," Joey throws in, "the patient is rotated to the right quite a bit. Just have a look at the trachea and the unfolded aortic arch! This is one poorly taken radiograph. The rotation is another reason for the increase in density." "OK, OK, I've got the message," mumbles Hannah, "and which one of you smart alecs can tell me now why the patient is short of breath?" A long silence ensues, then Ajay replies softly: "Hannah, I would worry about that large air-filled structure in the heart shadow. How about this being a large hiatal hernia or even an 'upside-down-stomach'! That could explain the dyspnea."

Pleural Effusion

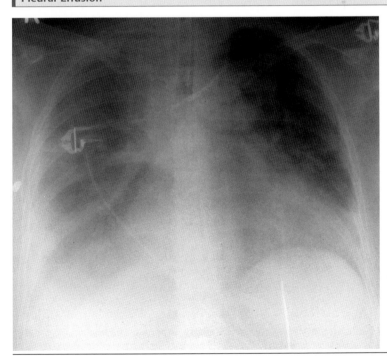

Fig. 6.**29** This large right-sided and smaller left-sided pleural effusion extends far superiorly in this portable chest film obtained from a recumbent patient in bed. For this reason the complete lung appears homogeneously opacified. The interface between diaphragm and lower lobe is obliterated on the right side—go ahead and compare it to the left side. The vessels close to the hilum are enlarged and their margins are unsharp. The bronchi can be traced far into the lung core. The heart appears enlarged, even for a portable supine study. This is compatible with cardiogenic pulmonary venous congestion with subsequent edema.

Hemothorax

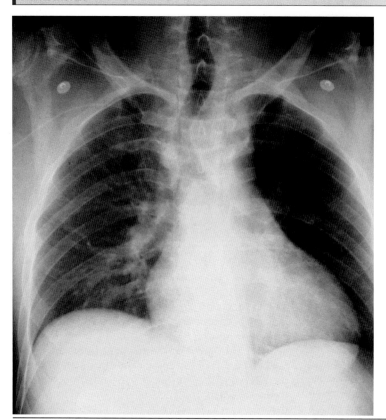

Fig. 6.**30** The right-sided loss of normal radiolucency is due to a hemothorax that is subtle but is a consequence of a severe deceleration trauma in a motor vehicle accident (MVA). The upper mediastinum is widened, indicating a possible large-vessel rupture, which was in fact the case in this patient.

Swyer–James Syndrome

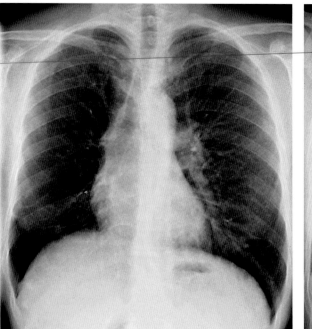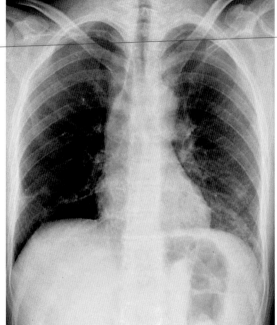

Fig. 6.**31** These CXRs in inspiration (left) and expiration (right) show decrease in vasculature in the right hemithorax (also compare both hila) and hyperinflation of the right lung (also called "air trapping"). The right hemidiaphragm does not move at all.

All are impressed—a real team effort. Hannah jots down the preliminary report. "Well, I should be depressed. But thanks anyway. Talking about gastrointestinal stuff," she goes "I'm starving. Let's go for lunch!"

6.3   Acute Pulmonary Changes

Acute Diffuse Linear, Reticular, Reticulonodular (Interstitial) Pattern

Checklist: Acute Diffuse Interstitial Pattern

- Are the increased markings linear, reticular, or made up of small nodules?
- Are they associated with segmental or lobar consolidation?
- Do the vessels appear unsharp or enlarged cranially?
- Can you detect air bronchograms?
- Are the increased lung markings more evident centrally or basally?
- Are there areas of increased radiolucency and decreased vascularity?
- Are the bronchi dilated, their walls thickened?
- Is the heart enlarged?
- Are the hila plump in appearance?

Patterns of Evil

David Shortbreath (57) has been brought to the emergency room. He has had chest pain at work several times over the past few weeks; it has been just absolutely awful because he felt severely short of breath at the same time. His colleagues at the construction site grabbed him, sat him in the car, and rushed him to the hospital, breaking all speed limits on the highway. During that ride Mr. Shortbreath could breath in more easily when he held his head out of the window and breathed against the airstream with his mouth open. Now the ER docs are taking care of him, studying the laboratory parameters and getting an ECG. A chest radiograph is also done (Fig. 6.**32**). Paul stands close to the lightbox to get a quick first glance at the image.

➜ What Is Your Diagnosis?

Left ventricular failure with pulmonary venous congestion: Pulmonary venous congestion is a typical consequence of left ventricular dysfunction, for example, after coronary infarction. The mounting pulmonary venous pressure is reflected on the CXR by a number of specific findings:

- *Pulmonary venous redistribution:* The first reaction of the pulmonary vasculature to an increase in vascular pressure is to make use of the vessels' reserve capacity. In this process the blood is redirected from the basal lung vessels, which normally hold more blood owing to the hydrostatic pressure gradient, to the cranial pulmonary vessels (see Fig. 6.**1**). This phenomenon is also called pulmonary venous redistribution.

The Case of David Shortbreath

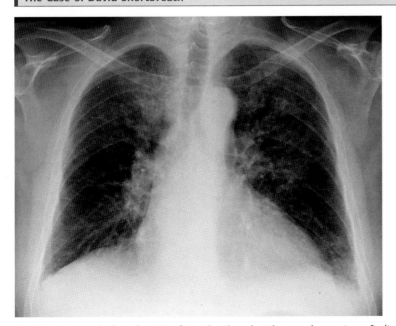

Fig. 6.**32**   Have a look at the CXR of Mr. Shortbreath. What are the pertinent findings?

! The normal size relation of the basal to the cranial vessel calibers is about 2 : 1 (at identical distance from the hilum).

The basal vessels may even contract a little during this process. Naturally these changes are only noticeable if the patient is upright at the time the CXR is taken (hydrostatic pressure!) (Fig. 6.**33**). In the recumbent patient the pulmonary venous redistribution cannot be diagnosed because the vessel calibers even out; the vector of the hydrostatic pressure gradient has now changed to the anterior–posterior direction, which is not visible on a frontal supine radiograph (see Fig. 6.**3**)!

- *Fluid exudation into the interstitium:* If the reserve capacity of the vessels is exhausted, fluid begins to leak into the interstitium. This process can be observed on the CXR if one looks for these four different structures:

1. *The interlobular septae:* Fluid in the radially oriented interlobular septae is best appreciated where the septae are parallel to the x-ray beam and where they cannot be mistaken for vessels. This is the case in the peripheral 1 cm of the parenchyma of the lung where vessels are so small that they are beyond the limits of radiographic visualization. The resulting linear structures on the CXR are called Kerley lines: Kerley B in the basal periphery (these are the most important ones, Fig. 6.**34a**) and Kerley A in the cranial periphery. If the thickening is so pronounced that it becomes visible as a reticular pattern in the central perihilar lung, this is called the Kerley C pattern. Kerley C lines are rarely seen in pulmonary venous congestion but do occur when the interstitium is infiltrated by malignant cells. This dreaded but frequent complication of, for example, advanced breast carcinoma is called lymphangitic spread or carcinomatosis (Fig. 6.**34b**).

2. *Fissures:* Interlobar fissures are made up of two layers of pleural lining and thus two layers of interstitium as well. Furthermore, a little fluid may enter the pleural space between the two pleural linings. If the fissures appear particularly prominent or thickened on the CXR, the reason may be fluid overload in the interstitial space (Fig. 6.**34a**).

3. *Bronchial wall:* The thickness of the interstitium can also be evaluated by looking at the walls of the larger bronchi in the neighborhood of the hilum that are running parallel to the x-ray beam and therefore appear

Upper Lobe Pulmonary Venous Redistribution

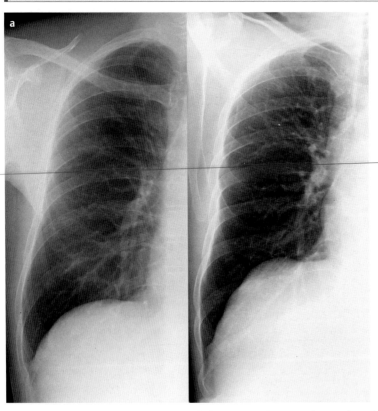
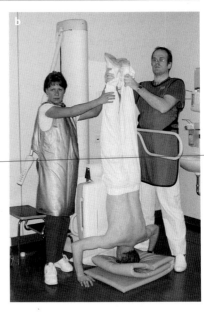

Fig. 6.**33 a**   On the left you see a normal chest exposed in the standard erect position. Compare the vessel calibers at the same distance to the hilum both at the lung base and apex. The size relation of the basal vessels in comparison to the upper lobe vessel is about 2:1. On the right, the same volunteer has changed body orientation, with a subsequent redistribution of the pulmonary perfusion. Check the vessel calibers!
b The documented position is not unusual at large academic institutions and reverses the natural hydrostatic pressure gradient.

Kerley Lines

a Kerley B lines

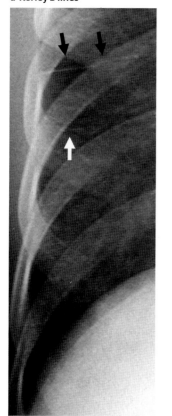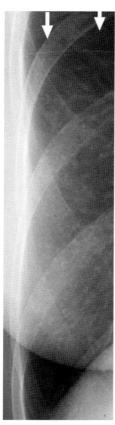

b Kerley C lines

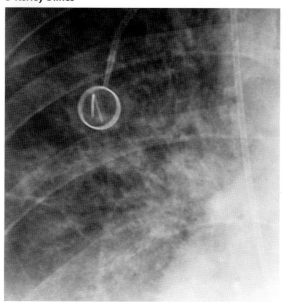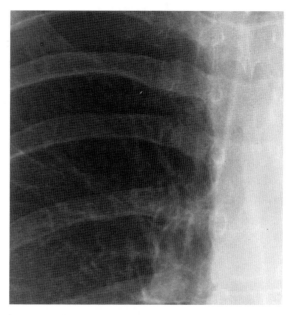

Fig. 6.**34 a** On the left you see a section of a CXR in severe lung edema. Note the thickening of the minor fissure (black arrow) and the horizontal interlobular septae (white arrow) in the pulmonary periphery. Vessels do not normally show in this parapleural stripe. Compare to a normal section below.

b On the left is a section of an erect CXR. The lung interstitium with the vessels, bronchi, and the surrounding fibrous tissue is irregular, micronodular, and reticular in pattern. This is a case of lymphangitic carcinomatosis in a breast cancer patient. The tumor cells grow along the interstitium and form knotty cell nests. Compare to a normal anatomy below.

"Bronchial Cuffing"

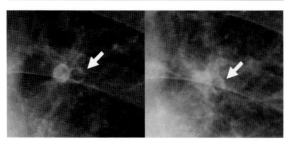

Fig. 6.**35**   Bronchus and artery appear in a typical "number 8" configuration when imaged head-on or "down the barrel." The bronchial wall normally does not exceed 1 mm (left section, arrow). In pulmonary edema the thickness of the interstitium around the bronchial wall and the artery increases (right section, arrow) rendering their contours unsharp.

as ringlike structures when imaged "end-on" ("down the barrel"). The normal bronchial wall is about 1 mm thick and barely perceptible. If its thickness increases and its contours become unsharp, this is called "bronchial cuffing" (Fig. 6.**35**).

! You can recognize a bronchus by searching for the accompanying artery: The combination of the two structures looks like an "8" with one ring of it filled.

4. *Vascular wall:* Naturally, the same occurs in the vessel walls but it cannot be observed that well. (Do you know why?) Eventually the caliber of the vessels increase and their contours become hazy (Fig. 6.**35**).

• *Fluid leaking out of the interstitium into the alveolar space:* If the pulmonary venous pressure remains high or continues to increase, the interstitial lymph drainage is eventually overwhelmed and the fluid is pressed into the alveoli. The subsequent corresponding radiographic pattern is that of patchy and confluent density; this is also called an alveolar pattern. Radiographically the lung tissue now appears much denser than the bronchi, which is why they now become visible against the backdrop of the alveoli. This phenomenon is also called "air-bronchogram" and is typical for alveolar disease (Fig. 6.**36a**). Frequently, fluid exudation begins in the perihilar region and then expands toward the periphery. It may do so simultaneously in both lungs, sparing the lung periphery: a "butterfly distribution" or "bat's wing" pattern (Fig. 6.**36b**) results that is the hallmark of severe alveolar edema. In patients who are severely compromised, perhaps in the intensive care unit, who have been lying on one side for a prolonged period of time, the distribution of alveolar fluid may be asymmetric. Furthermore, patients with severe inhomogeneously distributed bullous emphysema can only produce the radiographic appearance of alveolar edema in the "good" portions of their lung, because the remainder of the lung is made up of large air-filled spaces with very few if any blood vessels.

Acute Alveolar Pulmonary Edema

a "Air bronchogram"

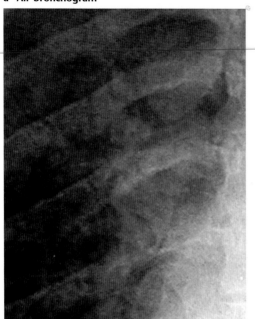

b "Butterfly or batwing edema"

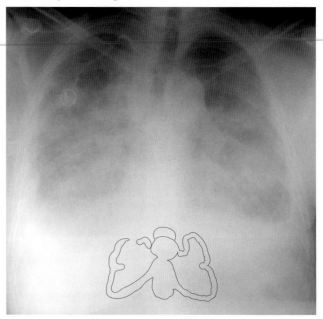

Fig. 6.**36 a**   If the bronchial tree can be traced from the hilum to the central lung parenchyma, this is also called "air bronchogram." **b** The edema spares the lung periphery initially. The typical butterfly or batwing configuration results.

The First Descriptor of Pulmonary Lines
Peter James Kerley was an Irish radiologist who trained in Vienna during the Golden Twenties of the last century. He later worked in London at the Westminster Hospital. The Royal College of Radiologists named a lecture in his honor. He is said to have been a witty fellow with a flair for extravagant diagnoses. As a normal human being, you should try for the former and avoid the latter.

Viral pneumonia: The interlobular septae can also become engorged in some viral pneumonias, for example, in CMV pneumonia (Fig. 6.**37**). Again, you see the infamous Kerley lines. Of course, the pulmonary venous redistribution typical of pulmonary venous congestion is usually absent and the clinical presentation is quite different from pulmonary edema.

Miliary tuberculosis: Acute widespread small nodules in the lungs of a patient with clinical signs of an infection point to a miliary tuberculosis (Fig. 6.**38a**) but can also be caused by a variety of endemic fungal infections such as histoplasmosis, coccidioidomycosis, and blastomycosis, depending a little on which part of the world you work in. If this disease is overcome, the little granulomas tend to calcify (Fig. 6.**38b**).

→ **Diagnosis:** Paul finds enough signs of pulmonary congestion on the CXR and is convinced that the symptoms are so straightforward that he does not hesitate to diagnose cardiogenic interstitial lung edema. The follow-up CXR supports his interpretation because it shows the progression into typical alveolar edema (Fig. 6.**39**). The registrars have by now been able to confirm their suspicion of a myocardial infarction with ECG and laboratory findings and have initiated the appropriate therapy. They are still puzzled, however, about the "breathing out of the car window" bit of the history. Paul has already discussed the issue with Joey and both have the same explanation: Being driven at high speed, Mr. Shortbreath breathed against the airstream and thus simulated a PEEP (positive end expiratory pressure) respiration, which serves to keep the terminal airways open. That helped him a lot. (Go ahead and try it out on your way home—but make sure your seatbelt is fastened, stay clear of other cars, and dodge insect swarms!)

Viral Pneumonia

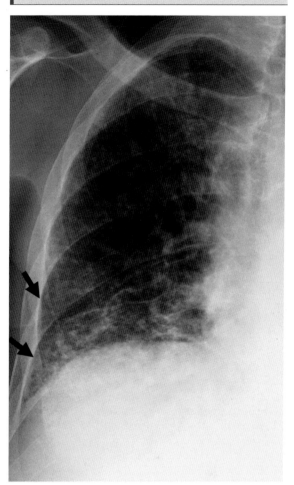

Fig. 6.**37** This is a section of the CXR of a patient with a cytomegalovirus (CMV)-induced pneumonia; the interlobular septae are thickened. This patient was immunosuppressed after organ transplantation.

If you ask different people "Does this patient's CXR show pulmonary edema?" you frequently get different answers—the decision is not always that simple. Try to use the above-mentioned criteria and listen closely to the clinical impression of the registrars in charge of the patient. After a little while you and your perception will be adequately tuned to diagnose this condition with some certainty.

Miliary Tuberculosis

a Active

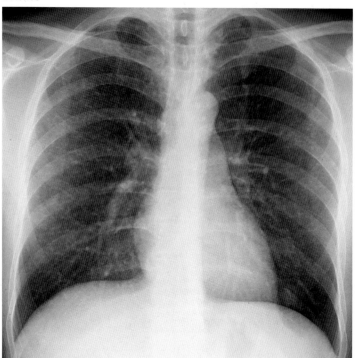

b Inactive

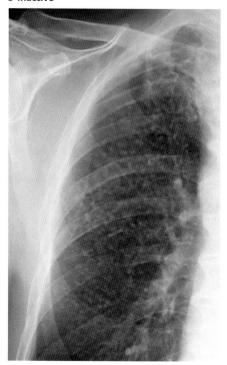

Fig. 6.**38 a**   This immunosuppressed HIV patient developed an active miliary tuberculosis. **b** The tiny, very dense nodules on this radiograph are typical for an inactivated miliary tuberculosis (milium= millet or sorghum). This patient had been admitted for a replacement of his total hip arthroplasty.

The Case of David Shortbreath

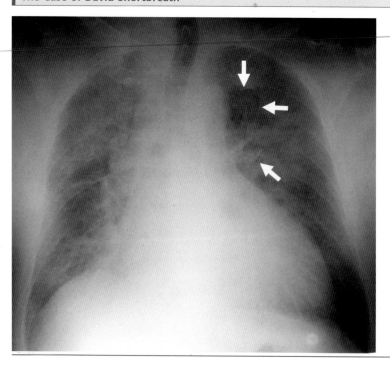

Fig. 6.**39**   This is the follow-up study of Mr. Shortbreath—a portable radiograph that shows an increase in pulmonary venous congestion. In the perihilar region the exudation of fluid into the alveoli is documented by spotty and/or cloudy opacities. The heart is significantly enlarged.

Acute Diffuse Acinar, Confluent (Alveolar) Pattern

Checklist: Acute Diffuse Alveolar Pattern

- Is the consolidation predominantly central or peripheral?
- Do the vessels appear unsharp or cranially distended?
- Are the perceptible bronchial walls thickened?
- Is the heart enlarged?
- Are there symptoms of a myocardial infarction?
- Could the fluid balance be positive (patient on hemodialysis, intensive care setting, infusion therapy)?
- Are there signs of infection?
- Could an allergic or toxic reaction be present (organic dusts, gas, drugs)?

Something is Filling Up

Mary Chang (57) has been brought to the emergency room straight from her apartment in Bondi. Her neighbor called the ambulance after having found her wheezing at her front door. Currently Mrs. Chang cannot be questioned because the ambulance medics had to sedate and intubate the distressed patient. Giufeng tries to get some information from the friendly neighbor who accompanied her to the hospital: Yes, she overheard a loud argument and the slamming of doors in Mrs. Chang's apartment quite a while before she

found her. But she is not really close to her next-door neighbor. Giufeng is a little perplexed as she returns to her viewbox where the CXR and Hannah are already waiting for her (Fig. 6.**40**). Hannah has spotted a policewoman together with a detective in the emergency waiting area.

→ What Is Your Diagnosis?

Pulmonary edema: A lung edema due to an increase in the pressure of the pulmonary circulation could certainly be present (see Fig. 6.**36b**, Fig. 6.**39**). This could be due to a myocardial infarction, which must be excluded in this case. A patient with renal insufficiency in dire need of a dialysis could also present with an image like that.

Pulmonary hemorrhage: In pulmonary hemorrhage, as may occur in Wegener granulomatosis or in Goodpasture syndrome, the alveoli fill with blood (Fig. 6.**41**).

Hypersensitivity pneumonitis due to exogenous allergens: The inhalation of many different allergenic organic substances such as bird excrement, the dust of bird feathers, moldy hay or barley, paper or sawdust can initiate a massive pulmonary hypersensitivity reaction including exudation of fluid into the alveoli.

Pneumocystis carinii pneumonia: In an AIDS patient with the symptoms of a pulmonary infection, *Pneumocystis carinii* pneumonia is very probable (Fig. 6.**42**).

The Case of Mary Chang

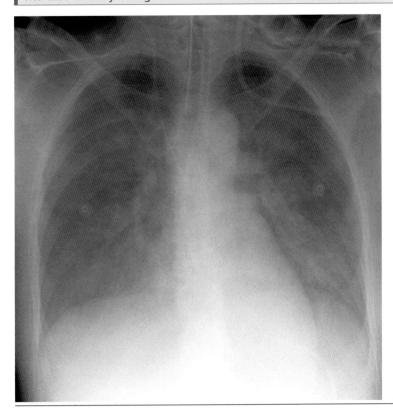

Fig. 6.**40**   Observe the CXR of Mrs. Chang. Which diagnoses must be discussed?

Lung Hemorrhage

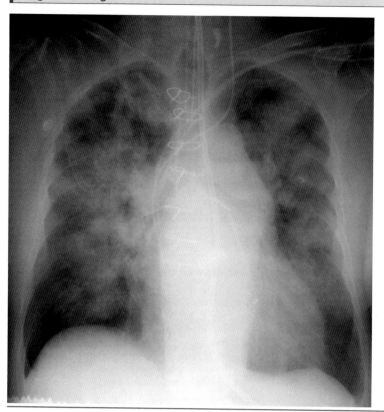

Fig. 6.**41**   This elderly lady had a heart valve implanted. Postoperatively a fulminant pulmonary hemorrhage resulted that led to this remarkably dense opacification (hemosiderin content!) of both lungs.

Pneumocystis carinii Pneumonia

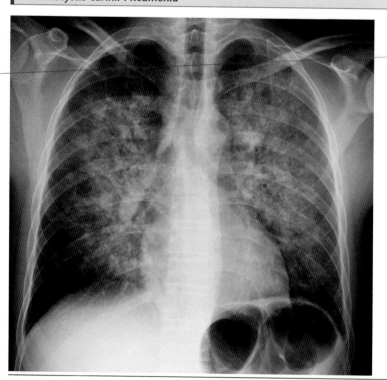

Fig. 6.**42**   A severe *Pneumocystis carinii* pneumonia occurred in this HIV patient. Changes are much more subtle in most other patients. In these less obvious cases a high-resolution CT (HRCT) is recommended.

Asbestosis

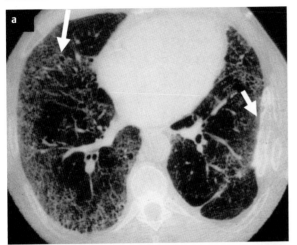

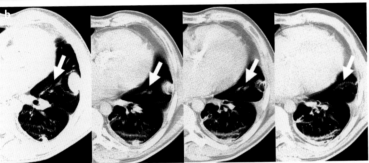

Fig. 6.**47 a**   In asbestosis, peripherally accentuated pulmonary fibrosis with scarring, small bullae, and bronchiectasis (long arrow) develops. The pathognomonic extensive pleural plaques often have a calcified flat and smooth top (short arrow), also called "Tafelberg" (tophats).
b In recurring and chronic pleural effusions, lung components may collapse and spiral up into a special kind of atelectasis: the so-called "round atelectasis," which must be differentiated from malignant lesions. The typical comet-tail sign (arrows) that shows the spiral course of the pulmonary vessels into the lesion helps in the differentiation. If the radiographic appearance suggests rounded atelectasis, simple follow-up imaging may be scheduled to assess stability or resolution over time.

Sarcoidosis

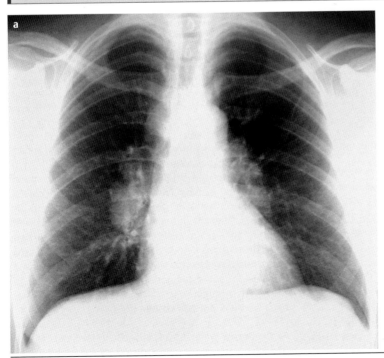

Fig. 6.**48 a**   The central lung parenchyma (also see **b**) has an abnormal micronodular appearance. The hilum is notably enlarged—lymph nodes full of noncaseating granulomas are the cause of the change.

Sarcoidosis

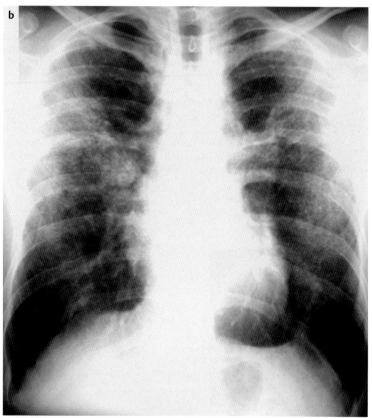

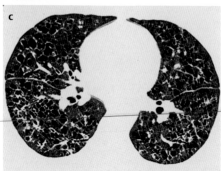

Fig. 6.**48 b**   A late complication can be pulmonary fibrosis.
c Scattered areas of honeycombing are seen, which are hallmarks of end-stage lung disease. The bullous structures are best appreciated in HRCT.

particularly of UIP, lung transplantation is the only treatment option.

Cystic fibrosis: If Mr. Coalfire were younger, severe generalized changes of the lung architecture could point to cystic fibrosis (Fig. 6.**50**).* The rather typical pattern is due to dilated bronchi some of which are plugged with viscous mucus.

*Only state-of-the-art constant mucolytic and antibiotic therapy lets these patients reach adulthood. They suffer from recurring bouts of pulmonary infections.

Lymphangioleiomyomatosis: Lymphangioleiomyomatosis is a disease that occurs almost exclusively in young women, characterized by proliferation of atypical smooth muscle in pulmonary lymphatic vessels, blood vessels, and airways. Gradually progressive interstitial lung disease, recurrent chylous pleural effusions, and recurrent pneumothoraces are among the sequelae of this disease, which leads to the demise of the patient unless lung transplantation is performed. There is a multitude of other special diseases of the pulmonary interstitium. They are difficult to discriminate and, as a student and nonpulmonologist, you will not be asked to do so.

→ **Diagnosis:** Hannah and Paul are a little exhausted after browsing through the differential. They have agreed that

Idiopathic Lung Fibrosis

a "Usual interstitial pneumonitis" (UIP)/idiopathic pulmonary fibrosis (IPF)

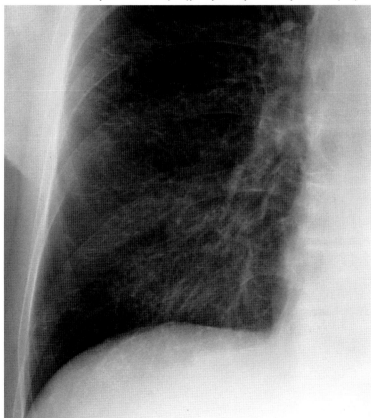

b "Desquamative interstitial pneumonitis" (DIP)

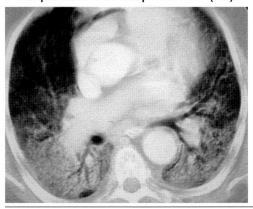

Fig. 6.**49 a** The fine linear and reticular structures in the periphery—much like Kerley lines—indicate changes of the interstitium in pulmonary fibrosis. The heart is small, the vascular filling is normal, and there are no clinical signs of pulmonary venous congestion.
b Additional alveolar opacities in desquamative interstitial pneumonitis (DIP) point to an active process potentially responsive to therapy with corticosteroids.

this could very well be a case of idiopathic lung fibrosis. They have talked to the patient and have not found anything in the way of an occupational risk: Mr. Coalfire was a bricklayer all his life and has always enjoyed the fresh air—OK, OK, he has smoked quite a bit but quit about 8 years ago. An HRCT will verify the diagnosis and determine whether therapy with steroids has a fair chance of success.

❗ Generations of gray-haired radiologists plus the WHO have committed themselves to the classification of micronodules in CXRs—mainly to classify findings in occupationally exposed workers with lung disease to determine their entitlement to worker's compensation. High-resolution chest CT has facilitated this effort enormously. Fortunately, the number of exposed workers decreases continuously as occupational legislation is improved and enforced and as technology moves on.

Cystic Fibrosis

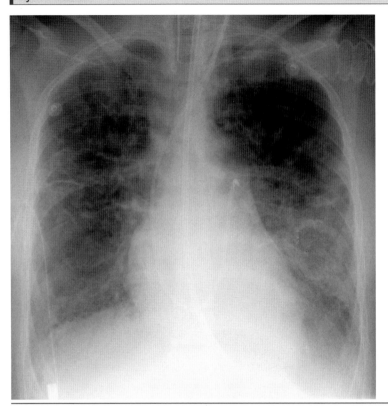

Fig. 6.**50** The generalized, irregularly dilated bronchi in cystic fibrosis produce the characteristic bullous pattern. This patient is currently in the intensive care unit for a relapsing pneumonia.

6.5   Pulmonary Symptoms without Correlating Findings in the Chest Radiograph

Checklist: Pulmonary Symptoms without Correlating Findings in the CXR

- Was a myocardial infarction ruled out?
- Has the possibility of a pulmonary embolus been considered?
- Are the symptoms suggestive of an aortic dissection?

But Those in the Dark Remain Unseen

Undira Candi (65) complains about sudden tremendous chest pain and increasing shortness of breath. An ECG and the laboratory tests have been ordered in the emergency room but the results are not out yet. The CXR is ready for inspection (Fig. 6.**51**). Giufeng scrutinizes it with great care while Ajay looks over her shoulder. At first glance she cannot find any abnormality. Ajay agrees. Based on their observations they rule out a relevant pulmonary venous congestion as a consequence of left heart failure in myocardial infarction. Doc Reginald, the registrar on call covering the emergency room, stops by and scratches his head: He worries about a pulmonary embolism, which is the most serious cause of unexplained dyspnea. He wants a venogram or a Doppler ultrasound of the lower extremities and a ventilation/perfusion scan, possibly a pulmonary angiography after that—and he wants Giufeng and Ajay to organize all of it. Giufeng gives him her best irritated look and suggests bringing Mrs. Candi to the CT scanner at once to answer all questions with just one examination—a "one-stop-shop" procedure. That one examination would suffice to cover the whole differential, she declares. Ajay is really impressed and Reginald complies after just a little resistance.

→ What Is Your Diagnosis?

Pulmonary embolism: Pulmonary embolism is a frequent disease and also frequently overlooked—in excess of 50%; the CXR tends to be normal.

! Most pulmonary embolisms are not diagnosed because the entity is not considered at all.

Only in extensive lung embolism are platelike atelectases (Fig. 6.**52**), lung infarctions (Fig. 6.**53a**), and associated pleural effusions seen on the standard CXR. Owing to the lack of perfusion, the pulmonary vessels may constrict ("Westermark" sign), a phenomenon best appreciated in

The Case of Undira Candi I

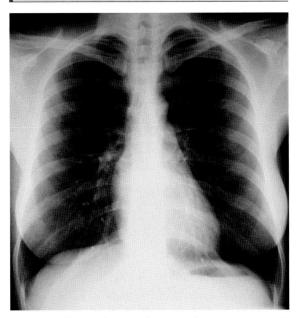

Fig. 6.**51**   Observe the CXR of Mrs. Candi. Do you agree with Giufeng and Ajay?

Pulmonary Embolism: Chest Radiograph

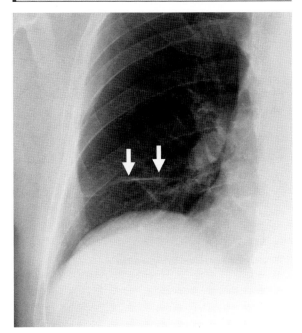

Fig. 6.**52**   Note the typical basilar platelike atelectasis that is seen in patients with pulmonary embolism but is certainly also a frequent finding in all patients unable to take a deep breath in (for example, after abdominal surgery). The most common finding in patients with pulmonary embolism is a normal CXR.

CT (Fig. 6.**53a**). The ventilation-perfusion scan shows a discrepancy between intact ventilation and missing perfusion to the affected segment of lung, also called "mismatch" (Fig. 6.**54a**).

> ! A comprehensive CT protocol for pulmonary embolism nowadays encompasses a CT angiography of the pulmonary arteries (Fig. 6.**53b**) and a CT venography (performed immediately afterwards and without the need for additional contrast medium administration) starting at the level of the knee joint and proceeding to the confluence of the common iliac veins at the bottom of the vena cava (Fig. 6.**53c**). Above that level, thrombosis is very rare. Patients with venous thrombosis below knee level do not require treatment with anticoagulation, therefore detection would not alter management significantly.

Aortic dissection: An aortic dissection starts with an intimal tear, frequently in the ascending aorta just above the valvular level, through which blood enters the aortic wall and separates the aortic wall layers. Aortic dissection occurs frequently in patients with arterial hypertension and those with Marfan syndrome. Excruciating pain and dyspnea occur as often as in pulmonary embolism. If the dissection blocks the origin of a coronary artery, myocardial infarction may ensue. CT angiography of the pulmonary vessels also depicts the aorta in a contrast medium phase that will also demonstrate aortic dissection. In order to exclude both entities in one scan session on a fast multidetector-row CT scanner, the scan delay after beginning of the contrast injection in the CT scanner may need to be increased compared to the exclusion of pulmonary embolus alone, or you need to scan twice in rapid succession in order to ensure that there is sufficient contrast in the aorta. It is very important to determine the involvement of the ascending aorta in aortic dissection (type A), because of the risk of myocardial infarction (Fig. 6.**55a**, **b**). A type A dissection thus requires immediate surgery. Fortunately, the cervical vessels exiting the arch often prevent the retrograde extension of dissections originating in the descending aortic arch into the ascending aorta (type B, Fig. 6.**55c**). Type B dissection is less dangerous and is most often managed conservatively unless relevant organ arteries are occluded. If this happens, the vascular surgeon or the interventional radiologist swings into action: The occluding dissection membrane is perforated with a special technique and/or a stent is applied to restore perfusion (Fig. 6.**56**).

Pulmonary Embolism: Diagnosis by CT

a Chest CT

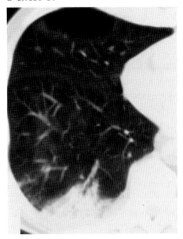
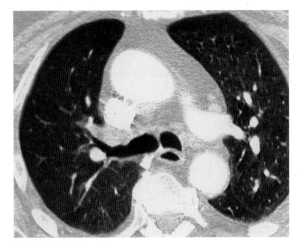

b CT angiography

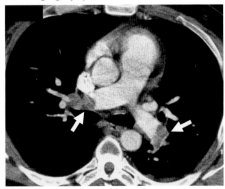

Fig. 6.**53 a**   The opacity in the lower lobe shows the typical triangular shape of a vascular territory. This is a classic pulmonary infarction due to pulmonary embolism (left). The reduced perfusion of the right lung is also suggested by the loss of vascular markings (right). **b** The fresh embolic material is appreciated in both pulmonary arteries as central filling defects in the vessel and outlined by the administered intravenous contrast (arrows). An older embolus tends to cling to the vascular wall molded along its circumference. **c** CT venography shows the presumptive cause of the embolism—a thrombus in the left femoral vein (left) that extends up into the inferior vena cava (right). Only the more expensive and cumbersome MR venography rivals the reliability of CT for thrombus detection.

c CT venography

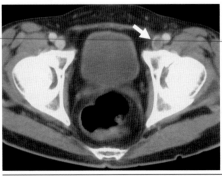
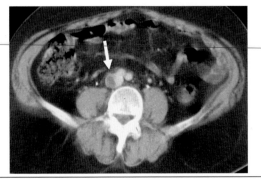

Pulmonary Embolism: Ventilation/Perfusion Scintigraphy

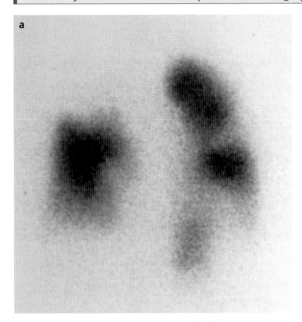

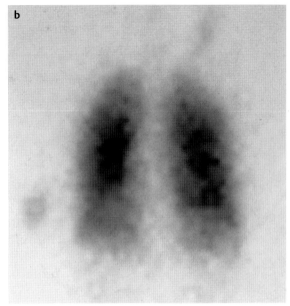

Fig. 6.**54 a** There is notable absence of radiotracer activity in the right upper lobe on perfusion imaging. **b** On ventilation images, aerosolized radiotracer is normally distributed to the right upper lobe. This mismatch of ventilation and perfusion images points to a pulmonary embolism. With the advent of advanced spiral CT protocols, the importance of this method in the diagnosis of pulmonary embolism is decreasing continuously. As opposed to CT, the sensitivity of scintigraphy is also hampered by any coexisting pulmonary parenchymal abnormalities such as pneumonia or atelectasis, which are common findings in many patients at increased risk for pulmonary embolus.

Aortic Dissection

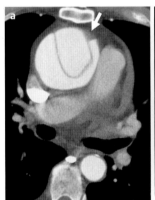

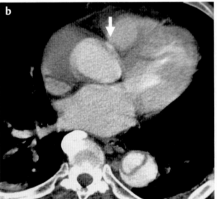

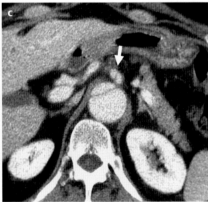

Fig. 6.**55 a** On this scan the dissection membrane is clearly visible within the dilated ascending aorta: It is the detached intima. Along its margins, the intimal flap is still partially connected to the supporting adventitia by arclike fibers (arrow), a phenomenon that helps to decide which is the false lumen. In this case the false lumen is the outer lumen. **b** The large vessels tend to exit from the false lumen. Vessels may also be obstructed, however. In this patient the outflow of the coronary arteries is still detectable (arrow), but an immediate surgical intervention was necessary. By the way, the aortic dissection is also visible—as in **a**—in the descending aorta. **c** Lastly, the dissection may also extend into larger branch vessels, such as the superior mesenteric artery (arrow).

Therapy of Aortic Dissection

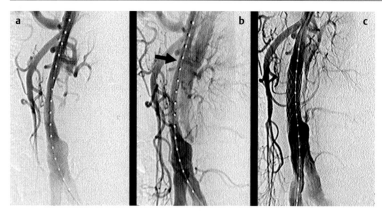

Fig. 6.**56**   You see an abdominal aortic angiogram of a patient with an iatrogenic type B dissection complicated by extensive claudication. **a** The contrast-filled true lumen is compressed by the unopacified false lumen. The renal arteries are also not opacified. **b** After fenestration of the dissection membrane (arrow) with a balloon, the renal arteries are reperfused. **c** Because the patient remained symptomatic, the dissection membrane was reapproximated to the vessel wall by deploying a stent (a small expandable wire-mesh tube) distal to the fenestration. This procedure finally provided symptomatic relief.

Non-Hodgkin Lymphoma

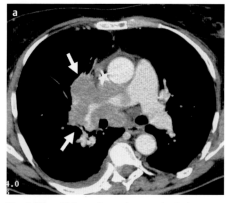

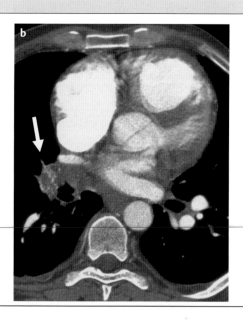

Fig. 6.**57 a**   This patient also reached the emergency room with the preliminary diagnosis of pulmonary embolism. The documented tumor masses around the right main bronchus proved to be non-Hodgkin lymphoma. **b** It could, of course, also have been an extensive bronchial carcinoma (arrow) such as in this patient.

Pneumonia: Pneumonia can demonstrate similar symptoms and may be all but invisible on plain CXRs—for example, if it is located in the dense retrocardiac area or if the patient is grossly overweight and difficult to image (see Fig. 6.**11a**). Again, CT will also diagnose this entity without problems.

Mediastinal/pulmonary tumor: A mediastinal or pulmonary tumor may also cause clinical symptoms that resemble pulmonary embolism (Fig. 6.**57**).

➜ **Diagnosis:**   Giufeng has persuaded Doc Reginald. The immediate CT examination reveals the true problem in this case (Fig. 6.**58**). A type A aortic dissection is present that needs surgical attention "stante pede" (that is: while standing on this foot, immediately, on the double). Reginald is relieved to have the diagnosis and contacts the thoracic surgeon on call. The senior medical consultant, who has also been alerted, inquires who this bright young lady in the chest imaging unit might be.

The Case of Undira Candi II

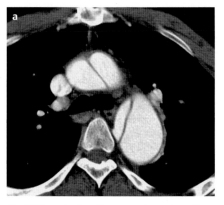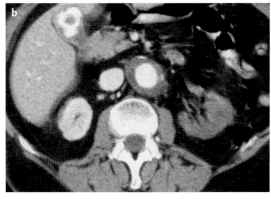

Fig. 6.**58 a**　A dissection membrane is well appreciated in the ascending as well as the descending aorta. The coronary arteries are in acute jeopardy. **b** In the abdomen, another problems becomes evident: The left kidney is no longer perfused.

6.6　Lesions in the Mediastinum

Widening of the Upper Mediastinum

Checklist: Widening of the Upper Mediastinum

- Was the patient positioned straight?
- Is the trachea narrowed and/or displaced?
- Does the mass pulsate under fluoroscopy?
- Is the mass located anteriorly or posteriorly?

! With regard to the etiology of masses in the anterior upper mediastinum, the famous "4 T rule" applies: thyroid, teratoma, thymus, and . . . terrible lymphoma.

Truly Large or Just a Matter of Unfortunate Perception?

Robert Waggoner (36) has recently noticed a swelling of his neck. While jogging in the morning he becomes short of breath pretty early these days. The enlarged veins at the neck get in the way of his wet shave. His family doctor has sent him for a chest radiograph on short notice. Joey studies the CXR together with Hannah (Fig. 6.**59**). The upper mediastinum is definitely widened—Mr. Waggoner has been perfectly positioned for the film. The trachea is stenosed. Both students contemplate the range of differential diagnoses.

The Case of Robert Waggoner I

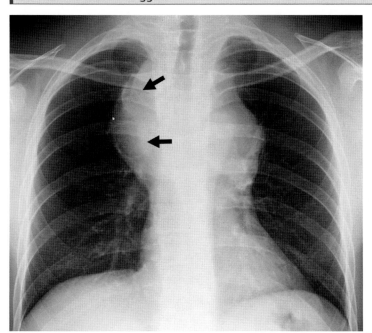

Fig. 6.**59**　Analyze the CXR of Mr. Waggoner. Which diseases do you have to consider?

Goiter

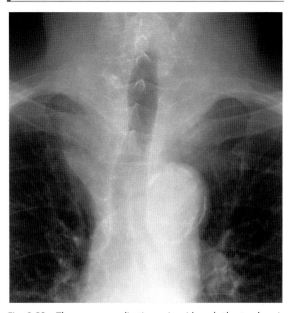

Fig. 6.**60**   The upper mediastinum is widened, the trachea is compressed by the goiter. Calcified thyroid nodes are not seen.

➔ What Is Your Diagnosis?

Goiter: Enlarged thyroids are the most frequent masses in the upper mediastinum (Fig. 6.**60**). They can become enormously large, displace and narrow the trachea, and lead to dyspnea on exertion. Typically they move up and down during swallowing. Frequently nodules develop inside the goiter that calcify coarsely and can become visible on the CXR.

Lymphoma: Lymphomas may occur in the upper mediastinum, where they displace the trachea and the vessels. Occasionally a superior vena cava syndrome results that needs therapy fast (and best after sufficient histological samples have been collected by CT-guided core needle biopsy). Naturally, enlargement of the lymph nodes may also be due to inflammatory processes, for example, tuberculosis or sarcoidosis.

Teratoma: Teratomas may consist of all elements of the blastodermic layer and therefore can contain fat, rudimentary teeth, and bones (Fig. 6.**61**). If you unequivocally find any or all of these features on a CT, the diagnosis is a quick and solid one.

Teratoma

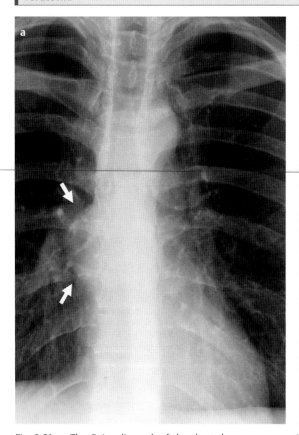
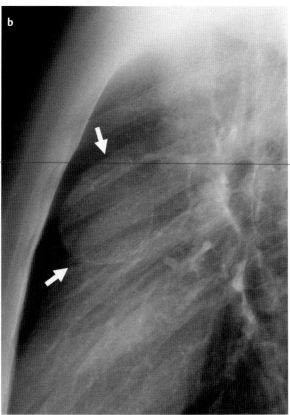

Fig. 6.**61 a**   The P-A radiograph of the chest shows a mass projecting below the azygos angle (arrows).
b The lateral view reveals the anterior location of this partially calcified lesion (arrows). Even if we do not see any teeth, this is a teratoma.

Right Heart Enlargement

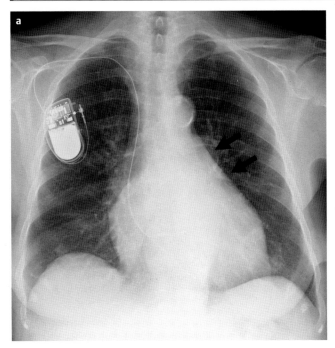

Fig. 6.**69**   The flattening of the heart concavity (**a**, arrows) and the enlarged contact area to the sternum (**b**, arrows) suggest right ventricular enlargement (see Fig. 6.**1**).

Constrictive pericarditis: Constrictive pericarditis is a postinflammatory entity characterized by pericardial calcifications visible especially in the periphery of the heart shadow (Fig. 6.**67**).

Valvular calcifications: Calcifications of the heart valves are best appreciated on the lateral views of the chest and can be assigned to the individual valves (see Fig. 6.**2b**).

Left heart enlargement: Left heart enlargement causes an abnormal but smooth bulge of the left lower heart contour. It occurs in left ventricular hypertrophy, as is seen, for example, in chronic arterial hypertension or in aortic valvular stenosis (Fig. 6.**68**), and in left ventricular dilatation, for example, in patients with aortic valve insufficiency or decompensated left heart failure, often due to severe coronary insufficiency. In arterial hypertension the left ventricular hypertrophy is frequently associated with an elongation of the aortic arch.

Right heart enlargement: Right heart enlargement manifests itself as a flattening or a bulge of the normally concave left upper heart contour. In this location, the pulmonary artery is displaced upward and laterally by the enlarged right ventricle. The enlarged right ventricle occupies the retrosternal space, which is well appreciated on the lateral CXR (Fig. 6.**69**). If the ventricle is hypertrophic but not enlarged as in pulmonary hypertension due to pulmonary fibrosis, the pulmonary artery is dilated centrally. The result is the typical appearance of a *cor pulmonale* (see Fig. 6.**75**).

Left ventricular aneurysm: A left ventricular aneurysm may develop after an extensive coronary infarction. It appears as a circumscribed bulge of the heart contour (Fig. 6.**70**).

Aneurysm of the Cardiac Wall

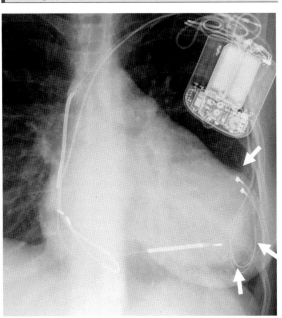

Fig. 6.**70**   The balloonlike bulge of the left heart contour (arrows) is a left ventricular aneurysm complicating extensive myocardial infarction.

Funnel Chest

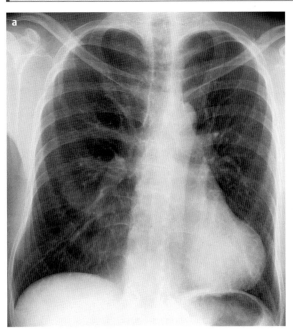

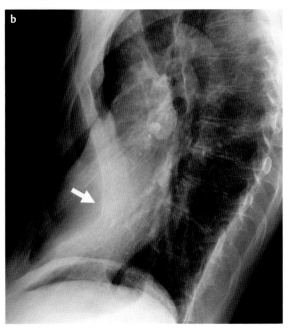

Fig. 6.**71 a**   The atypical shape of the heart (do you see the bulge of the left heart contour?) and the obliteration of the right heart contour ("silhouette sign"?) make sense only after inspection of the lateral film.

b The sternum (arrow) is located a few centimeters ventral of the spine in funnel chest (pectus excavatum). Of course, the heart is heavily deformed to fit into this chest.

Funnel chest (pectus excavatum): A funnel chest can deform the heart silhouette significantly; the underlying sternal deformity can best be identified on the lateral CXR (Fig. 6.**71**).

Hiatal Hernia

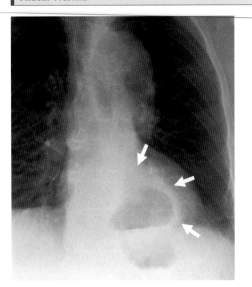

Fig. 6.**72**   The air-filled thick-walled structure is projecting over the heart shadow (arrows). This is a large hiatal hernia.

Hiatal hernia: This entity is the most frequent incidental mass in the retrocardiac space (Fig. 6.**72**). Owing to its air content and thick wall it is recognized with ease in most cases. If verification is needed, a lateral chest radiograph after ingestion of a small amount of barium will prove the hernia. It must, however, be differentiated from diverticula of the lower esophagus.

➙ **Diagnosis:** Giufeng has already seen some hiatal hernias and, as a matter of fact, did not really consider any alternative diagnosis in this case. For Mrs. Myers there won't be any consequence if she has no related complaints.

! The analysis of a complex heart configuration on a CXR needs a lot of time and brains and is hampered by a large number of variables. It is a first-rate intellectual challenge. Fortunately for all of us who do not play chess, echocardiography offers answers in less time and with more reliability. In the good ol' days there was more time for analysis—and no alternative. The typical heart configuration on a CXR should, however, be recognized and called by its right name.

Ben Felson and the Role of Funnel Chests in the Differential Diagnosis
Benjamin Felson was a grand American lecturer and a witty, inspiring radiologist. If you ever get a chance to read his book on chest radiology, go for it. In it he narrowed down a rather long radiological differential to two entities. Of these he picked one because the other one was "about as rare as a funnel chest in the Italian film colony." Which tells you a lot about humor and Italian movies in the sixties.

6.7   Enlargement of the Hila

Checklist: Enlargement of the Hila

- Is the enlargement unilateral or bilateral?
- Does the hilum in question have a lobulated configuration?
- Are there any hilar calcifications?
- Are there associated pulmonary parenchymal changes (fibrosis, micronodules)?
- Does the mass pulsate during fluoroscopy?

Just a Few Excess Curves

Hillary Frimpton (42) has called upon her doctor because she has felt unwell for several days and has been suffering from a dry cough. Her doctor has sent her for a chest radiograph. Paul and Giufeng cover the chest imaging unit as Mrs. Frimpton's image pops up on the viewing monitor (Fig. 6.**73**). The hilar enlargement is obvious.

→ **What Is Your Diagnosis?**

Sarcoidosis, lymphoma, tuberculosis, silicosis: Bilateral hilar lymph node enlargements can be caused by sarcoidosis, lymphoma, tuberculosis, and silicosis. It is the additional findings—clinical and radiological—that help differentiate these entities. In *sarcoidosis* interstitial micronodules are often present in the lung (see Fig. 6.**48a**, **b**). In *lymphoma* lymph nodes in other locations are also frequently enlarged (see Fig. 6.**59**). *Tuberculosis* must be considered particularly in immunosuppressed patients and patients who come from underdeveloped countries. In *silicosis* the enlarged lymph nodes tend to develop characteristic calcifications (see Fig. 6.**46a**).

> ⚠ A unilateral enlargement of a hilum is indicative of a bronchial carcinoma until proven otherwise (Fig. 6.**74**).

Pulmonary hypertension: Pulmonary hypertension, for example, as a consequence of pulmonary fibrosis or severe chronic obstructive airways disease (Fig. 6.**75**), triggers dilation of the pulmonary artery as a reaction to the increased vessel resistance. The hila become enlarged accordingly. A contrast-enhanced CT will easily verify the purely vascular nature of the increase in hilar size.

→ **Diagnosis:** Paul checks the CXR very carefully but cannot find any evidence of pulmonary fibrosis or emphysema. The bilateral hilar enlargement is most likely caused by enlarged lymph nodes. Giufeng hopes for sarcoidosis as a cause and the odds are in her favor. If other clinical parameters do not support this diagnosis, a tissue sample will have to be taken—best by way of a bronchoscopy.

The Case of Hillary Frimpton

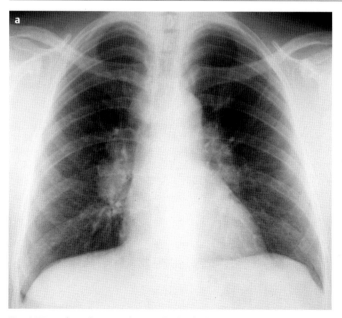
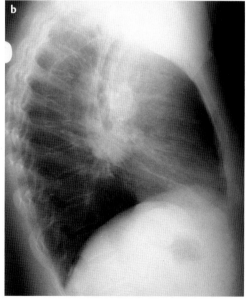

Fig. 6.**73**   What diseases do you think of when looking at Mrs. Frimpton's films?

Bronchial Carcinoma

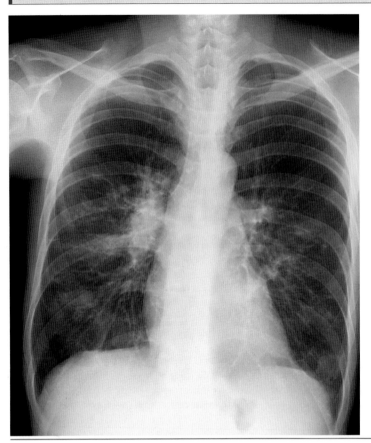

Fig. 6.**74**   The right hilum is definitely enlarged with an irregular margin. This turned out to be a bronchial carcinoma.

Pulmonary Hypertension

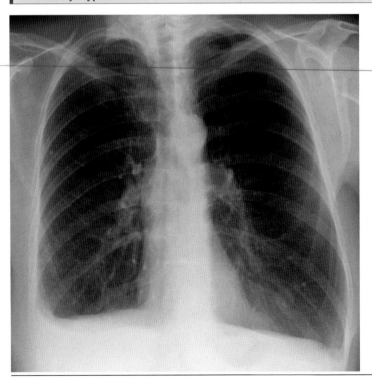

Fig. 6.**75**   The lungs are massively overinflated and the diaphragms are flattened accordingly; the vessels show an irregular course. This is severe emphysema that has led to pulmonary hypertension. The pulmonary artery is consequently dilated and there is a significant step in vascular caliber between the hilum and the lung parenchyma.

6.8   The Ultimate Exam

Paul celebrates his last day in the chest unit and has brought along a large box of cookies. It is late in the afternoon and Giufeng eats one biscuit after the other while sipping her cappuccino and listening to Paul's bright future plans with great amusement. Suddenly Gregory comes around the corner holding a pack of films in his hands. He senses the very special occasion and whips some of his films on the viewbox. "How about a tiny test, Paul?" he roars and pats him on his shoulder. Giufeng stops sipping her coffee and puts the cookies down with a smile, looking forward to a little entertainment. "Histoire

Test Cases

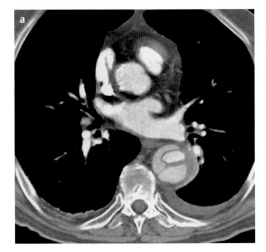

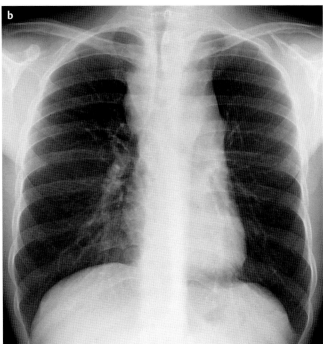

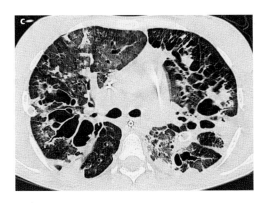

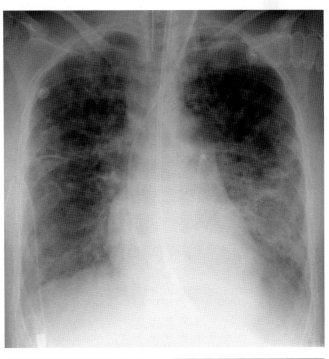

Fig. 6.**76a–h**
a Sudden severe chest pain is the symptom in this patient.
Don't stop with the basic diagnosis! Classify it further.
b This patient comes with dyspnea of two days' duration.
c History is withheld.

Test Cases

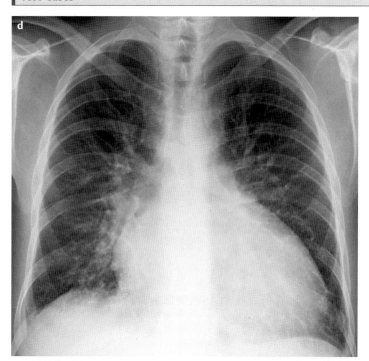

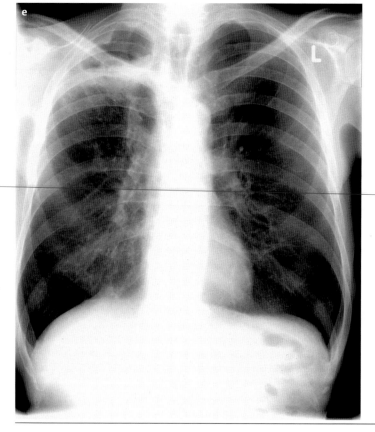

Fig. 6.**76a–h**
d A case that just came in.
e This young patient has not been feeling well lately.

inconnue," adds Gregory with an awful accent (meaning: history withheld)—he has been showing off his French since he stayed in Paris for a three-month neurointer-

ventional course last summer. "You'd better polish up on your pronunciation," Giufeng says casually. Gregory's smile freezes. Giufeng's own French is pretty good.

Test Cases

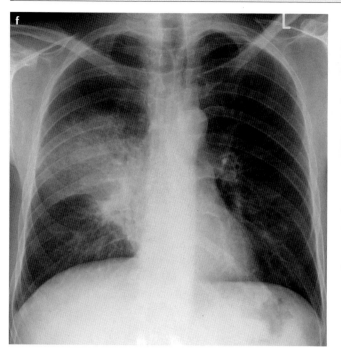

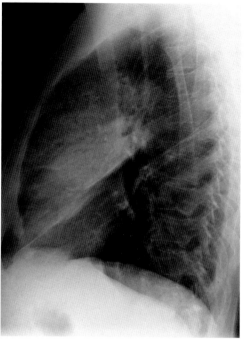

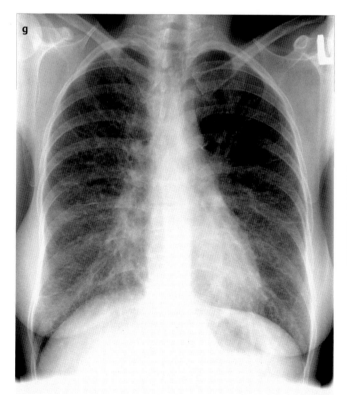

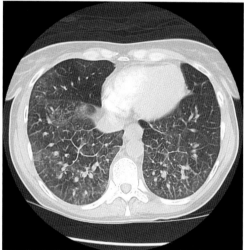

Fig. 6.**76a–h**
f This one is also unwell.
g This lady has been a regular visitor to the hospital.

Much to his disappointment, Gregory has not yet heard her speak in her soft Mandarin mother tongue. Paul sits up and focuses on the films: It is now or never. Gregory has a little surprise stowed away for the two interns (Fig. 6.**76a–h**). Why don't you go ahead check it out yourself.

Test Cases

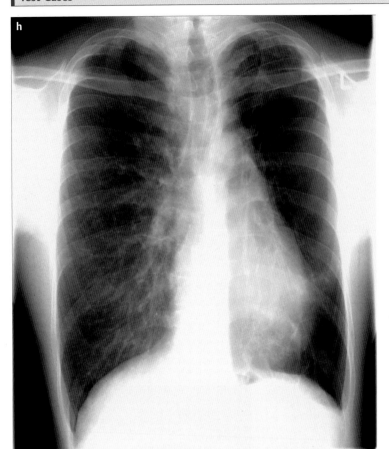

Fig. 6.**76a–h**
h This patient sits in front of you and smiles. He knows his diagnosis—do you?

Implantation of a Port

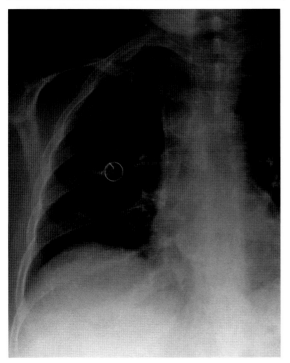

Fig. 7.**14** The port reservoir with inserted port needle is located on the pectoral muscle and the tip of the port tube is visualized in the cava at the correct level, that is, just superior to the right atrium.

mage to the lid using dedicated special tip needles (port needles). Foxhenry tunnels the skin from the pocket to the puncture site with a flexible blunt rod and pulls the port tube through. "Now check this out," he grins to Giufeng. "How do we get rid of the sheath?" Giufeng gives him a helpless glance. "We call this the 'banana-peel-technique.' You pull the sheath out of the vessel, then grab those two lashes at its end and pull them apart. The sheath is split in two halves and the port tube is freed. Cunning, isn't it?" The tube is cut to the correct length, tube and reservoir are connected, and both skin openings are sutured. Foxhenry tests the function of the port using that dedicated port needle and a little contrast and is quite satisfied with the end result (Fig. 7.**14**).

! A vascular port may only be punctured with a so-called port needle. Normal needles cause leaks! After use, the port must be filled with heparinized saline to prevent clotting of the port tube.

7.7   Embolization

Checklist: Embolization

- Is the region to be embolized dependent on an end artery?
- Does the vascular territory to be embolized feed other crucial vessels?
- Is there a danger of preexistent collaterals into vulnerable regions opening during the embolization?

This Vascular Bed is Put to Rest!

Sid McFlennan (64) had his left kidney removed six months ago because of a renal cell carcinoma. Now he has developed a large swelling in the right thigh after an awkward movement. The radiograph has shown a pathological femur fracture just below the trochanter (Fig. 7.**15a**). The trauma surgeons want to stabilize the fracture but they fear the large hypervascularized metastatic mass in the area. For that reason they have asked for the preoperative embolization of the mass. Dr. Chaban looks at the images together with Paul and Ajay.

➔ **Procedure:** Chaban punctures the femoral artery in the groin in antegrade direction and performs an angiogram of the vascular territory in question (Fig. 7.**15b**). The large hypervascularized mass lights up with contrast right away—the trauma surgeon's call for help seems justified. Over a selective catheter Chaban injects tissue glue into the feeding vessels and puts some endovascular coils on top (Fig. 7.**15c**). "Now it is the surgeon's game," he nods to Paul. Ajay wonders where else the technique can be used. "Embolizations of this kind can be performed in all kinds of tumor bleeds. You can, for example, also treat uterine leiomyomas like that. Angiomas and arteriovenous malformations [Fig. 7.**16a**, see also p. 249] are also dealt with in that fashion. But the action can become extremely tricky if you work in vital vascular territories like, for example, the spinal cord. Obstruction of important vessels with dislodged embolic material or by iatrogenic dissections is the most relevant and consequential complication," Chaban says with an earnest look on his face. "Fascinating," says Ajay. Paul is impressed. He has seen enough—intervention is just not his cup of tea.

! Embolizations had better be done by cold-blooded pros.

Embolization of a Metastasis

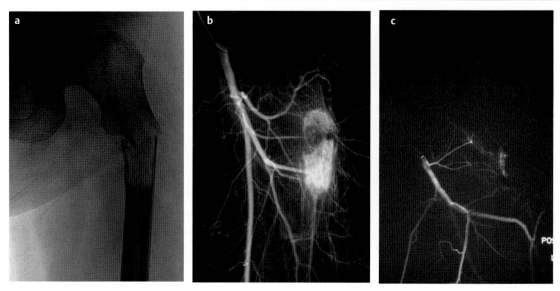

Fig. 7.**15 a** This metastasis has destroyed the cancellous bone and eroded the cortex. The fragments are scattered around in the adjacent tissue. **b** Selective angiography of the femoral artery shows the tumor's vascular bed supplied by branches arising from the deep femoral artery. **c** The final run after embolization shows only little residual vascularization within the tumor.

Embolization of Arteriovenous Malformations

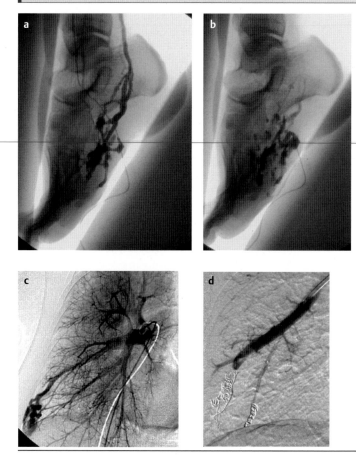

Fig. 7.**16 a** This young man has a vascular malformation of the foot that is the cause of increasing problems: for a start, his shoes do not fit anymore. After percutaneous puncture of the vascular mass with a butterfly needle, the whole extent of the lesion is visualized angiographically. **b** Subsequently, tissue glue mixed with contrast is injected under fluoroscopy. The mass will shrink in the weeks and months to come and with a little luck the symptoms will dwindle. **c** The arteriovenous malformation depicted in this pulmonary angiogram caused relevant shunting. **d** The obstruction of the feeding vessel with a few coils settled the problem.

7.8   Neural Blockades

- Has conservative pain therapy been given a real chance?
- Has the source of the pain been correctly identified?

The Pain Relievers Don't Do Their Job Anymore

Hank Podgorny (68) has been a "window shopper" for quite a while, suffering from severe arteriovascular disease. Dilations and stent implantations in his femoral arteries have already been done but they did not really solve his problem. Lately the narrowed small peripheral arteries—those that cannot be dilated with a balloon—have been the cause of his pains. And, well, OK, smoking is the last real pleasure in his life, he says, as his wife sits by his side scowling. The right leg hurts almost constantly and his toes on that side have already turned blue. His family physician has arranged this appointment for him. As Dr. Schaeffer calmly briefs a nervous Podgorny about potential complications such as neuralgia, hypotension, impotence, or failure of ejaculation, his wife leaves the room snorting. Schaeffer turns to Ajay to explain everything about the procedure in the CT control room.

→ Procedures

Block of the lumbar sympathetic nerve: "Mr. Podgorny will get a lumbar plexus block. This is a combination of vascular and pain therapy. We block the sympathetic plexus on the right side, thus in effect dilating the peripheral vessels and also treating the pain. Let's measure the temperature of the calf before the intervention." Mr. Podgorny is already positioned prone on the CT table. The thermometer shows 26.5 °C at the medial side of the right lower leg. On the left the temperature is few degrees higher. On a limited CT, Schaeffer has found just the right approach at the level of the L3/4 vertebral bodies. She disinfects the puncture site about 7 cm lateral to the spinous process and injects a local anesthetic. She then advances a long, thin needle along the lateral side of the vertebral body and positions its tip neatly in front of the spine (Fig. 7.**17a**). She injects a little lidocaine mixed with contrast and waits for 5 minutes (Fig. 7.**17b**). "Why don't you measure the temperature once more," she asks Ajay. But Podgorny feels a change already and comes alive: "Sumthin's happenin', Doc," he declares. The temperature has indeed risen to 32 °C. Schaeffer smiles and administers 15 ml of a solution of absolute alcohol mixed with lidocaine and contrast to make the block a definitive one. The final distribution of the mixture is documented once again by CT (Fig. 7.**17c**). Podgorny is satisfied: "Dad leg ha'n been dis warm for ten years. No pain no more. You ge'me to walk now Doc an' I'm in heaven." While Podgorny joins his wife who has been chatting animatedly with Magdalena in postinterventional monitoring, Schaeffer explains to Ajay a few other pain therapy interventions that can be elegantly and safely done with CT guidance.

Block of the celiac plexus: Block of the celiac plexus is performed in severe pain in the region of the celiac trunk—mostly due to invasive pancreatic carcinomas. The target of the injection that can be done via a dorsal or ventral approach is the celiac plexus around the arterial celiac trunk. After a test injection of lidocaine, approx. 20 ml of a strong alcoholic solution is administered.

Infiltrations with lidocaine and corticosteroids: Lumbar nerve root blocks are performed in patients with radicular pain. Peridural infiltrations of the spinal canal are done in cases of spinal canal stenosis. Infiltrations of the intervertebral and iliosacral joints are also possible. All these interventions are best performed with CT guidance.

Block of the Lumbar Sympathetic Nerve

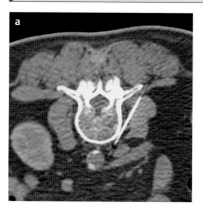 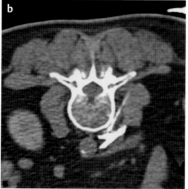 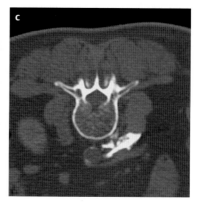

Fig. 7.**17 a**   The needle tip is located inside the lumbar plexus directly anterior to the vertebral body. **b** The injected fluid, a mixture of lidocaine and contrast, spreads in the target area. **c** In a second step, 15 ml of a strong alcoholic solution is injected to inactivate the plexus permanently. The final scan documents the sympatholytic fluid in the lumbar plexus.

7.9   Gregory's Test

Giufeng, Ajay, Joey, and Paul sit around enjoying cup of coffee with some cookies as their day draws to an end. Suddenly Hannah turns around the corner: "You have got to have a look at this," she smiles at them. "Segner is just now taking Gregory apart for good. Greg is all excited and tense." "We should go listen, perhaps we can learn a thing or two," suggests Joey. "Oh, for heaven's sake, why don't you leave them alone. Gregory probably wouldn't appreciate a crowd right now," says Giufeng. "Now, there is a good reason!" Paul grins, and moves to the door together with Joey. "Let's move, mates!"

"This could have gone all wrong and it still may, Gregory," shouts Segner as our students turn the corner. Gregory crouches on the procedure table, his scrubs clinging to his chest like a wet mop. Segner ignores the interns' arrival and continues his yelling sermon with swollen neck veins. "If you do an elective intervention you cannot brief the patient on the table, dammit! When and where must this happen? And then you did not check the clotting! Just how stupid can one be! Which parameters do you need to know and what are the minimum or maximum levels? And then you had someone inexperienced compress the puncture site—Gregory, you must have had a blackout! Don't tell me about a long intervention! Let me tell you what a long intervention is. You'd better pray that inguinal hematoma does not get larger or get infected. The guys in intensive care will laugh their heads off. Listen, Greg, this is my outfit and this is radiology, not cardiology. You'd better get your act together before you touch another catheter in this department." Segner storms out the door. Gregory takes a deep breath and remains silent—of course he knows that Segner is right. Giufeng pushes the others out of the room "Get lost now, all of you!" she says and returns into the dark room closing the door behind her. Gregory was pretty careless. Giufeng knows why: he learned today that one of his articles has been accepted for publication in *Radiology*. He was absolutely out of it. The hype did not do him any good. Can you help Gregory with the answers to Segner's questions?

8 Bone and Soft Tissues

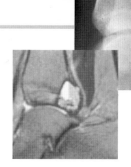

Imaging of skeleton and soft tissues is the cradle of radiology. Here the technology had the greatest therapeutic impact in the early decades. Even today seasoned radiologists are faced with major challenges in this field and must prove their mastery. They share this interest with a sizable number of clinical specialists from other fields with whom—in their own and the patient's best interest—they must be competent partners. Decades of experience, a strong interest in the science behind imaging phenomena, a substantial library—the most voluminous book on the subject fills about 5000 pages in small print—and an inexhaustible passion for the great interesting case make up a real "bone radiologist." It is thus nothing to turn into overnight. Students and young colleagues need to constantly search for and learn the key findings to improve their skill in this field. A sound knowledge of the proper clinical indications for the available imaging modalities is a good start (Table 8.1).

Table 8.1 **Suggestions for diagnostic modalities in musculoskeletal imaging**[1]

Clinical problem	Modality	Comment
Bone pain	XR	Gross assessment of symptomatic areas.
	NM	Bone scan indicated if symptoms persist and plain XRs are negative. Shows number of lesions.
	MRI	Appropriate if symptoms persist and conventional XR and NM fail to diagnose disease.
Suspected primary bone tumor	XR	May help to characterize the lesion; sufficient in many cases; should be carried out when bone pain does not resolve. If XR is suggestive of primary bone tumor, referral to a specialized center is advised.
	MRI	Useful for further characterization and necessary for local staging; should be performed before any biopsy.
	CT	Can show bony detail better at some sites (e.g., spine) and helps analyze internal matrix in some tumors (e.g., osteoid osteoma); easily demonstrates calcification/ossification. Chest CT if CXR is negative to assess pulmonary metastases for many primary malignant lesions. CT-guided biopsy should be carried out in specialized bone tumor centers.
Osteomyelitis	XR	Initial modality of choice, can be normal for first 2–3 weeks.
	NM	Two- or three-phase skeletal scintigram is more sensitive than XR but nonspecific. Labeled white cell scintigraphy may distinguish infection from other lesions.
	MRI	Accurately demonstrates infection, especially in the spine.
	CT	Used to identify bony sequestrum.
Known primary tumor/suspected skeletal metastases	MRI	Primary modality of choice. More sensitive and specific than NM, especially for marrow-based lesions and in the axial skeleton. May underestimate number of peripheral lesions.

CT, computed tomography; DXA, dual-energy x-ray-absorptiometry; MRI, magnetic resonance imaging; NM, nuclear medicine; US, ultrasound; XR, radiography.

Table 8.1 Suggestions for diagnostic modalities in musculoskeletal imaging[1] (Continued)

Clinical problem	Modality	Comment
	XR	Only for specific focal symptomatic areas; correlation with positive NM (exclusion of degenerative disease) and to determine stability.
	NM	Sensitive test but correlative imaging is needed to increase specificity. Useful for overall assessment for skeletal metastases as long as the tumor causes sufficient local bone turnover to become detectable.
Suspected myeloma	XR skeletal survey	For staging and identifying lesions that may benefit from radiotherapy. Survey of limited value for follow-up and to assess response to therapy.
	MRI	Very sensitive, even when limited to spine, pelvis, and proximal femora. Particularly useful in nonsecretory myeloma or in the presence of diffuse osteopenia. Can be used for tumor mass assessment and follow-up under therapy.
	NM	Insensitive test in myeloma.
Osteomalacia	XR	To establish cause of local pain or equivocal lesion on NM.
	NM	Skeletal scintigraphy can show increased activity and some local complications such as pseudofractures. Bone densitometry may be needed.
Metabolic bone disease	XR	May be helpful to differentiate new from old vertebral fractures or to identify different causes of pain. Correlation with NM will be required.
	NM	Skeletal scintigraphy may be useful for differentiating causes of hypercalcemia (metastases, hyperparathyroidism) and of raised alkaline phosphatase (Paget disease).
	DXA	DXA or quantitative CT quantifies bone mineral content.
Arthropathy, presentation	XR affected joint	May be helpful to determine cause, although erosions are a relatively late feature.
	XR hands/feet	In patients with suspected rheumatoid arthritis, XR of feet may show erosions even when symptomatic hands appear normal.
	US or NM or MRI	All accurately show acute synovitis. NM can show distribution. MRI can assess articular cartilage and early erosions.
Arthropathy, follow-up	XR	Needed by rheumatologists to assist management decisions.
Hallux valgus	XR	For assessment before surgery.
Spinal problems		
Pain, suspected osteoporotic collapse	XR	Lateral views will demonstrate compression fractures. NM or bone densitometry (DXA or quantitative CT) provide objective measurements of bone mineral content; can also be used for metabolic bone disease.
	MRI	More useful in distinguishing between recent and old fractures and can help exclude pathological fractures. Excellent modality to assess for extraosseous soft tissue mass in pathological fractures.
Cervical spine		
Neck pain, arm pain, suspected degenerative change	XR	Neck pain generally improves or resolves with conservative treatment. Degenerative changes begin in early middle age and are often unrelated to symptoms.

CT, computed tomography; DXA, dual-energy x-ray-absorptiometry; MRI, magnetic resonance imaging; NM, nuclear medicine; US, ultrasound; XR, radiography.

Table 8.1 Suggestions for diagnostic modalities in musculoskeletal imaging[1] (Continued)

Clinical problem	Modality	Comment
	MRI	Consider MR and specialist referral when pain affects lifestyle or when there are neurological signs. Myelography (with CT) may occasionally be required to provide further delineation or when MRI is unavailable or impossible to obtain.
Thoracic spine		
Pain without trauma: suspected degenerative change	XR	Degenerative changes are invariable from middle age onward. Imaging is rarely useful in the absence of neurological signs or pointers to metastases or infection. Consider more urgent referral in elderly patients with sudden pain to show osteoporotic collapse or other forms of bone destruction. Consider NM for possible metastatic lesions.
	MRI	May be indicated if local pain persists or is difficult to manage or if there are long tract signs.
Lumbar spine		
Chronic back pain with no pointers to infection or neoplasm	XR	Degenerative changes are common and nonspecific. Main value in younger patients (e.g., less than 20 years), spondylolisthesis, ankylosing spondylitis, etc., or in older patients >55. In cases where management is difficult, negative findings may be helpful.
	MRI	First-choice method when symptoms persist or are severe or where management is difficult. Imaging findings are to be interpreted with caution because abnormalities are frequent and not necessarily related to clinical signs. Negative findings may be helpful.
Back pain with possible serious features such as: ■ Onset <20 years ■ >55 years ■ Sphincter or gait disturbance ■ Saddle anesthesia ■ Severe or progressive motor loss ■ Widespread neurological deficit ■ Previous carcinoma ■ Systemic illness ■ HIV ■ Weight loss ■ Intravenous drug abuse ■ Steroids ■ Structural deformity ■ Nonmechanical pain	MRI	Together with urgent specialist referral, MRI is usually the best modality. Imaging should not delay specialist referral. NM is also widely used for possible bone destruction, and in cases of chronic pain or where infection is suspected.
	XR	"Normal" plain XR may be falsely reassuring but XR should be done to exclude spondylolisthesis or spondylolysis.
Acute back pain: suspected disk herniation; sciatica with no adverse features	XR	Acute back pain usually due to conditions that cannot be diagnosed on plain XR (osteoporotic collapse and spondylolisthesis are the exception). "Normal" plain XRs may be falsely reassuring.
	MR or CT	Imaging disk herniation requires MRI or CT: MR is generally preferred. Correlation of clinical and imaging findings is important as a significant number of disk herniations are asymptomatic. Either MR or CT is needed before intervention (e.g., epidural injection). MRI is better than CT for postoperative problems.

CT, computed tomography; DXA, dual-energy x-ray-absorptiometry; MRI, magnetic resonance imaging; NM, nuclear medicine; US, ultrasound; XR, radiography.

Table 8.1 **Suggestions for diagnostic modalities in musculoskeletal imaging**[1] (Continued)

Clinical problem	Modality	Comment
Shoulder problems		
Painful shoulder	XR	Not indicated initially. Degenerative changes in the acromioclavicular joints and rotator cuff are common.
Shoulder impingement	MRI	Although impingement is a clinical diagnosis, imaging is indicated when surgery is being considered and precise delineation of anatomy is required. Degenerative changes are also common in the asymptomatic population.
	US	Subacromial and acromioclavicular joint impingement are dynamic processes that can be assessed by US.
Shoulder instability	CT/MRI arthrography	Glenoid labrum and joint space are well delineated by both techniques. Some gradient echo MR techniques can show the labrum well without arthrography. Arthrography (with or without CT), US, and MRI may all be used in the diagnosis.
Rotator cuff tear	Arthrography, US, or MRI	MRI provides the best global assessment and has highest accuracy when combined with arthrography.
Knee problems		
Knee pain: without locking or restriction in movement	XR	Symptoms frequently arise from internal derangement of ligamentous or cartilaginous structures and these will not be demonstrated on XR. Osteoarthritic changes are common. XRs needed when considering surgery.
Knee pain: with locking, restricted movement or effusion (loose body)	XR	To identify radiopaque loose bodies.
Knee pain: arthroscopy being considered	MRI	Can assist the management decision whether to proceed with arthroscopy. Even in those patients with definite clinical abnormalities, warranting intervention, surgeons find preoperative MRI helpful in identifying unsuspected lesions.
Pelvic and hip problems		
Sacroiliac (SI) joint lesion	XR	May help in investigation of seronegative arthropathy. SI joints is usually adequately demonstrated on A-P lumbar spine or pelvis.
	MRI, NM, CT	MR or CT or perhaps NM when plain XRs are equivocal; earlier detection with MRI, particularly after contrast. MRI is advantageous in children and adolescents.
Hip pain: full or limited movement	XR	Symptoms often transient. Only if symptoms and signs persist or history is complex (e.g., chance of avascular necrosis) or if hip replacement might be considered.
	MR	Useful to demonstrate inflammation. MR arthrography to evaluate acetabular labral tears.
Hip pain: suspected avascular necrosis	XR	Abnormal in established disease.
	MR	Most sensitive in the detection of early avascular necrosis and will demonstrate extent.
Painful prosthesis	XR	To detect loosening.
	NM	Normal skeletal scintigraphy excludes most late complications. Labeled white cell scintigraphy can help distinguish loosening from infection.

CT, computed tomography; DXA, dual-energy x-ray-absorptiometry; MRI, magnetic resonance imaging; NM, nuclear medicine; US, ultrasound; XR, radiography.

Table 8.**1 Suggestions for diagnostic modalities in musculoskeletal imaging**[1] (Continued)

Clinical problem	Modality	Comment
In the child		
Nonaccidental injury/child abuse	XR	Age 0–2 years: skeletal survey and head CT mandatory. Age >2 years: XR clinically suspect area. XR should be performed by radiographers trained in pediatric radiographic techniques.
	NM	Skeletal scintigraphy in children >2 years if skeletal survey is equivocal. Findings must be correlated with other patient data.
Irritable hip	US	Will confirm presence of effusions that can be aspirated for diagnostic and therapeutic purposes. Cannot differentiate septic from transient synovitis.
	XR	XR, which may include frog lateral view, is required if slipped capital epiphysis or Perthes disease is suspected and if symptoms persist. If symptoms persist, follow-up should be as for limping child.
Limping	US	Will confirm presence of effusions that can be aspirated for diagnostic and therapeutic purposes. Cannot differentiate sepsis from transient synovitis.
	XR	Proper clinical assessment needed. If pain persists or localizing signs are present, XR is indicated. If slipped epiphyses are likely, lateral XRs of both hips are needed. Gonad protection should be used routinely unless shields obscure area of clinical suspicion.
	MRI	According to local policy, expertise, and availability.
Clicking hip; suspected dislocation	US	XR may be used to supplement US examination. XR is indicated in the older infant.
Osgood–Schlatter disease		Bony radiological changes are visible in Osgood–Schlatter disease but overlap with normal appearances. Associated soft tissue swelling should be assessed clinically rather than radiographically.
Back or neck pain	XR/MRI/CT	Persistent back pain in children may have an underlying cause and justifies investigation. Choice of imaging following consultation. Scoliosis and neurological findings merit MRI/CT. MRI defines spinal malformations and excludes associated thecal abnormality.
Short stature/growth failure	XR for bone age	Only in children >1 year: Nondominant hand only.
Soft tissue problems		
Soft tissue mass/ suspected tumor	MRI	Provides best local staging and tissue diagnosis in a proportion of patients.
	US	Can differentiate between solid and cystic tumors, is good for biopsy, and can monitor progress of benign masses such as hematoma.
	CT	Has greater sensitivity for calcification; good for biopsy.
Possible recurrence	MRI	Modality of choice.

[1]Modified after: RCR Working Party. *Making the best use of a Department of Clinical Radiology. Guidelines For Doctors*, 5th ed. London: The Royal College of Radiologists, 2003.

CT, computed tomography; DXA, dual-energy x-ray-absorptiometry; MRI, magnetic resonance imaging; NM, nuclear medicine; US, ultrasound; XR, radiography.

8.1   How Do You Analyze a Bone Image?

The analysis of a bone image should always differentiate between assessment of the bone itself, the joints, and the surrounding soft tissues.

Bone

Every bone has a typical absolute and age-dependent size as well as a configuration and an axis of orientation typical for its function. Comparison with the contralateral side may be very helpful to the radiologist in ambivalent cases, especially in children.

The bone consists of the outer solid cortical bone and the inner cancellous bone. The **bone cortex** is dense like ivory and is perforated by occasional nutrient vascular channels. Its exterior and interior margins are rather smooth. In hyperparathyroidism or if aggressive metastases infiltrate from the outside, the bone cortex becomes permeated. In metastases of the cancellous bone or multiple myeloma this occurs from the inside. The normally smooth outer contour becomes unsharp when the periosteum reacts to injuries (periosteal callus formation; periosteal reaction), inflammations, and neoplastic lesions.

The **cancellous bone** with its very location-specific architecture gives the bone stability while its weight remains low. The very well vascularized bone marrow rests in its interstices. It normally has a high fat component except if hematopoiesis is increased, such as in children and women with strong menstrual bleeds. Inflammatory and neoplastic diseases frequently occur here and destroy the

typical radiological pattern of spongiosa. In thick bones or where air- and feces-filled intestines are superimposed over the bone, such as the over the iliac bone, large defects of the cancellous bone may go undetected. Other modalities can help in these cases: bone scans visualize the increased regional or focal bone turnover and MRI shows—among other things—the displacement of the fatty bone marrow. With age (*carpe diem*—seize the day: age begins at 35 here) the bone density decreases slowly. Corticosteroids accelerate this process, which typically increases the risk for vertebral body and femoral neck fractures. During extended phases of physical inactivity (after fractures and other injuries; space missions—lack of gravity) the bone density decreases, particularly in the vicinity of the joints. As physical activity is resumed, an altered, coarser trabecular pattern may remain.

Joints

A joint consists of the articulating bones, the cartilage, any additional special fibrous cartilage (i.e., menisci), ligaments, tendons, and the joint space, which is lined by the synovial membrane and contains synovial fluid. Conventional radiographs demonstrate only a limited number of these structures. The configuration of the articulating bones is one major radiographic finding. Only magnetic resonance tomography depicts all joint components.

In osteoarthritis, the *degeneration* of a joint over time, one can observe formation of osteophytes in the periphery of the joint, an eccentric loss of joint space in the area of heaviest physical load, sclerosis, and subchondral cyst formation. In a primary *inflammation* of the joint, also termed inflammatory arthropathy, subchondral demineralization, a generalized concentric loss of joint space, bone erosions in the joint periphery close to the synovial insertion, and occasionally even ankylosis may occur. Small osseous fragments, so-called "loose bodies" can be detected in the joint. Joint effusions may become evident by the displacement of fat pads adherent to the joint capsule or located directly in the joint (such as the Hoffa fat pad in the knee). Articular recesses that are normally collapsed become visible small opacities when the joint is fluid-filled and they are surrounded by fatty tissue planes.

Soft Tissues

The soft tissues—muscles, ligaments, tendons, fat planes, nerves, and vessels—are difficult to evaluate with plain radiographs. Of course, severely calcified vascular walls in atherosclerosis are easy to appreciate and should be commented upon. Anatomical interfaces between fat and other soft tissues can be very helpful in radiography (i.e. to diagnose lipomas or joint effusions). An optimal evaluation of the soft tissues, however, is possible only with MRI owing to its superb soft tissue contrast (see Fig. 4.4a, p. 20).

▌ A Diagram of Bone

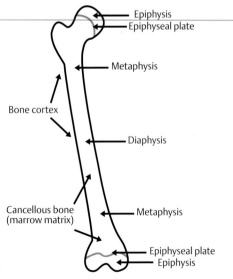

Epiphysis
Epiphyseal plate
Metaphysis
Bone cortex
Diaphysis
Cancellous bone (marrow matrix)
Metaphysis
Epiphyseal plate
Epiphysis

See the main terms used in bone anatomy.

I See an Abnormality—What Do I Do Now?

Follow the scheme described below and try to answer the following questions:
- Is it a focal process of the bone or is it there generalized osseous change?
- Is the osseous lesion lytic (bone structure is lost) or blastic (bone structure becomes denser)?
- Is the key symptom articular pain?
- Is the key symptom back pain?
- Is there an associated soft tissue mass?

The acute traumatic findings will be dealt with in the chapter on trauma (Chapter 14). Now let us have a look at the first case.

8.2   Diseases of the Bone

Focal Bone Lesions

Checklist: Focal Bone Lesions

- How old is the patient?
- Are there clinical symptoms?
- Where in the bone is the lesion?
- What is its biological behavior (Table 8.2)?

There Ain't No Class without Gwilym Lodwick

Boris Packer (22) has bruised his knee joint severely during one of his international tennis tournaments. Looking at the radiographs, Paul is pretty sure that there is no fracture. He has, however, searched the image with great care and has found a circumscribed lesion in the distal femur (Fig. 8.1). Boris has never had any complaints in this area before the tournament. It is undoubtedly an incidental finding. Has Paul saved Boris's life by detecting a little malignant lesion so early that it can be resected without any further harm? Or is this a benign lesion that should best be ignored to spare Boris the risks of more invasive diagnostic procedures? Paul remembers good ol' Gwilym Lodwick's time-honored classification of bone lesions (Table 8.2). He defines the lesion as a Lodwick grade IA, which indicates a benign nature.

Who is Gwilym Lodwick?

Gwilym Lodwick was a famous American bone radiologist. After leaving his chair at the University of Missouri at Columbia, he and his gigantic collection of skeletal cases moved into a little office at the Massachusetts General Hospital of the Harvard Medical School. There he continued to teach for a long time. He was not easy to get along with but was a full-blooded, dyed-in-the-wool radiologist.

Table 8.2 Classification of bone lesions according to Gwilym Lodwick[1]

Criteria of the lesion \ Grading	IA	IB	IC	II	III
Pattern	Geographic	Geographic	Mandatory geographic	Moth-eaten or geographic	Mandatory permeative[2]
Contour	Regular Lobulated Multicentric, (but sharp)	Regular Lobulated Multicentric Ragged/poorly defined	Regular Lobulated Multicentric Ragged/poorly defined Moth-eaten (<1 cm)	Edge characteristic if geographic, mandatory moth-eaten edge >1 cm	Any edge
Cortex penetration	None/partial	None/partial	Mandatory total	Total by definition	Total by definition
Sclerotic rim	Mandatory	Optional	Optional	Optional but unlikely	Optional but unlikely
Cortical expansion	Optional, expanded cortex ≤1 cm	If sclerotic rim present, expanded cortex >1 cm	Optional expanded cortex	Optional but unlikely	Optional but unlikely
Malignancy	More likely to be benign				More likely to be malignant

[1] Lodwick et al. Determining growth rates of focal lesions of bone from radiographs. Radiology 1980; 134: 577–583.
[2] Infiltrating the cortex.

The Case of Boris Packer

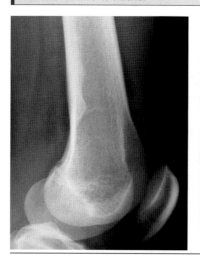
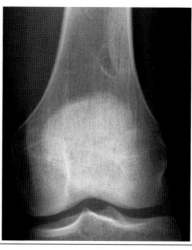

Fig. 8.1 You see a magnified view of the knee radiograph of Boris Packer. Is there anything abnormal?

→ **What is Your Diagnosis?** These are frequent benign bone tumors in childhood and adolescence:

Enostosis: The enostosis, also called "bone island," is an island of cortical bone within the cancellous bone. Radiologically it appears as a focal, mostly round or oval sclerosis of the cancellous bone without any response in the surrounding bone (Fig. 8.2). The enostosis often does not show activity on bone scans and can thus be differentiated from osteoblastic metastases in ambivalent cases.

Osteoma: An osteoma consists of very dense bone and occurs most often in the paranasal sinuses (Fig. 8.3). It can be associated with intestinal polyposis (Gardner syndrome).

Osteoid osteoma: This tumor is most often located in the bony cortex of the femur and tibia but also in the axial skeleton. It consists of a severe periosteal reaction with new bone formation around an often rod-shaped nidus that contains a neurovascular bundle (Fig. 8.4). Nocturnal pain that is relieved by low-dose acetylsalicylic acid is a typical symptom. The interventional radiologist can treat this lesion by inserting a radiofrequency needle into the nidus and ablating the neurovascular bundle by electrical coagulation or by alcohol instillation.

Enchondroma: An enchondroma is a cartilaginous, lobulated tumor within the marrow space of cancellous bone, frequently in the hand bones (Fig. 8.5). It tends to

Enostosis

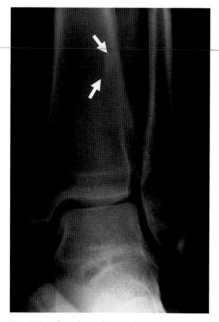

Fig. 8.2 This dense bone island (arrows) is located in the distal metaphysis of the tibia close to the cortex.

Osteoma

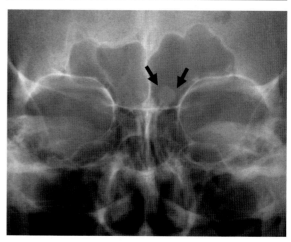

Fig. 8.3 This pea-sized dense sclerotic lesion (arrows) sits in the left frontal sinus. It is an osteoma in a typical location.

Osteoid Osteoma

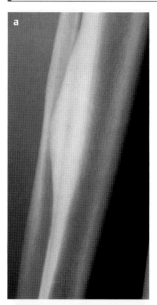

Fig. 8.**4a** The dorsal cortex of the tibia is significantly thickened—a nidus can only be suspected. **b** CT gives more information. The reactive new bone formation around the nidus is well appreciated. This nidus must be resected/drilled out by the surgeons or ablated with alcohol or coagulated electrically by the interventional radiologist.

have a sharp margin, can erode the cortex, and occasionally contains "popcorn" shaped calcifications. If symptoms arise, especially in older patients, a malignant transformation into a *chondrosarcoma* must be excluded. If endchondromas arise at multiple locations, an *enchondromatosis*

Enchondroma

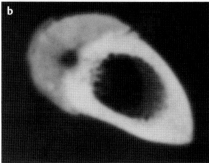

Fig. 8.**5** A number of typical enchondromas are depicted in the proximal and middle phalanx of this finger. They can cause fractures.

(syn.: *Ollier disease*) may be present that may lead to fractures in affected bones during childhood and malignant transformation in adulthood (up to 30%). If soft tissue hemangiomas are also seen, *Mafucci syndrome* is present.

Osteochondroma

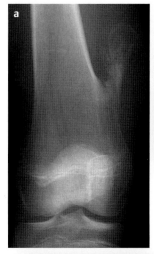
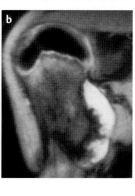

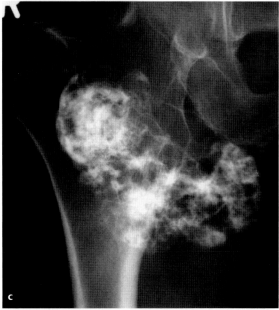

Fig. 8.**6a** This typical cartilaginous exostosis extends medially and takes the bone cortex with it. If these lesions reside in the direct vicinity of a neurovascular bundle, mechanical impairment may develop. They may fracture, as this one has at its base. **b** This is a broad-based osteochondroma of the proximal metaphysis of the humerus in a young patient (the epiphyseal cartilage is still visible). It shows a thick cartilaginous cap. With increasing age, this chondral cap will lose its thickness. This MR sequence is a dedicated T2-weighted chondral sequence on which the cartilage demonstrates a very high signal. **c** Chondromatous tumors may turn into malignant chondrosarcomas such as this one. The popcorn-like structure of the cartilaginous calcifications is quite typical for this entity. These are tumors of the older patient.

Nonossifying Fibroma

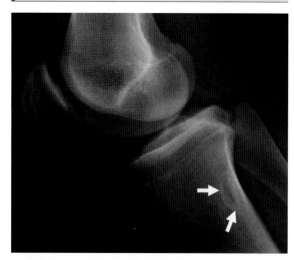

Fig. 8.**7** Have a look at the bubbly bone lesion (arrows) in the dorsal proximal tibia hugging the bone cortex. It has a sclerotic margin. This is a typical nonossifying fibroma that should best be left untouched. It heals on its own come adulthood.

Osteochondroma: An osteochondroma or a osteocartilaginous exostosis (Fig. 8.**6a**) is a frequently stalked protrusion of the metaphyseal bone with a cartilaginous cap (Fig. 8.**6b**) that can calcify and normally decreases in thickness as the skeletal growth comes to an end. The exostoses can cause restrictions of movement as well as injuries to the vessels and nerves. If the thickness of the cap increases again, or if new symptoms arise, a malignant transformation to a *chondrosarcoma* (up to 25 %) must be excluded, especially if multiple osteochondromas are present (Fig. 8.**6c**).

Nonossifying fibroma: This tumor has a bubbly, grapelike appearance with a sclerotic margin and is found immediately adjacent to the inner surface of the metaphyseal cortex of mostly long tubular bones. With increasing skeletal age it moves toward the epiphysis (Fig. 8.**7**). It

is a frequent incidental finding in children and adolescents.

Giant cell tumor: The giant cell tumor occurs in early adulthood (never during childhood) and usually lodges close to the knee joint (approx. 50 %). It is often associated with an eccentric osteolysis that can erode or expand the cortex (Fig. 8.**8a**). Infiltration of the soft tissues is possible and emphasizes the semimalignant character of the tumor. In sectional imaging modalities, fluid–fluid interfaces are occasionally visible inside the tumor (Fig. 8.**8b**).

Paul must, however, also exclude some other diagnoses:

Fibrous dysplasia: In this bone malformation, which can occur as a single lesion or multiple lesions (associated with café-au-lait skin lesions and precocious puberty as part of the McCune–Albright syndrome), the tubular bone is expanded and often bent, and the bony cortex is often eroded but not completely perforated. The inner structure of the bone has a "ground glass" appearance (Fig. 8.**9a**) on CT. In the skull the irregular sclerosis and the expansion of the bone dominate the picture (Fig. 8.**9b, c**), which can lead to an injury of cranial nerves.

Bone cyst:
Simple bone cyst: The simple bone cyst becomes symptomatic when the weakened cortical bone fractures at its site. It is a bubbly lesion located in the metaphysis of cancellous bone close to the epiphysis, often with a sclerotic margin. The lesion is fluid-filled and expands the cortex slightly. If it fractures, hemorrhage into the cyst may occur and a cortical fragment often falls inside the lesion. This is as typical a sign for a bone cyst as there is in radiology and is called the "fallen-fragment sign" (Fig. 8.**10a**).
Aneurysmal bone cyst: This lesion is an osteolytic process and consists of a blood-filled cavity. The aneurysmal bone cyst is located eccentrically in the metaphysis of tubular bones. The cortex may be expanded and perforated. For that reason differentiation from malignant lesions is not always possible. On MRI or CT fluid–fluid interfaces may be seen within the cystic fluid (Fig. 8.**10b**).

Giant Cell Tumor

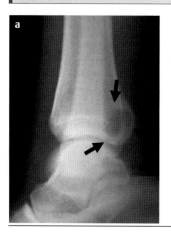

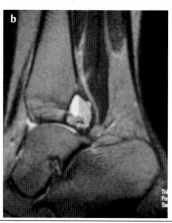

Fig. 8.**8 a** The margins of this bone lesion (arrows) are very irregular and ill defined. The cortex has clearly been destroyed. This is a typical giant cell tumor. **b** On MRI the same lesion shows a fluid–fluid interface. You can also appreciate a focal defect of the cortex.

The Case of Agatha Kristeeze

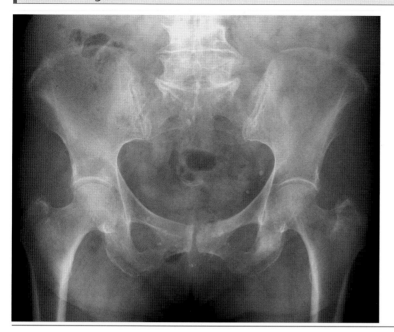

Fig. 8.**17** You are looking at the pelvic radiograph of Agatha Kristeeze. Do you agree with Giufeng?

Metastases

a Osteolytic metastases   **b, c Osteoblastic metastases**

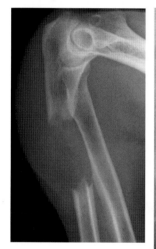

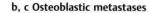

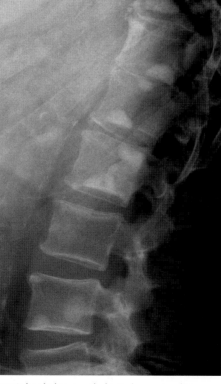

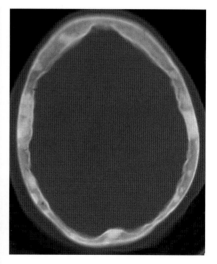

Fig. 8.**18 a** This osteolytic metastasis has led to a pathological fracture of the ulna. The defect is very irregular in its margin and a large soft tissue component seems to be present as well. The patient had a renal carcinoma of which this was a peripheral metastasis. **b** The lumbar vertebrae show multiple very dense regions indicating osteoblastic metastases. This man had a prostate carcinoma. Had the patient been a woman, one would have had to consider primarily underlying breast cancer. **c** The bone windows of the head CT in this same patient show the osteoblastic lesions in the skull.

Multiple Myeloma

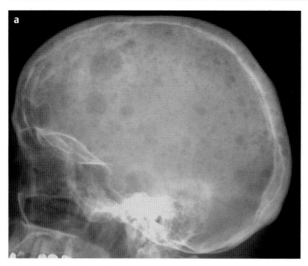 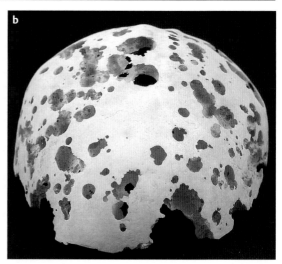

Fig. 8.**19 a, b**   The radiograph of the skull (**a**) shows multiple patchy defects. An extensive infiltration of the cancellous bone with abnormal myeloic cells is likely. This historic specimen (**b**) emphasizes the degree of destruction that may be present in myeloma. (Thanks to the Berlin Museum of Medical History for permission to use this photograph.)

under way to use whole-body MRI to screen for metastases, which may be more sensitive overall. Targeted radiographs then exclude degenerative changes as a cause of the increased bone turnover and may help define the risk of fracture before radiation therapy or a surgical treatment is initiated.

Multiple myeloma: Multiple myeloma is a disease of the elderly. Typically, osteolytic lesions arise in the long tubular bones and the axial skeleton—osteoblastic lesions are rare. An early radiographic sign is erosion of the cortical

Osteopoikilosis

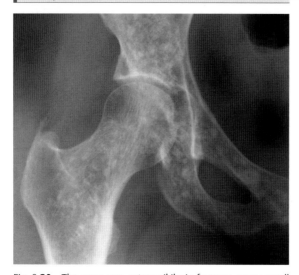

Fig. 8.**20**   The very rare osteopoikilosis features many small bone islands within the cancellous bone.

bone from the within the marrow space (Fig. 8.**19**). If the cortex is permeated by the tumor, a large soft tissue component may develop. In the axial skeleton the bone structure may turn very coarse in diffuse disease. Multiple myeloma is primarily diagnosed on the basis of laboratory parameters. Its extent and the course of the disease as well as the fracture risk are well documented in an elaborate series of radiographs of the axial skeleton and the proximal extremities. MR is more sensitive than radiography in detection of disseminated disease foci; its success is mostly based on the ability to image bone marrow displacement due to the disease and bone marrow edema. Bone scans are not indicated in myeloma because they may fail to demonstrate the sites of involvement in a large number of patients.

Some other, nonneoplastic diseases also have to be considered by Giufeng:

Osteopoikilosis: This is a benign, asymptomatic disease that features multiple small sclerotic bone lesions, mainly in the pelvis (Fig. 8.**20**) and the tubular bones. Bone scans show no abnormality in osteopoikilosis.

Paget disease: Paget disease (syn.: osteitis deformans) is a regional disease of the skeleton in the elderly. Its pathogenesis remains obscure. It is quite frequent in the British Isles, is seen in up to 10% of those above 80 years old in Central Europe and North America, and is almost unknown in China. The altered bone is enlarged; its texture becomes rather coarse and fibrous ("woven bone," Fig. 8.**21**). Cortical thickening is a prominent feature often associated with the sclerotic phase of the disease. Despite the apparent increase of cortical thickness, the overall stability of the bone decreases because the new bone is of

Paget Disease

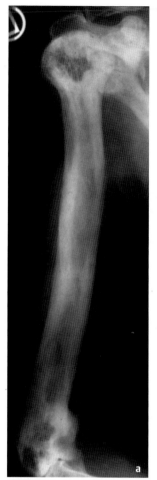

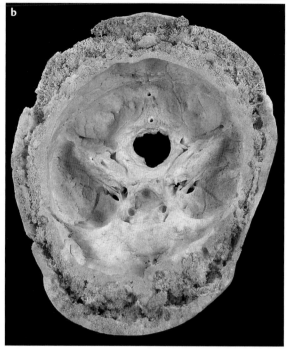

Fig. 8.**21 a, b**   The radiograph of the humerus (**a**) shows an enlargement of the whole bone with thickening of the cortex and an extreme coarseness of the cancellous bone pattern—so-called woven bone. This is a typical case of Paget. The view of a skull base specimen from above (**b**) illustrates the "textile" character of the bone in Paget disease and makes clear why the cranial nerves may eventually be compressed and why patients used to come to their physicians for advice because their hats would no longer fit. (Thanks to the Berlin Museum of Medical History for permission to use this photograph.)

inferior quality. Patients therefore are often afflicted with fractures and bending of the bone. In the early phase of the disease, osteolytic foci occur and the disease may have a rather aggressive plain radiographic appearance. The risk of a malignant transformation into an osteosarcoma is around 5%; this diagnosis should be suspected if patients develop pain in the absence of evidence of a fracture. Bone scans show a very high bone turnover.

Do You Know about Paget?

Sir James Paget was a prominent surgeon and pathologist in London during the late 19th century. He was the personal medical attendant to Her Majesty Queen Victoria. Several disease entities have been named after him, the most frequent being the osteitis deformans. One of his most important mottos is still true today and you as a doctor should probably also follow it at least when you converse with colleagues: "To be brief is to be wise."

Brown tumor (osteoclastoma):   This phenomenon is associated with hyperthyroidism; it is an osteolytic lesion (Fig. 8.**22**) that occasionally expands the bone. It owes its name to the hemosiderin content visible macroscopically when dissected by the pathologist. Laboratory parameters and the other radiological signs of hyperparathyroidism (see p. 36) can help in the differentiation from malignant osteolytic lesions.

→ Diagnosis: Giufeng is quite sure she knows what is going on. Mrs. Kristeeze suffers from osteoblastic metastases. The most probable primary tumor is a breast carcinoma. Now it is important to get a tissue sample of that primary tumor. First of all, the referring physician, who knows the patient best, is contacted and the further steps are agreed upon. Whether and how you inform the patient about a devastating condition depends on a lot of factors. If you decide to talk to your patient about such a diagnosis with far-reaching consequences, time, compassion, and a solid helping of empathy are needed. Giufeng has a look in the waiting area. Mrs. Kristeeze is completely absorbed by the latest book by Patricia Highsmith. Her personal doctor will tell her the diagnosis and guide her through the coming difficult times.

Brown Tumor

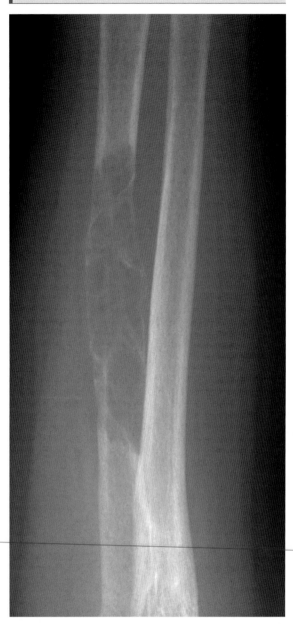

Fig. 8.**22**   An extensive osteolytic focus is seen in the diaphysis of the radius of this patient with hyperparathyroidism.

⚠ The more consequential a diagnosis is for the patient, the more carefully must the breaking of the news to the patient be prepared. It is generally the referring physician who knows the patient best and who should cautiously inform, explain, and support. A mature and responsible patient must, however, also be treated as such by the radiologist.

Generalized Bone Diseases

Checklist: Generalized Bone Diseases

- Is the bone density increased or decreased?
- Are the trabeculae of the cancellous bone unsharp, sharp, or coarsened?
- Is the bone already fractured?
- Are there osseous defects?

Little Old Lady

Hetty Vord's (72) golf handicap has recently deteriorated. She has noticed that her swing has changed: in order not to hit the ground she must grab the club a little lower. The pain in her back has also increased. Her 27-year-old grandson—a psychiatrist in training—has told her that she is shrinking. She told him to mind his own business and to stop growing himself. It is because of her pain that she has now come for a radiograph of the lumbar spine. Paul and Ajay look at the radiograph together (Fig. 8.**23**).

The Case of Hetty Vord

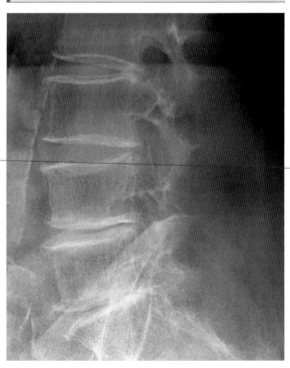

Fig. 8.**23**   Can you call the diagnosis on the basis of these lumbar spine films of Mrs. Vord?

Congenital Bone Diseases

a, b Osteogenesis imperfecta

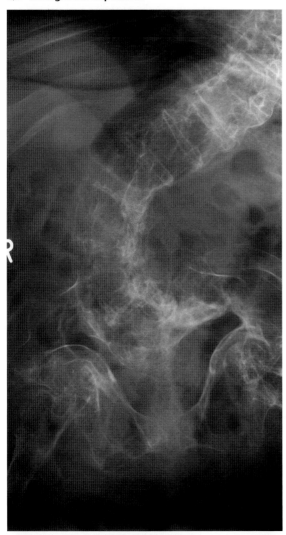

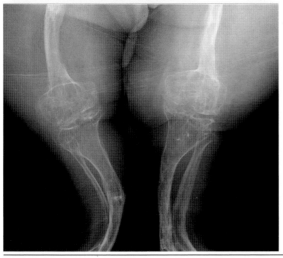

c Osteopetrosis

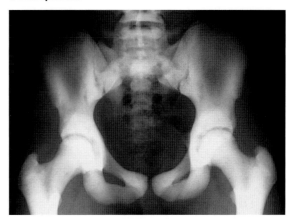

d Camurati–Engelmann-disease

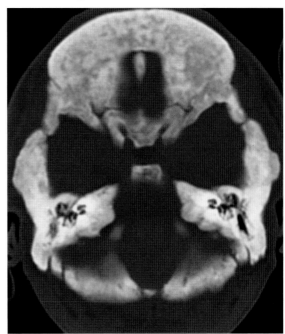

Fig. 8.**30 a, b** Observe the severely decreased bone density and the deformation of the bones in osteogenesis imperfecta. Scoliosis and short stature result. **c** In osteopetrosis the whole bone is increased in density. **d** Camurati–Engelmann disease is characterized by an obliteration of the cancellous bone and an expansion of the bone. This sectional CT of the skull base at the level of the sella shows the stenosis of both optical canals (arrows). The patient was already blind on one side.

Hypertrophic Osteoarthropathy

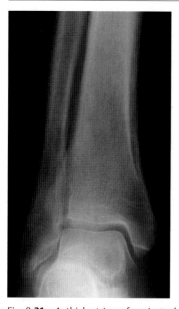

Fig. 8.**31** A thick stripe of periosteal new bone formation is visible along the cortex of the tibia and also the fibula. This is reason enough for a smart radiologist to start a diagnostic work-up for pulmonary disease, which would prove that the initial finding in the tibia was indeed hypertrophic osteoarthropathy. Severe venous insufficiency and burn injury of a limb can also set off this kind of periosteal reaction.

The Case of Hikka Meckinen

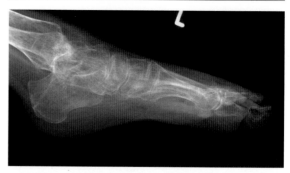

Fig. 8.**32** This radiograph shows the foot of Mr. Meckinen. Which disease entities do you have to consider?

! If we are finished with the image analysis and the clinical information of the referring colleagues is not sufficient, we go ahead and do what no one has dared to do before: We talk to the patient!

Disuse Atrophy

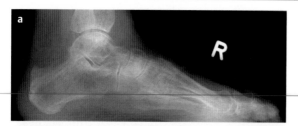

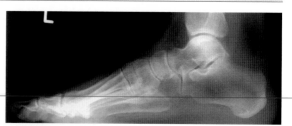

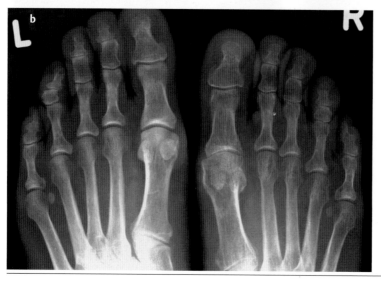

Fig. 8.**33 a** This patient was immobilized for quite a while because of a fracture of the femoral shaft. The inactivity led to an atrophy of the immobilized bone. Radiographically, significantly decreased density and severely coarsened trabecular structure of the bone are seen (left). A view of the contralateral leg shows the normal appearance for comparison (right).
b Compare the osseous structure of the right and left feet. The bone density on the left is markedly decreased and the spongiosal structure is coarsened. There is no soft tissue swelling. This patient was immobilized for a very long time because of a complicated lower leg fracture.

Sudeck Disease

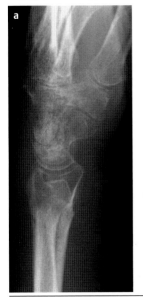
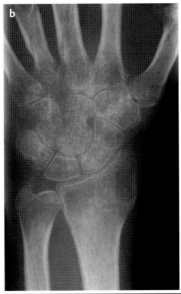

Fig. 8.**34**   This hand is severely demineralized owing to Sudeck disease. The swelling of the hand can be appreciated on the lateral view (**a**). In the anteroposterior radiograph (**b**) there is sharp demarcation of the demineralized bone from the more normal forearm at the level of the radiocarpal joint.

Consequences of an Accident

Hikka Meckinen (35) found himself in the middle of a heap of tires after a pretty exciting and problem-riddled trial with a new race car a few months ago. He suffered a femoral shaft fracture that is all but completely healed now. His left foot, however, continues to worry him. It is swollen, warmer than his right foot, and painful. Joey and Paul analyze the radiograph of the foot (Fig. 8.**32**). They notice the diffuse demineralization of the foot skeleton. The soft tissues are not well enough appreciated on the radiograph.

→ **What is Your Diagnosis?**

Disuse atrophy: Skeletal disuse atrophy, caused by the immobilization of an extremity after trauma or during space flight, is an often patchy periarticular loss of bone mineralization (Fig. 8.**33a**). It begins subchondrally. As the extremity is put to use again, the bone recovers its density. If the atrophy was so severe that the bone matrix was reduced, the ensuing remineralization appears coarser than normal (Fig. 8.**33b**) because the remaining trabeculae of the cancellous bone become thicker and denser.

Sudeck disease: Sudeck disease is caused by a malfunction of the autonomous nervous system after a trauma, or may be idiopathic. The diagnosis is made on the grounds of symptoms and clinical findings such as swelling and hyperthermia of the limb in question. It is verified radiologically by the demineralization of the bone (Fig. 8.**34**).

→ **Diagnosis:** Joey is quite sure of his diagnosis after having talked to the patient and having examined his foot: This is real Sudeck disease.

8.3   Diseases of the Spine

Checklist: Diffuse Back Pain

- Is the general configuration of the spine intact?
- Is the alignment of the vertebral bodies normal?
- Are the intervertebral disk spaces normal?
- Are the vertebrae complete and symmetrical?
- Are there transitional vertebrae?
- Are the sacroiliac joints normal?

It's the Backbone Over and Over Again

For years Will Walton (45) has been suffering from severe back pain that, off and on, has tied him to his bed for days in a row. As a self-employed truck driver, father of three, and builder of a new family home, he is looking for rapid relief. For the last three days now he has not been able to walk owing to the pain. Ajay and Paul review the radiographs of his lumbar spine (Fig. 8.**35**). Are there any visible signs of degeneration?

→ **What is Your Diagnosis?**

Osteochondrosis: Osteochondrosis is the degenerative loss of height of the intervertebral disk, which ends in the destruction of the central disk and the formation of a central "gas" pocket (also called "vacuum phenomenon"). In addition, osseous protuberances—spondylophytes—are formed at the rims of the vertebral end plates; these may become very large and eventually bridge the intervertebral gap (Fig. 8.**36**). Degenerative osteophytes may also develop around the posterior facet joints. The

The Case of Will Walton

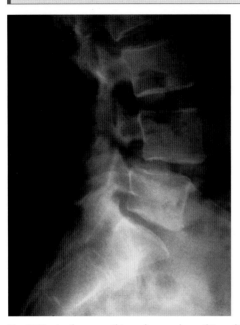

Fig. 8.**35**   Is there anything abnormal on this radiograph of Will Walton's lumbar spine?

combination of spondylophytes, osteophytes, and the loss of disk height may narrow the neuroforamina and eventually cause nerve compression syndromes.

Vacuum in the Body?

The vacuum phenomenon is quite reliable when degenerative changes of the disk space need to be differentiated from infectious ones. But is it really a vacuum? Some researchers have sampled diskal "vacuums" with needles and reported a high content of nitrogen. See Figure 8.**36b** and **c** for proof that some sort of biomechanical phenomenon is at work: In **b** the spine is flexed forward—no pocket is seen. As the spine is flexed backward in **c**, the pocket appears out of nowhere.

Intervertebral joint osteoarthritis: Intervertebral or facet joint osteoarthritis can cause a narrowing of the spinal canal and the neuroforamina. As the integrity of the joints decreases, intervertebral misalignment may ensue that further encroaches on the spinal canal and the foramina—the so called pseudospondylolisthesis or degenerative spondylolisthesis (Fig. 8.**37**).

Osteochondrosis

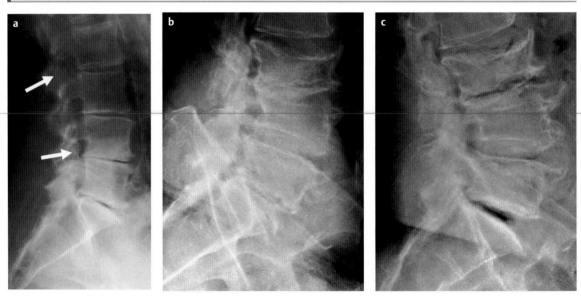

Fig. 8.**36 a–c**   The lower lumbar spine (**a**) is affected by extensive degenerative disk disease and associated typical osseous changes. The uppermost visible intervertebral disk has normal height—all others are reduced in height. The disks are all but destroyed. Dark stripes are seen within the residual disk. This "vacuum phenomenon" is a sure indication of a degenerative process. The vertebral end plates are sclerotic. Their margins show osseous protuberances—spondylophytes. The deterioration of the disk decreases the strength of the spinal architecture, leading to malalignments such as seen at the L5/S1 level on this radiograph. Note how the loss of disk height also diminishes the size of the neuroforamina (arrows). The foramen has a normal diameter at the L2/L3 level but at the L5/S1 level it is much smaller. A nerve root must squeeze through there! Functional radiographs of the lumbar spine bent forward (**b**) and backward (**c**) performed within seconds of each other prove that the phenomenon is indeed due to vacuum: the stripes develop out of nothing in (**c**).

True Spondylolisthesis (Spondylolysis)

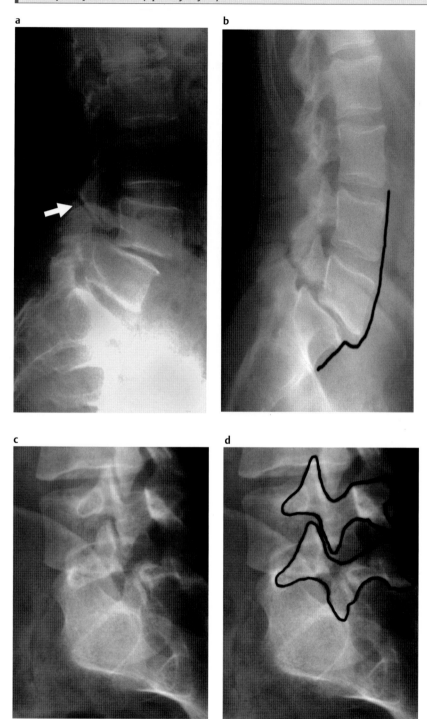

Fig. 8.**43 a**   This radiograph shows the slippage of L4 relative to L5 to good advantage. The listhesis is classified as a Meyerding grade I–II. The defect in the pars interarticularis is also well seen in this patient (arrow). **b** That is not always the case. Draw one line along the anterior margin of the vertebral bodies and another along the posterior edge of the spinous processes (compare degenerative spondylolisthesis, Fig. 8.**37b**). The lines prove that the malalignment is one vertebral level higher posteriorly compared to ventrally—the spinous process and its vertebral body are disconnected. **c** On the oblique view, the silhouette of two "Scottie dogs" is visible. **d** In this case the upper dog runs around unrestrained while the lower dog wears a "leash"—the radiographic lucency that corresponds to the defect in the pars interarticularis of the affected vertebral body.

Ankylosing Spondylitis

a Sacroiliitis

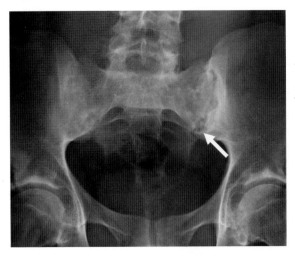

b "Bamboo spine"

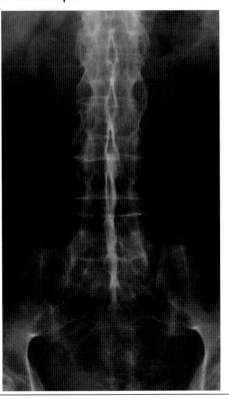

Fig. 8.**44 a**   The right iliosacral joint is already fused in its lower part. The left iliosacral joint shows pronounced periarticular sclerosis along erosions of the bone (arrow). This is a rather typical pattern of ankylosing spondylitis. **b** In the final phase and with maximal expression of Bechterew disease (as ankylosing spondylitis is also called), the paraspinous ligaments become ossified, giving rise to the so-called "bamboo spine." The intervertebral spaces are completely bridged by ossified tissue, which reduces the flexibility of the spine to nil. Any deceleration trauma may have dire consequences in this setting.

Did You Know That . . .?

Wladimir von Bechterew was a neurologist and psychiatrist in St. Petersburg around 1900. His psychiatric ideas and models were highly speculative, but his neuroanatomical scientific work is relevant to this day. He was one of the first to comprehensively describe ankylosing spondylitis. One of his colleagues and major rivals in St. Petersburg was Ivan Pavlov, whose experiments we all know. In 1927 the leader of the Soviet Union, a certain Comrade Stalin, sought his medical advice. The 70-year-old Bechterew diagnosed a grave paranoia and did not hesitate to tell the dictator. Bechterew survived the diagnosis by a whole day.

→ Diagnosis: After analyzing the malalignment of Mr. Walton's lumbar spine, both Paul and Ajay come to the same conclusion: there is an osseous defect in the pars interarticularis of L4. This is a true spondylolysis with associated spondylolisthesis and is the most likely explanation for the patient's complaints.

Could an additional disk herniation have aggravated the situation? Of course. If there are nerve root symptoms and surgery is considered as an option, an additional MRI is indicated and could verify the disk herniation.

The radiograph of the lumbar spine can allow diagnosis of osteochondrosis, malalignment, instability, spondylolysis and ankylosing spondylitis. It should always be the first imaging modality to be used in back pain.

8.4   Diseases of the Joints

Checklist: Articular Pain

- Are the symptoms monoarticular or polyarticular?
- Are the joints in question weight-bearing and prone to degeneration?
- Is the configuration of the joint normal?
- Is the joint space narrowed? If so, only in the weight-bearing zone (eccentrically) or everywhere (concentrically)?
- Is the periarticular and subchondral bone increased or decreased in density?
- Are there any periarticular cysts?
- Is the soft tissue of normal appearance?
- Are there clinical signs of inflammation?

Joints of the Upper Extremity

When the Shoulder Goes on Strike

André Aklassi (32) has been troubled lately by shoulder pain that slowly ruins his serve. He needs a diagnosis and therapy rapidly because the season is in full thrust and the Australian Open is approaching. His wife accompanies him. Hannah is rather excited, while Joey, a baseball fanatic, could not care less. A standard radiograph of the shoulder has already been performed elsewhere and apparently showed no abnormal finding. The students go ahead and analyze the MR image of the shoulder (Fig. 8.**45**).

→ What is Your Diagnosis?

Degeneration of the shoulder joint: The rotator cuff is a group of fused flat tendons that arcs over the humeral head and inserts into the greater tuberosity of the humerus. It thus forms the roof of the shoulder joint. Forward elevation of the arm and overhead motion pinches the cuff and the subacromial bursa against the overlying acromion and the acromioclavicular (AC) joint. This can lead to a chronic injury—also called impingement—which is most pronounced when there is coexisting *osteoarthritis of*

The Case of André Aklassi

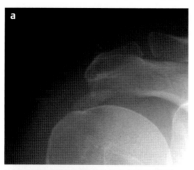

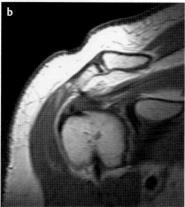

Fig. 8.**45** The radiograph (**a**) and the diagnostic MR image (**b**) of Mr. Aklassi's shoulder joint. Can you call the diagnosis already?

the AC joint (Fig. 8.**46c**), which can form subacromial spurs. Extensive calcification of the bursa (Fig. 8.**46a**) or even a rupture of the rotator cuff (Fig. 8.**46b**) may ensue. Eventually a full-blown *osteoarthritis of the shoulder joint* (Fig. 8.**46d**) develops with the typical signs of degeneration such as eccentric loss of joint space, periarticular osteophytes, and subarticular sclerosis of the articulating bones.

Shoulder dislocation: A shoulder dislocation is often accompanied by ligamentous or osseous injuries. Not only can the cartilaginous glenoid labrum be torn but small focal compression fractures of the humeral head (Hill–Sachs defect, Fig. 8.**47**) and avulsions of the inferior osseous glenoid labrum (Bankart lesion) are also possible and may need to be treated.

→ Diagnosis:
Hannah diagnoses a rupture of the rotator cuff. Joey has found calcifications in the subacromial bursa. Mr. Aklassi discusses the findings with his wife and they decide to seek the service of a good shoulder surgeon.

Dolor, Tumor, Rubor

Barbara Noosh's (78) hands have been hurting for quite a while, especially in the morning. She has had to quit knitting. Calling her son on her old red rotary dial phone has also been a pain. The finger joints are swollen. Paul has a short conversation with her and then turns his attention to the radiographs (Fig. 8.**48**).

→ What is Your Diagnosis?

Rheumatoid arthritis (RA): This entity is a rheumatic disease that is seropositive for the rheumatoid factor antibody in 70–80% of cases and runs a chronic relapsing clinical course. Regions most often affected are the radiocarpal joints, the styloid process of the ulna as well as the metacarpophalangeal and proximal interphalangeal joints (Fig. 8.**49**). In the first place the bone is demineralized close to the joint and there is periarticular soft tissue swelling. In a later phase there is a generalized loss of joint space in the absence of new bone formation (as you would see in osteoarthritis). Erosions of the bone develop in the articular periphery where cortical bone is not protected by overlying cartilage and is therefore exposed to the synovial inflammatory response. Eventually typical subluxations with ulnar deviation in the finger joints occur. Severe joint mutilations and fusions indicate end-stage disease.

Psoriatic arthritis: Seronegative psoriatic arthritis is a complication of psoriasis. It prefers the distal interphalangeal joints, but the iliosacral joints and the spine can also be involved. The skin manifestations, thick, pitted fingernails, and the impressive swelling of single fingers, which is also visible on radiographs ("sausage digit," Fig. 8.**50**), are pathognomonic.

Consequences of Degenerative Diseases of the Shoulder Joints

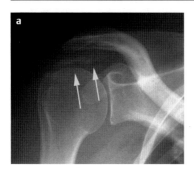

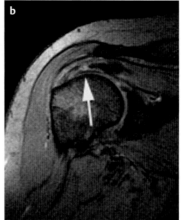

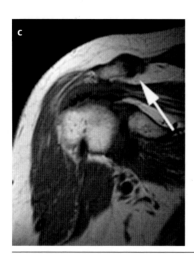

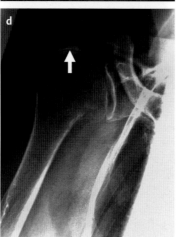

Fig. 8.**46 a** Calcifications in the subacromial bursa (arrows) indicate problems of the rotator cuff, which in turn can be due to osteoarthritis of the acromioclavicular joint, often when associated with a subacromial spur. **b** The rotator cuff, an arc of tendons of shoulder muscles, is low in water content and shows consistently low in signal in MRI for that very reason. On this image of a T2-weighted sequence, a fluid-filled defect (arrow) is visible in the cuff. This is a rupture of the rotator cuff. **c** The osteoarthritis of the acromioclavicular joint shown here (arrows) causes impingement that over time may contribute to rupture of the rotator cuff. **d** The advanced degenerative disease of the shoulder joint in this patient has completely used up the subacromial space (arrow)—bone rubs on bone. The osteophytes along the lower contour of the humeral head confirm the diagnosis.

Shoulder Dislocation

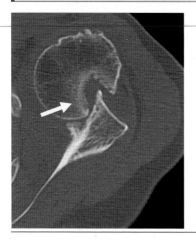

Fig. 8.**47** This CT section through the shoulder joint shows an anterior shoulder dislocation after trauma. During dislocation, the humerus banged against the anterior bony glenoid labrum, which caused an impression fracture of the humeral head—the so-called Hill–Sachs defect (arrow). The homogeneous bone sclerosis along the base of the groove and the osseous support rim at the neck of the scapula indicate that this dislocation has been present or has recurred regularly for quite some time.

The Case of Barbara Noosh

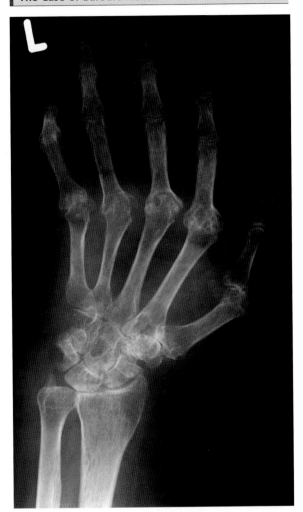

Fig. 8.**48** This radiograph of Mrs. Noosh's hand shows changes characteristic of a specific disease. Can you tell which one?

Rheumatoid Arthritis

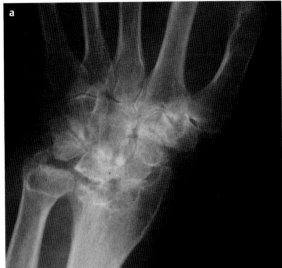

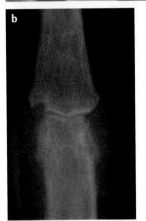

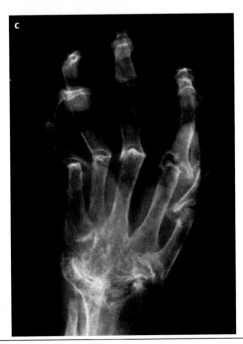

Fig. 8.**49 a–c**   Rheumatoid arthritis tends to start around the radiocarpal joint. Observe the loss of the joint space and the lytic defects in (**a**). Lytic defects also develop in the periphery of the finger joints (**b**). Advanced rheumatoid arthritis (**c**) is characterized by the almost complete joint destruction and ulnar deviation of the fingers. There are erosions of the periarticular cortex.

Psoriatic Arthritis

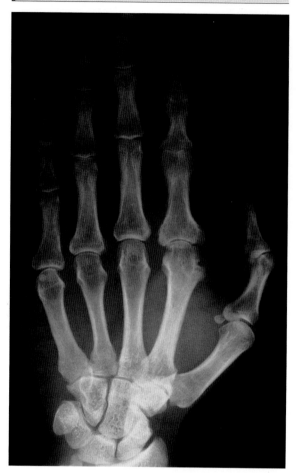

Fig. 8.**50**   The "sausage finger" (second digit) is a characteristic finding in psoriatic arthritis. The phalanges are plump, the joint spaces are diminished.

Heberden Type and Bouchard Type Osteoarthritis

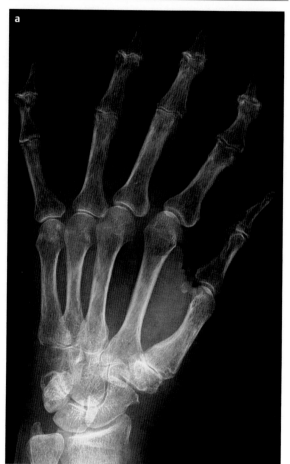

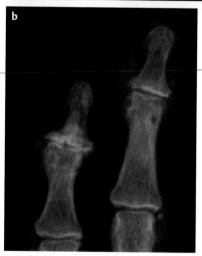

Osteoarthritis of the hand and finger joints: This condition preferentially affects the distal (*Heberden type*) and proximal interphalangeal joints (*Bouchard type*), the metacarpophalangeal joints, and the trapeziometacarpal joint of the thumb. In the example radiograph provided, the bases of the distal and middle phalanges show lateral and dorsal osteophytes, which give the joint something of a "bird in the sky" or "seagull wing" configuration (Fig. 8.**51**). Joint space loss is also seen.

→ **Diagnosis:** Paul has no doubt that Mrs. Noosh suffers from a textbook case of rheumatoid arthritis and he is right, of course.

Fig. 8.**51 a, b**   Changes in degenerative osteoarthritis dominate in the distal carpal joints and the distal finger joints (Heberden) (**a**). The degenerative changes are less pronounced at the level of the proximal interphalangeal joints (Bouchard). In addition there is degenerative change in the carpometacarpal joint of the thumb. The finger joint space (**b**) has the typical "bird in the sky" or "gullwing" configuration. Joint space loss is also seen. There is periarticular bone sclerosis and soft tissue swelling, resulting in the typical Heberden nodes.

Legg–Calvé–Perthes Disease

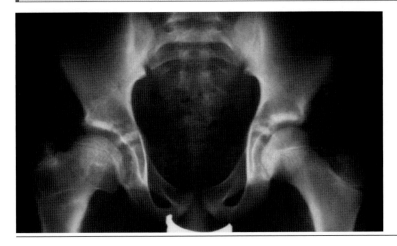

Fig. 8.**61** This is an image of the deformed femoral head of a child with Legg–Calvé–Perthes disease on the right. A corrective osteotomy has already been performed (do you see the traces of an osteosynthetic stabilization in the femoral metaphysis?) to halt or slow down the degenerative process.

much more effective in proving and excluding Legg–Calvé–Perthes disease, showing a signal loss along the femoral head margin. The entity frequently heals with a deformed femoral head (Fig. 8.61), which in turn causes osteoarthritis of the hip joint in the middle-aged adult.

A Truly International Group

Legg–Calvé–Perthes disease is a good example of an international scientific competition in the early 20th century—and how nicely it was solved. Arthur Thornton Legg was a pediatric orthopedic surgeon in Boston; Jaques Calvé worked as an orthopedic surgeon on the northern coast of France; and Georg Clemens Perthes was surgeon and radiologist in Leipzig and Tübingen. When naming this disease, do not forget to check your listeners' nationality, then put their countryman first.

Epiphysiolysis: Epiphysiolysis or slipped capital femoral epiphysis is the posterior and inferior subluxation of the femoral epiphysis due to an injury of the epiphyseal cartilage (Fig. 8.62). It tends to occur in late childhood, between ages 10 and 14, and is bilateral in 20% of cases. Pain in the groin, potentially extending into the knee joint, is typical. A short-term complication of epiphysiolysis is femoral head necrosis; a long-term complication is the deformation of the femoral head and subsequent osteoarthritis of the hip in early adulthood.

Hip dysplasia: Hip dysplasia is a congenital deformity of the acetabular bone and the femoral head. Less than two-thirds of the femoral head is covered by the acetabulum and the acetabular angle is too steep (Fig. 8.**63**). For that reason the femoral head has a tendency to recurrent dislocation. The diagnosis should be made in the first week of life, clinically or by ultrasound. If doubts remain, radiographs of the pelvis can prove the diagnosis. Therapy carries its own risks because it increases the risk of avascular necrosis of the femoral head and subsequent early-onset secondary osteoarthritis of the hip joint.

Epiphysiolysis

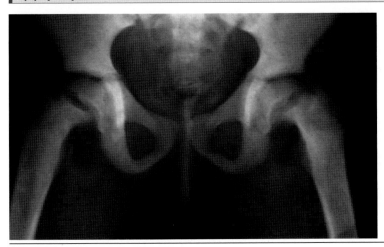

Fig. 8.**62** The medial slippage of the femoral epiphysis is obvious on both sides. In the early phase the surgeons try to halt the movement by inserting metal pins that traverse the epiphyseal cartilage.

Hip Dysplasia

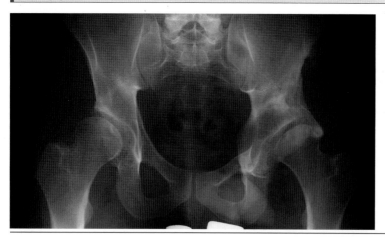

Fig. 8.**63** On the right a full-blown hip dysplasia is present. The acetabular angle is too steep, the femoral head is only partially covered. On the left a correction osteotomy of the acetabular bone has been performed. Now the head is covered to a greater extent but it is also flattened. Premature degeneration of this joint is very probable.

→ **Diagnosis:** The two students are quite sure that l'il Rumsfeld has a case of Legg–Calvé–Perthes disease on the right. If any doubt remained, MRI would bring certainty. But what on earth is the reason for Mrs. Hatburn's problem? None of the described infantile precursor diseases seems to have been present. Giufeng and Hannah are still staring at Mrs. Hatburn's radiograph and scratching their heads as Gregory turns the corner: "Hey, got any problems, the two of you?" he grins and plunges into a chair beside Giufeng. "Well, we have just been waiting for you, Greg Darling!" snorts Giufeng. "This doesn't look like a normal osteoarthritis to you, does it?" Gregory straightens up, collimates the radiograph on the viewbox with painstaking care, and contemplates the findings for a while. "Oh, Giu, you've learned so much from me in such a short time," he hums and leans back again. "You're quite right. This is indeed not a normal osteo of the hip. The joint is degenerated before its time because the bone is structurally weakened. Compare it to the other side and you see the typical textile or woven bone pattern of Paget disease on the abnormal side. Nice case, girls!" Giufeng does not know whether she should be thankful or close her eyes in disgust. Hannah makes an obscene gesture behind Greg's back. Let us leave the scene before Gregory gets into any more trouble. Had you thought of that diagnosis already?

The Case of George Tush

a

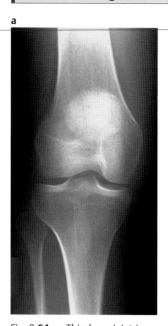
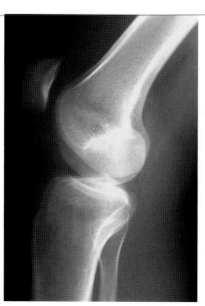

b

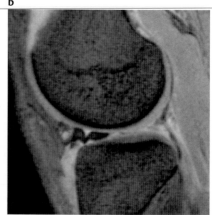

Fig. 8.**64 a**   This knee joint is completely normal radiologically. An effusion is not seen. **b** The finding is obvious on MRI, isn't it?

Osteoarthritis of the Knee

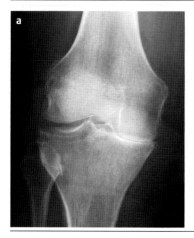

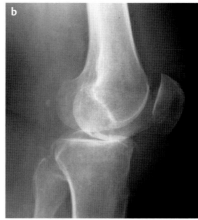

Fig. 8.**65 a** Loss of joint space width in the medial tibiofemoral joint compartment associated with osteophytes along the edge of the tibial plateau is pathognomonic for osteoarthritis (OA) due to a varus alignment of the lower extremity. The meniscal cartilage and hyaline cartilage covering the articulating bones is destroyed in the respective main weight-bearing zone. **b** A little osseous protuberance at the upper margin of the patella indicates patellofemoral osteoarthritis, which is often associated with OA of the tibiofemoral joint.

! Remember the "satisfaction of search" phenomenon: If you have your first diagnosis don't stop right there. Keep it in mind and then take another turn and look for other findings in the imaging study.

One Turn Too Many

While running the Sydney Marathon yesterday, George Tush (45) strained his knee on the Harbor Bridge, tripping over one of its security guards. Now it is swollen and painful and he is very worried. Paul looks at the radiograph of the knee in two projections first (Fig. 8.**64a**). It looks rather normal to him. The MRI examination of the knee shows the whole extent of the injury (Fig. 8.**64**b).

→ What is Your Diagnosis?

Osteoarthritis of the knee: Most of the time, advanced degenerative change of the knee joints can be diagnosed with standard radiographs (Fig. 8.**65**). Further imaging is usually not necessary.

Cruciate and collateral ligament sprain or tear: A full-thickness tear of *the anterior cruciate ligament* is best appreciated on T1-weighted MR images angled along the long axis of the ligament (Fig. 8.**66b**). The intact tendinous fibers seen in the normal knee (Fig. 8.**66a**) are no longer discernible. A *lesion of the posterior cruciate ligament* is well seen on straightforward sagittal images of the knee (Fig. 8.**66c**). The *collateral ligaments* are evaluated by looking at the coronal T1-weighted images.

Cruciate Ligament Injuries

a Normal anterior cruciate

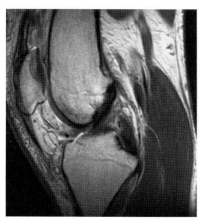

b Rupture of the anterior cruciate

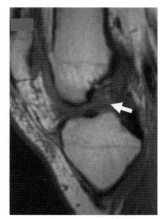

c Rupture of the posterior cruciate

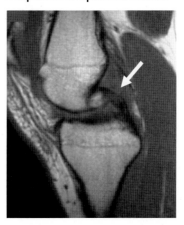

Fig. 8.**66 a** Observe this healthy knee joint with an intact anterior cruciate ligament. **b** The T1-weighted MR section along the axis of the anterior cruciate ligament should display the low-signal fibers of the ligament running from superior–posterior to inferior–anterior. Instead we see only a homogeneous gray mass because the anterior cruciate ligament is completely torn and edematous (arrow). **c** This T1-weighted sagittal MR section shows a defect in the course of the posterior cruciate ligament. This is also a full–thickness tear (arrow).

Meniscal Tear

a
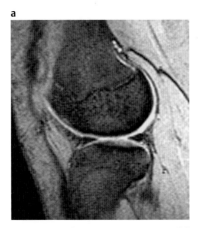

b
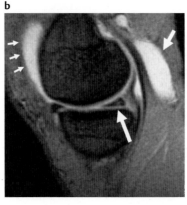

c
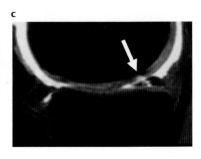

Fig. 8.**67 a**   These menisci are normal. **b** The posterior horn of the medial meniscus is torn. The tear reaches the undersurface of the meniscus (long arrow). There is an effusion in the suprapatellar bursa (small arrows), most likely hemorrhagic in nature. Arising from the posterior joint space, a synovial outpouching can develop filled with joint fluid—the rather frequent Baker cyst (short arrow), which is characteristically located between the tendons of the medial head of the gastrocnemius and the semimembranosus muscle. **c** Here you see a complete tear of the posterior horn of the meniscus. It is accompanied by a defect of the hyaline cartilage covering the femoral condyle (arrow).

Meniscal tear: This injury is best observed on T2-weighted coronal and sagittal images (Fig. 8.67). The cartilage is best visualized with dedicated cartilage sequences.

Baker cyst: The Baker cyst (Fig. 8.**67b**) is located posteromedially in the popliteal fossa, between the tendons of the medial head of the gastrocnemius and the semimembranosus muscle. It communicates with the joint via a slitlike connection and may cause compression syndromes or rupture. It is best detected on T2-weighted sequences. It may resolve on its own or is treated surgically.

→ **Diagnosis:** Paul diagnoses a tear in the posterior horn of the medial meniscus in Tush's knee. The posterior meniscus is dislodged ventrally and compresses the ventral meniscus—"kissing menisci" is the nice term for the phenomenon. This is an indication for surgery.

Occupational Disease?

Doris Goldberg (19) is an energetic young lady who has done a lot of footwork during her career: she is a ballet dancer. Now she has had pain in her ankle for a little while. The standard radiographs of her ankle show a region of increased density in her medial talus that needs further analysis. MRI of the ankle has been performed (Fig. 8.**68**). Giufeng and Joey analyze the image with care.

The Case of Doris Goldberg

a
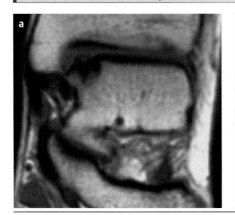

b
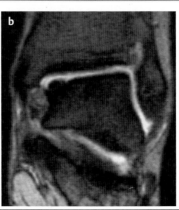

Fig. 8.**68**   Representative T1-weighted (**a**) and T2-weighted (**b**) MR sections of Mrs. Goldberg's upper ankle joint show an abnormality. Which entities do you have to consider?

von Recklinghausen Neurofibromatosis (NF1)

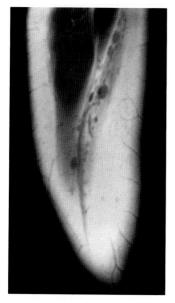

Fig. 8.**78** Multiple neurofibromas are located along the course of the neurovascular bundle.

margins, invades the neighborhood, and also contains fat (Fig. 8.**79**), a liposarcoma is probable and has to be ruled out through biopsy or excision. Lack of fat, however, does not exclude a liposarcoma.

Fibrosarcoma, malignant fibrous histiocytoma: Tumors with a high proportion of fibrous tissue such as fibrosarcoma (Fig. 8.**80**) or malignant fibrous histiocytoma (MFH) may show a relatively low signal on both T1-weighted and T2-weighted MR images. The reason is the paucity of protons in this tissue, which are needed for imaging in conventional magnetic resonance tomography. A low signal both in T1-weighted and T2-weighted

Liposarcoma

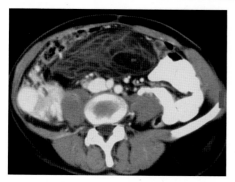

Fig. 8.**79** This CT image through the upper pelvis shows a large fatty tumor within the mesentery that is septated by fibrous strands of differing caliber. Histology confirmed the radiological suspicion of a liposarcoma.

Fibrosarcoma

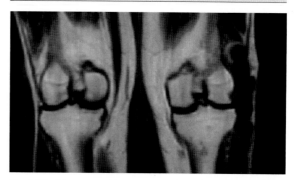

Fig. 8.**80** The coronal MR sections through both knee joints document a large signal-free structure along the left joint. This signal type is typical for fibrous, water-deprived tissue. Size, configuration, and signal suggest a malignant fibrous tumor here—a fibrosarcoma.

images can, however, also be caused by fast blood flow or calcifications in a tumor.

Myositis ossificans: The main characteristic of a myositis ossificans is the overshooting ossification of the soft tissues—frequently after a soft tissue trauma and resulting intramuscular hematoma. It is particularly pronounced if the patient has been in coma. The diagnosis is usually made from the plain radiograph (Fig. 8.**81**).

Myositis Ossificans (Heterotopic Bone Formation)

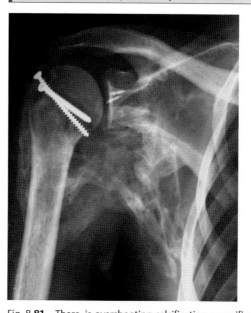

Fig. 8.**81** There is overshooting calcification or ossification of the soft tissues after a severe shoulder injury, often transforming a hematoma—myositis ossificans. The range of motion in this joint is naturally very limited. The patient also suffered a heavy brain injury and stayed in coma for three weeks. Comatose patients tend to develop particularly large areas of heterotopic bone formation.

Synovial Hemangioma

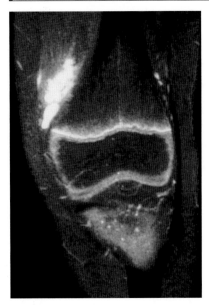

Fig. 8.82 This coronal MR section with fat saturation and after intravenous contrast administration displays a significantly enhancing structure lateral to the femoral metaphysis. Location and structure are typical for a synovial hemangioma.

Finally Joey considers lesions in typical locations:

Synovial hemangioma: This is a vascular lesion in the direct vicinity of the knee joint (Fig. 8.**82**).

Plantar/palmar fibromatosis: The plantar or palmar fibromatosis (better remembered as Ledderhose disease and Dupuytren disease, respectively) are nodular lesions of the fascia of foot and hand.

→ **Diagnosis:** Joey could not really get much more information out of the images. But he has got good news for Mr. Schwortenbakker. His tumor is definitely a lipoma, which can easily be resected by his plastic surgeon. Had the lesion fulfilled the above criteria of malignancy, Joey could have determined the most likely histological diagnosis by taking into account the age of the patient and the localization of the tumor. It would have earned him the special respect of the clinical colleagues.

8.7   Gregory's Test

Giufeng, Hannah, Paul, Ajay, and Joey sit in the skeletal imaging unit at the end of the day and are having a good time. As they dig into their quiche to order, Gregory opens the door. His face lights up as he notices the little crowd: "Apparently I came right on time," he roars and grabs the last piece of the quiche. "OK, who's ready for dessert? Come on, Joey, let's hear it!" He munches and whips a few films onto the lightbox (Fig. 8.**83**). Who can help Joey? Jot down your diagnoses. You'll find the answers at the end of the book (see p. 342).

Test Cases

Fig. 8.**83 a–l**

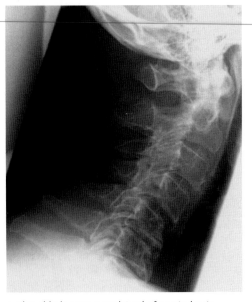

a This elderly man complained of cervical pain.

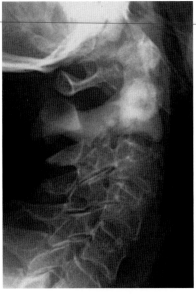

b This patient had the same problem.

Test Cases

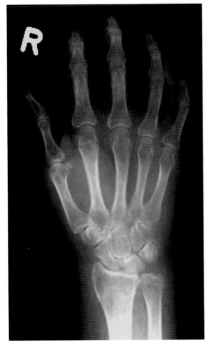

c This hand of a young woman was warm, swollen, and painful.

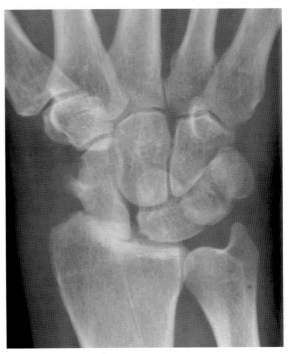

d This joint was painful.

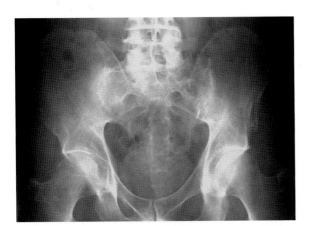

e This patient felt a little stiff and had unspecific back pain.

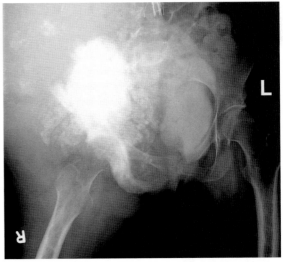

f A large swelling and pain in the right lower abdomen and pelvis was the problem here. Tell us the histology!

Test Cases

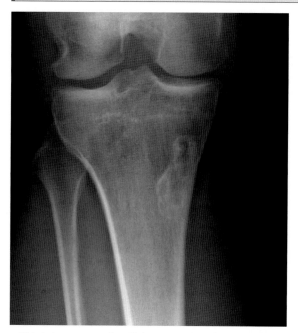

g This lad came straight off the soccer field.

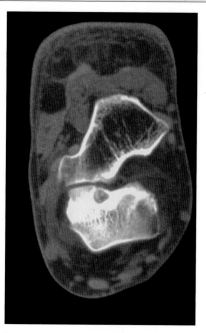

h The foot has been painful, especially at night.

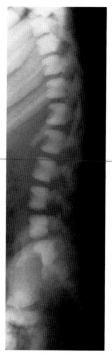

i This kid has a problem.

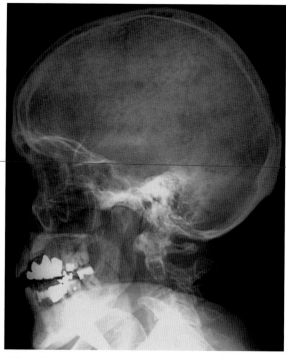

j This elderly patient has been sent by the internists.

Abdominal Film

c Chilaiditi syndrome

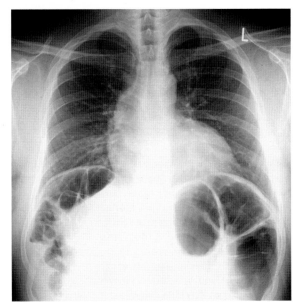

d Chronic pancreatitis

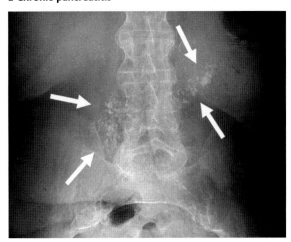

e "Sentinel loops"

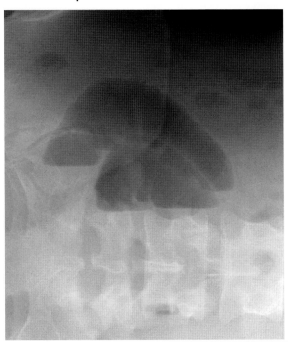

Fig. 9.**2a** This is a normal abdominal film. The liver shadow occupies the right upper abdomen. Its inferior margin can only be guessed on this film. The peritoneal fat stripe along the right lateral abdominal wall is visible, however. The spleen in the left upper abdomen is completely disguised by the splenic flexure of the colon. Almost the whole colon is filled with air. Stool is seen in the cecum, the descending colon, and the sigmoid colon. The small bowel is not visible at all. The gastric bubble is barely appreciated medial to the splenic flexure. In this slim patient the retroperitoneal fat is not abundant enough to clearly outline the contours of the kidneys and the iliopsoas muscle. **b** The lower margin of the liver, the contour of the kidney, and the border of the iliopsoas muscle are beautifully depicted in this patient. **c** In this patient, air-filled large-bowel loops are projecting over the liver. This entity is called Chilaiditi syndrome and tends to be an incidental finding without symptoms. **d** In chronic pancreatitis typical calcifications occur in the parenchyma (arrows) and have to be differentiated from atherosclerosis of the splenic artery **e** This cut-out of an abdominal radiograph of a patient positioned on the left side and taken with a horizontal beam shows air-filled small-bowel loops with air–fluid interfaces—so-called "sentinel loops." They indicate disturbances of the intestinal peristalsis. The difference in fluid level in the larger loop hints at peristalsis working to overcome an obstacle: this is a sign of a mechanical (dynamic) bowel obstruction or early obstructive ileus. The colon is devoid of air: the obstruction must be somewhere in the distal small bowel.

The structures of the retroperitoneum are easily distinguished as long as they have interfaces with the retroperitoneal fat: the contours of the **kidneys** and the **iliopsoas muscle** are regularly appreciated; the **pancreas** tends to be discernible only if its parenchyma contains punctate calcifications, for instance due to chronic pancreatitis (Fig. 9.**2d**).

The **urinary bladder** can be delimited in the lower pelvis if it is filled well. When fully expanded it tends to lift the intestines out of the pelvis.

Calcifications are frequently found in the following locations:

- Vascular walls: Particularly frequent in the aorta, the celiac artery and its branches, in particular the splenic artery and in the iliac arteries. Oval calcifications in the pelvis are often due to phleboliths in pelvic veins, particularly common in the veins next to the uterus and in the venous plexus around the bladder.
- Parenchymal organs: Kidneys (kidney stones), uterus (fibroids), liver and spleen (after granulomatous infec-

tions such as histoplasmosis), pancreas (chronic pancreatitis).

- Hollow organs: Particularly frequent in the gallbladder lumen (gallstones) or wall (porcelain gallbladder).
- Lymph nodes: Particularly frequent in the mesentery.

The **distribution of the intestinal air** and the thickness of the intestinal walls is of special importance. Air in the small bowel is rare in the healthy adult. It is an obligatory (regular) finding in neonates and frequent in small children. The stomach and the colon routinely contain varying amounts of air. The differences in caliber and wall structure (valvulae conniventes—or Kerckring folds—in the small bowel and haustral folds in the large bowel) make it easy to differentiate small and large bowel in most cases. Any air outside the intestinal lumen is abnormal and should prompt careful correlation with the patient's history: if surgery has recently been performed, free air may be related to the procedure. Careful comparison with prior radiographs is warranted if these are available, to ensure that this finding is not new or increasing

The **thickness of the bowel wall** is evaluated by observing the distance between two neighboring loops. In inflammatory and ischemic processes of the bowel, the thickness of the wall increases. If intramural gas (mostly in the form of small bubbles like a "string of pearls" or as streaks in the bowel wall, particularly in dependent parts of the bowel wall) is found, further diagnostic measures need to be taken. Although there is a benign condition termed "pneumatosis intestinalis," characterized by air in the bowel wall, this finding may also be associated with life-threatening conditions such as intestinal infarction or severe inflammation of the intestinum that need to be excluded.

The **amount and distribution of stool** throughout the colon should also be noted. Patients with severe constipation may present with acute abdominal pain.

Why Are You Interested in the Standard Chest Radiograph in a Patient with Abdominal Pain?

The areas under the diaphragm are of particular interest when confronted with abdominal symptoms: Air seen underneath the right hemidiaphragm (above and surrounding the liver) is intraperitoneal by definition. Free air in the peritoneum, of course, also reaches the underside of the left hemidiaphragm, but there the air in the stomach and in the splenic flexure of the colon may obscure it and can often not be distinguished from true free air, which leaves too much room for mistakes. For that reason, in patients unable to stand, the abdominal radiograph is performed with the patient turned all the way up on their left side: potential free air then rises to the right into the nondependent space between the diaphragm and the liver. Patients should remain in that position for at least 5 minutes before the radiograph is taken because it takes time for the air to rise into the right upper quadrant of the abdomen.

I See an Abnormality—What Do I Do Now?

First reflect on whether the perceived abnormality may be clinically relevant in that particular patient; put the observation into context with history and findings on clinical examination.

Most **calcifications** in the abdomen are of no clinical significance for the health of the patient. Exceptions are the calcifications seen in the expected location of the pancreas (chronic pancreatitis) and the ureter (renal colic). The combination of clinical findings and history in a given patient will often guide the diagnostic process toward the dominant clinical problem.

Free intraperitoneal air is very relevant finding and indicates the perforation of a hollow viscus. (Just a few milliliters of air is detectable!) But be aware: It may also be seen in patients who have undergone recent abdominal surgery, a common situation in a hospital setting. As mentioned above, careful comparison with prior postoperative radiographs is warranted, if these are available, to ensure that this finding is not new or increasing. In case of doubt, a phonecall to the clinician taking care of the patient is good practice and will often clarify the significance of the finding as well as help determine the need for further imaging or even surgical intervention. So do not ring the grand alarm bell right away.

Air in the retroperitoneum is always pathological. The contours of the kidneys, the pararenals, and the iliopsoas muscle become very distinct. Reasons may be the perforation of a retroperitoneal bowel segment (duodenum, parts of the colon and rectum) or the transit of air from the mediastinum into the retroperitoneal space in mediastinal emphysema.

The analysis of the **distribution of bowel gas** can help in the diagnosis of a number of entities:

An air-distended stomach is frequently found after *resuscitation* and may point to an earlier false intubation. It doesn't hurt to mention the distended stomach to the referring physician, because placement of a nasogastric tube can often provide relief to the patient.

Wide, air-filled small-bowel loops indicate a disturbance of the bowel peristalsis and are due to either a partial or complete ileus or small-bowel obstruction.

> **!** Differentiation between an ileus and a small-bowel obstruction is most readily afforded by auscultation: the absence of bowel sounds suggests an ileus (or extremely advanced obstruction), while high-pitched active bowel sounds suggest a mechanical bowel obstruction. Remember that even (!) radiologists may consider using the stethoscope every now and then to help make the right diagnosis.

The actual image appearance of the air- and fluid-filled small-bowel loops—also called "sentinel loops"—(Fig. 9.**2e**) hints at the character of the disturbance: If a mechanical obstruction is present, the intestinal peristalsis continues and tries to force the bowel content across the point of obstruction. A characteristic sentinel loop shows air–fluid interfaces at significantly different levels.

The air-filled bowel segments are naturally located proximal to the point of obstruction because the air distal to it is absorbed in time.

If the peristaltic problem is due to a paralysis or if the obstructed bowel is eventually exhausted, the air–fluid interfaces in the sentinel loops tend to remain at the same level: an adynamic ileus is present. (To observe the potential difference in fluid levels, the patient must remain motionless in the above-described positions for a few minutes.) Bowel sounds are typically absent in this situation. Extremely dilated air-filled large-bowel segments may be seen in **toxic megacolon**, in **large-bowel obstruction due to tumor**, or in **volvulus** (torsion of the bowel around its mesenteric root). The more chronic the problem, the larger the intestines can appear.

Now let us try this out on the first patient.

9.2   Patient with Acute Abdominal Pain

Checklist: Acute Abdomen

- Is the patient standing up or positioned on the left side, and is the x-ray beam horizontal?
- Do you see air outside of the gastrointestinal tract?
- Is the air within the gastrointestinal tract normally distributed?
- Are "sentinel loops" with air–fluid levels of differing height present?
- Are there characteristic calcifications present?

Mutiny in the Belly

The paramedics found Melissa Stonegrave (51) helpless on a park bench. Passersby had noticed her as she was lying on her side wincing and calling for help. The paramedics noted that she complained of severe abdominal pain. In the emergency room she was carefully examined. A nasogastric tube was inserted because the patient had vomited. Giufeng is looking through some rather boring cases of the teaching file when x-ray technician Thomas brings Mrs. Stonegrave's radiographs over from the emergency room for her to review. Giufeng puts the chest radiograph on the viewbox first, but sees nothing abnormal and puts it to the side. Pulmonary problems such as a basal pneumonia as a cause of her symptoms do not seem to be present. She grabs the abdominal radiograph and begins a careful analysis (Fig. 9.**3**).

➜ What is your diagnosis?

Free intraperitoneal air: In case of free intraperitoneal air, the perforation of a hollow organ such as the stomach, the duodenum (in ulcer disease), or the large bowel (for example in diverticulitis), or a traumatic perforation must

The Case of Melissa Stonegrave

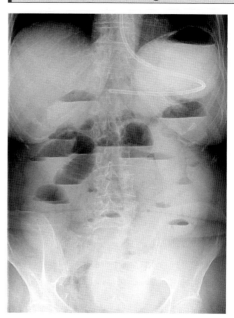

Fig. 9.**3**   Have a look at the abdominal radiograph of Melissa Stonegrave. Which finding grabs your attention right away?

be considered (Fig. 9.**4**). It may, however, also be residual air after a surgical intervention in the abdomen, which may persist for days and weeks.

Air in the retroperitoneum: Retroperitoneal air is much less frequent and occurs, for example, in perforations of retroperitoneal bowel segments such as the duodenum, colon, or rectum (Fig. 9.**5**). It can also occur in severe infections with gas-forming bacteria, e.g., emphysematous pyelonephritis in diabetic patients.

Air in the bowel wall: Air in the bowel wall can be observed in pneumatosis intestinalis (Fig. 9.**6a, b**), a benign asymptomatic condition, or in the late phase of bowel ischemia (Fig. 9.**6c**) that goes along with severe abdominal pain. In extreme cases the air reaches the portal venous system of the liver via the mesenteric veins (Fig. 9.**6d**). In the olden days this used to be a "signum mali ominis," an ominous sign indicating a deleterious course of the disease. In times of ubiquitous CT, the sign is much more often seen and is fortunately less prognostic.

Bowel obstruction (mechanical ileus): Also termed mechanical or dynamic ileus, this condition is characterized by a mechanical obstruction of the intestinal lumen (Fig. 9.**7a**). In the small bowel, postoperative fibrous bands, so-called adhesions, are the most frequent cause of obstruction followed by incarcerated hernias (inguinal, femoral, umbilical, and incisional). In children an intussusception may be the culprit. Gallstones that have perforated into the bowel lumen (Fig. 9.**7b**) may be a cause of obstruction that can be directly visualized on the radiograph. In the large bowel, colorectal carcinomas, volvulus of the

Free Intraperitoneal Air

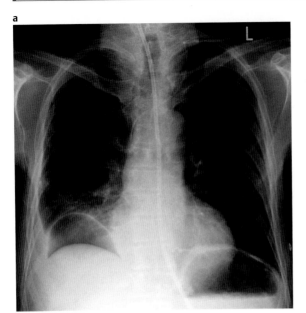

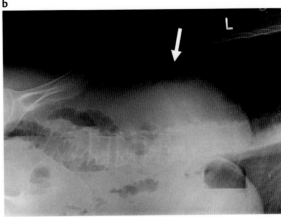

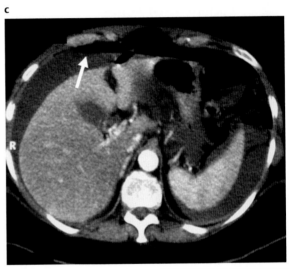

Fig. 9.4 a This upright chest radiograph shows an evident pocket of air underneath the right hemidiaphragm. The lungs themselves are clear. There is a small right-sided pleural effusion. This patient was brought into the emergency unit with an acute abdomen due to a gastric perforation. b In another patient positioned on the left side and imaged with a horizontal x-ray beam, an air depot is present between the liver, the diaphragm, and the abdominal wall (arrow). This patient underwent abdominal surgery two days before. An upright radiograph was still impossible to obtain. The air in some small-bowel loops indicates an additional disturbance of the intestinal peristalsis. c Free air in the abdomen is not quite that easy to diagnose by CT—if free fluid is also present the air–fluid levels are reliable proof (arrow).

Air in the Retroperitoneum

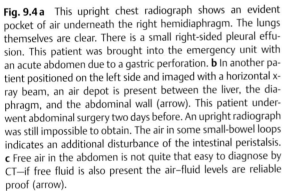

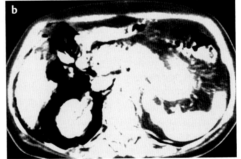

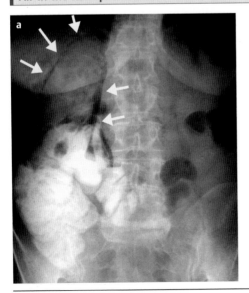

Fig. 9.5 a This abdominal radiograph shows the contour of the iliopsoas muscle (short arrows) and the right kidney (long arrows) extremely well, much better than normal. They are outlined by air that originated from a traumatic rupture of the duodenum. The colon is filled with some water-soluble contrast from a previous enema. b To confirm the diagnosis, this CT was windowed so the difference between fat (as it is seen in the subcutaneous tissues) and air (as it is present around the kidney) is amplified.

Air in Bowel Wall

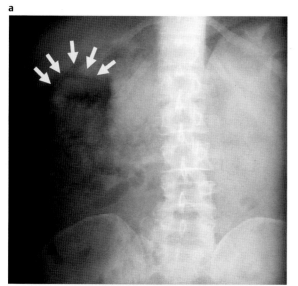

a

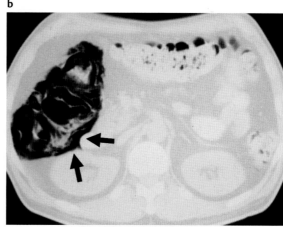

b

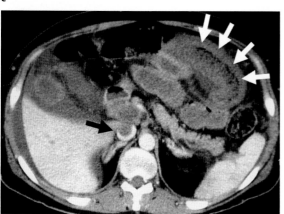

c

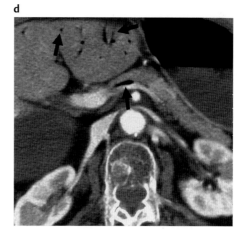

d

Fig. 9.6 a In the right upper abdomen several layers of air (arrows) are present around the intestinal lumen. **b** The CT confirms the presence of air in the bowel wall (arrows). This patient had an acute myelogenous leukemia (AML) but no intestinal symptoms whatsoever at that time and later. This turned out to be pneumatosis intestinalis. **c** The CT section in another patient with severe abdominal pain displays a marked thickening of the bowel wall with small air deposits in it—much like a "string of beads" (white arrows): This bowel segment is gangrenous.

In addition, thin rims of ascites are seen around the liver and also around the spleen. By the way: The contrast defect in the vena cava (black arrow) is not a thrombus but is a result of laminar flow! Blood rich with contrast medium from the kidneys flows along uncontrasted blood from the lower extremities. **d** Once there is air in the necrotic bowel wall, it can also enter the mesenteric veins and eventually the hepatoportal system (arrows).

sigma (Fig. 9.**7c**) or cecum and diverticulitis must be excluded as the cause of the ileus. Enemas with water-soluble contrast media are essential in the radiographic differentiation of these entities in the large bowel. CT of the abdomen with multiplanar 3D image reconstructions on a workstation can help determine the point of obstruction as well as provide clues to the underlying cause.

Paralytic ileus: The paralytic ileus may be due to a number of different conditions (Fig. 9.**8**). It is also the pathophysiological end point of a persisting untreated bowel obstruc-

tion. It may be seen after surgical interventions in the abdomen, after abdominal trauma, and in electrolyte imbalances, sepsis, peritonitis, or infiltration of the mesentery by tumor.

Acute pancreatitis: An acute pancreatitis is not normally diagnosed on the abdominal radiograph. The signs of recurring or chronic pancreatitis may, however, be visible and point the diagnostic work-up in the right direction (see Fig. 9.**2d**).

Mechanical Ileus

a Colon carcinoma

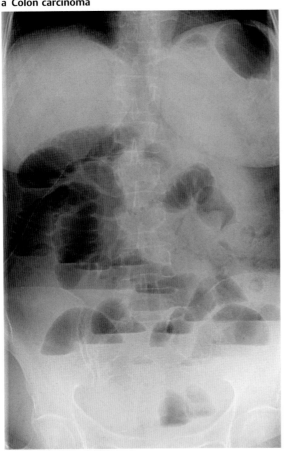

Fig. 9.**7 a** Numerous sentinel loops with air–fluid levels of varying heights indicate a mechanical (dynamic) ileus. The colon is essentially free of air. This was an obstruction due to a colon carcinoma. **b** Air is seen in the duodenum and proximal jejunum, almost none in the colon (left). This looks like a jejunal obstruction. The reason is a giant gallstone that has found its way into the jejunum. Can you see it above the left iliac crest? On its way into the jejunum the gallstone has created a communication (right) through which air seeps into the biliary system. Note the air-filled common bile duct coursing toward the distended duodenum! Air may also be seen in the biliary tract after the rather frequent therapeutic dilation of the papilla of Vater and must be differentiated from air in the portal system as an ominous sign of bowel ischemia. **c** In another patient an extremely dilated and air-filled bowel loop (left) is identified as sigmoid colon owing to its location and the obvious haustration. The colon is nicely outlined by air; the rectum shows no air at all. This is a sigmoid volvulus, a torsion of the sigma around its mesenteric root. The result is, of course, mechanical bowel obstruction. The configuration of the bowel in this entity is reminiscent of the underside of the "bean" that helps us through many a day: It is called the "coffee-bean sign." The volvulus is confirmed with the help of an enema with water-soluble contrast. We see a "bird's-beak" like configuration of the contrast column at the rectosigmoidal transition (right).   ▶

b Gallstone

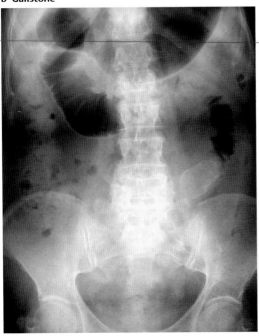

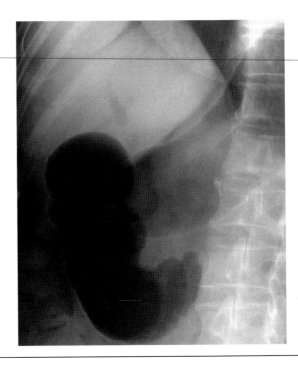

Mechanical Ileus

c Volvulus

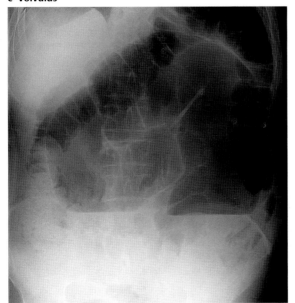

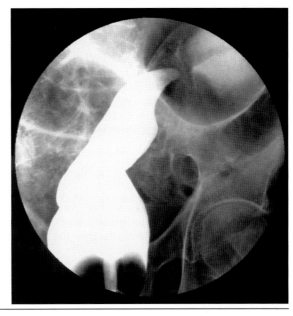

Paralytic Ileus

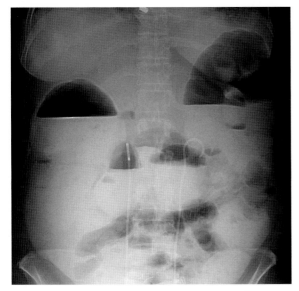

Fig. 9.8 In this cancer patient the diffuse spread of cancer in the retroperitoneum has necessitated stenting of both ureters to keep urine flowing from kidneys to the bladder. Now a paralytic ileus has developed on top of that: distended bowel loops with air–fluid interfaces that tend to have the same levels in one loop and that seem to be present everywhere. Note: Paralytic ileus is usually diagnosed with a stethoscope! Imaging is not really needed here.

→ **Diagnosis:** Giufeng has not found any free air in the peritoneum or retroperitoneum of Mrs. Stonegrave. However, she thinks that the distribution of air in the intestines is grossly abnormal. The colon is completely free of air, while the small bowel shows many sentinel loops with air–fluid levels of differing heights. It is quite clear to her that a mechanical bowel obstruction is present; air in the colon has been absorbed or passed. Giufeng diagnoses a dynamic, mechanical ileus on the basis of an obstruction of the small bowel or the proximal colon. As it turns out, Melissa Stonegrave had undergone a complicated cholecystectomy a few years earlier. During surgery, adhesions were found to be the cause of the small-bowel obstruction.

! Most bowel obstructions are actually treated conservatively with a nasogastric tube and observation. In fact, CT allows us to stratify patients into a surgical versus a non-surgical group by detecting the presence or absence of ischemia, portal venous gas, extraluminal disease, etc., which clearly represents an advance over the olden times when the clinical picture (signs of sepsis, shock, acidosis, etc.) was all we had in addition to the radiograph.

! Free intraperitoneal air and an ileus are best diagnosed on an abdominal radiograph with the patient standing or positioned on the left side and a horizontal x-ray beam. The infrequent retroperitoneal air and the cause of a mechanical bowel obstruction are often better appreciated on CT. Free fluid is detected most rapidly by ultrasound. Make a note of that: It is not always the most expensive modality that gives you the crucial information!

9.3   Diseases of the Esophagus

Checklist: Diseases of the Esophagus

- Does the patient choke or cough while eating or drinking?
- Does food get stuck when the patients is eating?
- Has a foreign body been swallowed?
- Does the patient complain about a lump in the throat, regurgitation of undigested food, or bad breath?
- Is swallowing painful for the patient?
- Has the patient had heartburn for extended periods?

The Steak Won't Go Down Easy

Jack Wiggle (86) comes to the radiology department for an examination because he has problems swallowing. He chokes quite often and feels a lump in the throat,

and his grandchildren have been complaining about grandpa's bad breath. He has brought one of them with him to help out with the test. Paul is just getting his first instructions on the art of fluoroscopy, the real-time x-ray examination of the intestinal tract. Dr. Llewellyn, a dyed-in-the-wool, old-school specialist in gastrointestinal imaging, watches him carefully while he sets out to do the examination. The clinical information given by Wiggle's general practitioner and the conversation with Mr. Wiggle as well as the young man who accompanies him have not provided any definite clues as to what is going on.

! If a functional swallowing disorder were suspected, dedicated videofluoroscopy of the swallowing act would be the examination of choice. Videofluoroscopy documents the different phases of the highly complex swallowing act in multiple video frames (Fig. 9.9). If, for example, the disturbance is due to the nonrelaxation of

---

Normal Swallowing

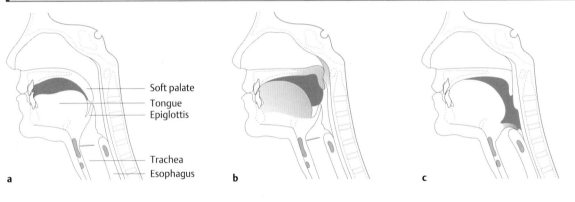

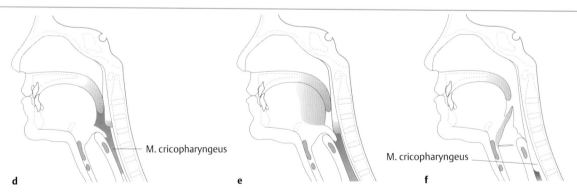

Fig. 9.**9**   This is what normal swallowing looks like. **a** The contrast bolus is held and formed between the tongue and the soft palate. **b** The tongue and the soft palate elevate to present the bolus to the oropharynx. In the process the soft palate seals the communication to the nasopharynx to prevent regurgitation. **c** The bolus moves dorsally and downward while the epiglottis seals the laryngeal introitus. **d** The soft palate descends even further and the cricopharyngeus muscle relaxes, permitting the passage of the bolus. **e** As the bolus has passed the cricopharyngeus muscle, the tongue base and the soft palate rise again. **f** As the bolus reaches the thoracic esophagus, the tongue base moves forward, the epiglottis flips up, and the larynx returns to its resting position. (From Richard M. Gore, Marc S. Levine, Igor Laufer, eds. *Textbook of Gastrointestinal Radiology*. Philadelphia: WB Saunders, 1994.)

the cricopharyngeal muscle, an injection of botulinum toxin may be considered. Specific other findings, such as weak stripping motion of the tongue, weakness of the soft palate, or food getting stuck in the valleculae or piriform sinus, can aid the speech pathologist in figuring out a new swallowing technique for the patient affected by these abnormalities.

Paul studies a frontal radiograph of the chest and upper abdomen that was obtained prior to the examination on Mr. Wiggle, which demonstrates no obvious abnormality To get oriented a bit, he has Mr. Wiggle take a little sip of a barium suspension and watches the barium pass through his esophagus under fluoroscopy. Subsequently he asks the patient to drink some more and obtains radiographs of the whole esophagus in two projections, both fully distended with the barium column and in double contrast technique to assess the mucosal lining of the esophagus. When he sees a narrow segment of esophagus, he hesitates and obtains some enlarged collimated views of this suspicious segment (Fig. 9.**10**).

→ **What is your diagnosis?**

Esophageal diverticula: These are circumscribed mucosal and submucosal outpouchings of the esophagus with little or absent muscular coverage. They are divided into traction and pulsion diverticula. Pulsion diverticula tend to

The Case of Jack Wiggle

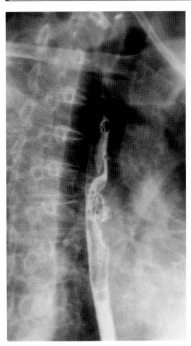

Fig. 9.**10**   Here you see the diagnostic film of the barium swallow of Jack Wiggle. Is there anything abnormal?

Diverticulum

a
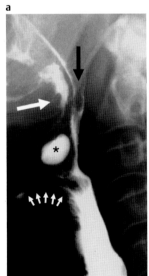

b
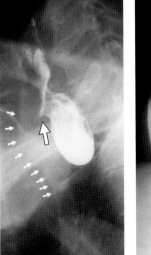

c
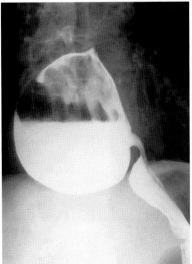

d
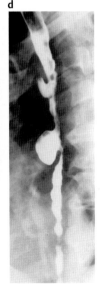

Fig. 9.**11 a**   This lateral view of the swallowing act shows the appearance after passage of the barium bolus into the esophagus. The soft palate is pressed against the dorsal pharyngeal wall (black arrow), thus preventing the regurgitation of food into the nasal cavity. The tongue base (large white arrow) has moved upward and backward; the epiglottis (small white arrows) seals off the laryngeal entrance. The bolus has entered the proximal esophagus. There is a diverticulum in the area of the epiglottic fold (star). It extends laterally from the tongue base. **b** In a Zenker diverticulum the depiction of the width of the diverticular neck (large arrow) is of particular importance to the surgeon. The esophagus and the trachea (small arrows) are displaced ventrally. **c** Another typical location of a pulsion diverticulum is the distal esophagus. **d** Traction diverticula tend to occur at the level of the pulmonary hila and are usually the consequence of inflammatory lymphadenitis in the mediastinum.

Achalasia

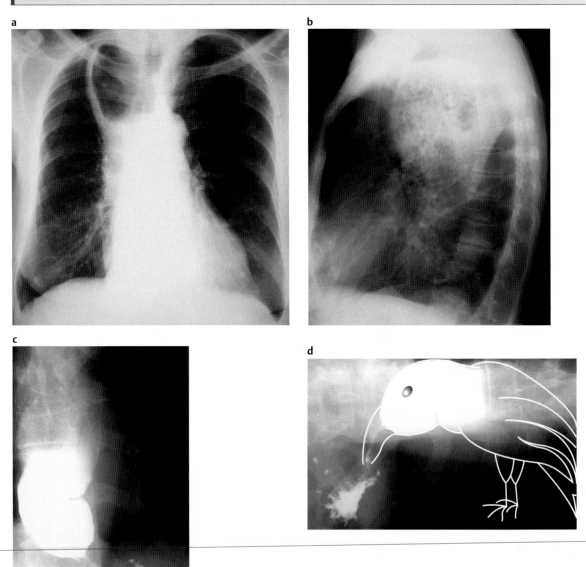

Fig. 9.**12 a**   The distended esophagus filled with remnants of food and air in this patient with achalasia is prominent up to the upper mediastinum. **b** The lateral projection of the chest displays the food impaction in the esophagus and the anteriorly displaced trachea with even greater clarity. **c** After the administration of oral contrast medium, the grossly dilated proximal esophagus and the narrowed ganglion depleted segment are outlined. This finding is also called the "bird's beak." **d** A little imagination helps, of course.

be cervical (Fig. 9.**11a**) and epiphrenic (Fig. 9.**11c**) and usually occur proximal to a relative point of obstruction such as the upper or lower esophageal sphincter or when a weak spot in the muscular wall of the esophagus gives way to the pressure. Traction diverticula due to pulling inflammatory processes (often in the mediastinum) occur almost exclusively at the level of the tracheal bifurcation (Fig. 9.**11d**).

The *Zenker diverticulum* is a pulsion diverticulum always located left of the pharyngoesophageal transition zone

(Fig. 9.**11b**). It may become extremely large and it can retain undigested food and can compress the esophagus. The food remnants give rise to the frequent symptom of halitosis (synonym for bad breath).

> **!** Esophageal diverticula can be overlooked during endoscopy, especially if they have a narrow neck, while widenecked diverticula may be mistaken for the esophageal lumen and be perforated when the endoscopist tries to advance the scope during the procedure.

Disturbances of the esophageal peristalsis:
Achalasia: In this neurogenic disorder those ganglion cells of the muscle layers of the distal esophagus that normally inhibit the contraction of the lower esophageal sphincter are decreased. It is rare in children and can occur throughout adult life. The disorder is characterized by a combination of absent peristalsis and a hypertensive lower esophageal sphincter, resulting in a functional obstruction at or close to the esophagogastric junction. Over time this can lead to a dilated esophagus, often filled with secretions and undigested food. The chronic irritation of the mucous membranes induces a chronic inflammation of the esophagus and is associated with a 10-fold higher risk of developing esophageal carcinoma. The diagnosis of achalasia may be suggested on a simple chest radiograph (Fig. 9.**12a**, **b**). The final confirmation is achieved by performing a barium swallow (Fig. 9.**12c**, **d**).
Diffuse esophageal spasm (DES): DES is due to a local neuro-degenerative process and it shows a completely different appearance: so-called "tertiary" (uncoordinated) contractions occur that may give the esophagus a "corkscrew" configuration; this kind of uncoordinated peristalsis is more frequent in the elderly (Fig. 9.**13**).
Scleroderma: Peristalsis of the esophagus is weakened or completely absent in scleroderma (Fig. 9.**14**). Delayed radiographs after a barium swallow may show residual contrast in the esophagus.

Diffuse Esophageal Spasm (DES)

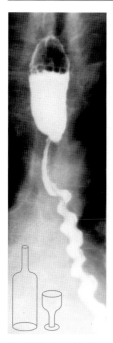

Fig. 9.**13** In elderly patients the peristalsis of the esophagus may become disorganized, losing its propulsive force. After barium has been given, the esophagus may look like a corkscrew in DES. This entity is not associated with alcohol abuse, however.

Scleroderma

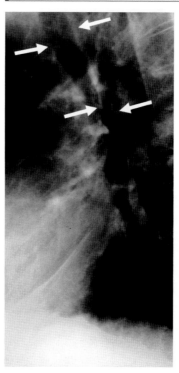

Fig. 9.**14** In extreme cases of scleroderma the rigid and dilated esophagus (thick arrows) may appear as a second air column behind the trachea (thin arrows)—the "double-barrel sign."

! Peristaltic disturbances are best diagnosed by a barium swallow examination.

Esophageal tumors: If the appearance on barium swallow suggests the possibility of an esophageal tumor, it must be considered to be malignant until proven otherwise. If the lesion is located in the very proximal esophagus, it is most likely a squamous cell carcinoma of the hypopharynx (Fig. 9.**15**) or of the esophagus (Fig. 9.**16a**); further distal the frequency of adenocarcinomas increases (Fig. 9.**16b**). These are particularly frequent if precursor diseases of the esophagogastric transition zone such as reflux esophagitis (Fig. 9.**17a**) or a Barrett esophagus (Fig. 9.**17b**) have been present.

Esophageal varices: Venous varices of the esophageal wall may develop as a consequence of portal hypertension due to liver cirrhosis (Fig. 9.**18**) or portal vein occlusion. The veins around the esophagus have connections to the portal system in the upper abdomen around the esophagogastric junction and drain into the azygos and hemiazygos venous systems in the posterior mediastinum, which are part of the systemic circulation. This pathway may be used by the body to decompress the portal venous system in the aforementioned conditions. Severe acute hemorrhage is the greatest risk associated with this condition.

Hypopharyngeal Carcinoma

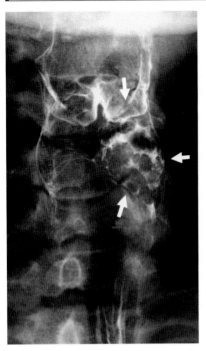

Fig. 9.**15** This polypoid growing hypopharyngeal carcinoma (arrows) is located in the left piriform recess, directly proximal to the entrance into the esophagus and directly distal to the epiglottis, which is nicely outlined by contrast medium. (Where was your anatomy book again?)

Esophageal Carcinoma

a

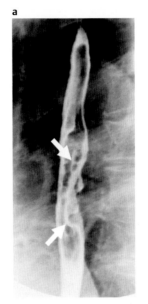

b

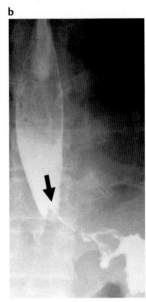

Fig. 9.16 a This esophageal carcinoma presents as an abnormal appearance of the esophageal wall contour (arrows), frequently with ulcerations. Submucosal lesions are also detectable in a barium swallow because they change the peristalsis of the esophageal wall; that is a real advantage in comparison to fiberoptic endoscopy. **b** A carcinoma of the distal esophagus like this one tends to involve the gastric cardia as well. Note the irregular proximal contour (arrow) and the distal margin of the stenosis.

Esophageal Carcinoma: Precursor Diseases

a Hiatal hernia

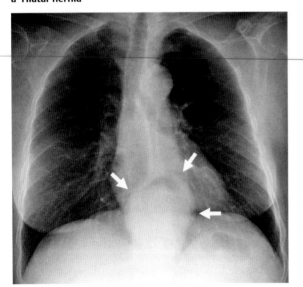

b Barrett esophagus

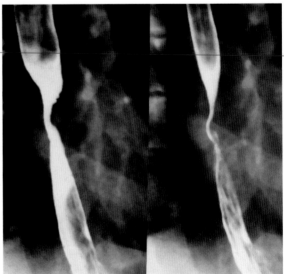

Fig. 9.**17 a** Hiatal hernias are recognized by their ringlike structure (arrows), frequently with air–fluid interfaces, in the mediastinum. To confirm the diagnosis, a small cup of barium is sufficient. **b** The leading characteristic of a Barrett esophagus is the stenosis or mucosal irregularity in the distal third of the esophagus, but often this precancerous abnormality is invisible to the radiologist. Distal to the stenosis, columnar epithelium replaces the normal stratified squamous epithelium in the esophagus as a result of chronic acid reflux into the distal esophagus.

Radiation Stenosis of the Rectum

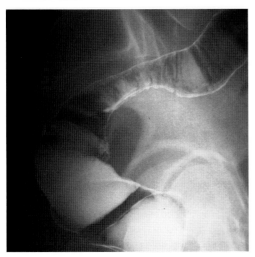

Fig. 9.**35** This woman had a pelvic malignant tumor and underwent radiation therapy. Now the rectum in the presacral region is fibrotic and stenosed.

Tapeworm in the Colon

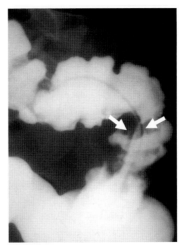

Fig. 9.**36** The two parallel lines within the bowel lumen (arrows) indicate the outer wall of the worm. The contrast medium between them is in the bowel of the tapeworm: bowel in bowel, so to say.

Ulcerative colitis: Ulcerative colitis is different from Crohn disease in that it has a different pattern of intestinal involvement. It begins in the rectum and progresses proximally in a continuous fashion (Fig. 9.**34**). Fistulas are hardly ever seen. Up to 10 % of all patients per year develop colon cancer, typically after several years of disease, which is why a total colectomy is often performed. Nowadays colorectal surgeons can preserve the patient's anal sphincter and build a new rectal pouch from small bowel, so that the patients can have a fairly normal life even without their colon and without the need for any external appliances.

Radiation colitis: Radiation colitis may develop after radiation therapy has been given to the abdomen and pelvis, for example, in pelvic tumors. Ulcerations and a bowel wall swelling arise that may ultimately result in a segmental bowel stenosis (Fig. 9.**35**).

The Ultimate Bleed

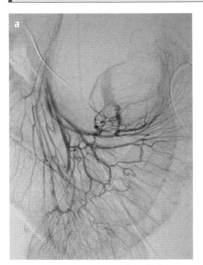
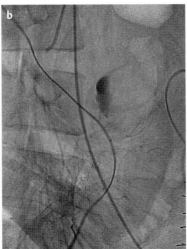
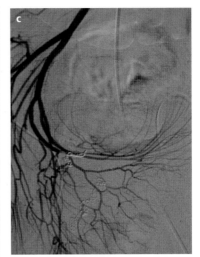

Fig. 9.**37 a–c** Arteriography of the mesenteric vessels is the modality of choice if the hemorrhage necessitates the infusion of packed red cells. The arterial phase (**a**) shows contrast extravasation into a jejunal loop (arrow). A later image after the clearance of vascular contrast demonstrates a persistent contrast depot in this location (**b**), which illustrates the force of the bleed. After several embolization coils have been deployed into the major feeding vessels, the bleeding is stopped (**c**).   ▶

Parasitosis of the colon: Parasites, for example, tapeworms (Fig. 9.**36**), may set up shop in the bowel as well and need to be considered in the differential diagnosis, especially if the patient has recently traveled to an endemic area or enjoys raw food.

➡ **Diagnosis:** Paul has checked the whole list of differential diagnoses, but the appearance, the patient's age, and sheer probability have led him to come to a straightforward conclusion: This is a sigmoid cancer that has led to a partial obstruction of the sigmoid colon. Diverticulitis could certainly produce a similar appearance, but the symptoms do not fit and other diverticula cannot be found. Llewellyn calls Mrs. Herbgarden's primary care physician. He arranges an urgent appointment for her in the surgical clinic during this conversation. Mrs. Herbgarden will visit her physician the next morning to find out about the result of the study and the treatment options.

Dr. Llewellyn takes a little time to tell Paul about the diagnostic handling of more intense and acute bleeds into the gastrointestinal lumen. "If endoscopy is impossible or does not yield any results, radiology comes into the picture. Basically it is the small and large bowel that need to be looked at in that setting. Angiography is the modality for really strong bleeds [Fig. 9.**37a–c**]. But if the patient does not require infusions of blood at the time of the intervention, chances are low of detecting the source of bleeding with a catheter-based contrast injection into a blood vessel: in that case don't even try an angiogram! On the other hand, if you find it you can embolize it right away! In lower intensity bleeds, nuclear medicine is your only chance: a blood pool scan will show bleeds of as little as 0.1 ml per minute. And you can image the patient over and over again in the first 24 hours after injection without giving more drug, so you can wait until they bleed again and then hunt for the source [Fig. 9.**37d, e**]."

9.6   Problems with Defecation

Checklist: **Disturbances of Defecation**

- Is the patient constipated?
- Is the patient incontinent of stool?
- Did the rectal digital examination reveal bleeding or a rectal prolapse?

An Embarrassing Problem

Samantha Pamper (68) has come to the department with a problem she does not really want to brag about: She has been stool incontinent for a few years and needs diapers when she leaves her home. She has given birth to three children and is grossly overweight. Her social life has suffered quite a bit. Finally she has found a female surgeon she trusts who specializes in incontinence and other rectoanal problems. For proper preoperative planning the surgeon needs to have functional information about the defecation process: she has ordered a defecography for Mrs. Pamper. Llewellyn is the specialist for this type of problem in the radiology department—he has all the utensils for it stowed away in a little cabinet: a camping toilet made of plastic and a large ruler with lead markings. He fixes the toilet to the footstand of the fluoroscopy unit and elevates it to a comfortable sitting position. After the rectal examination he cautiously introduces a large-lumen tube into Mrs. Pamper's rectum and injects a rather thick barium paste. The vagina is also lined with just a little contrast using a smaller tube. Mrs. Pamper is asked to squat on the toilet, ready to be fluoroscoped in a lateral projection with the lead ruler held tight between her thighs.

The Ultimate Bleed

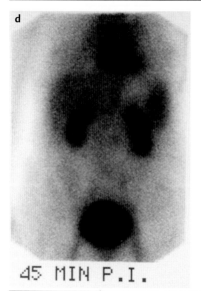
45 MIN P.I.

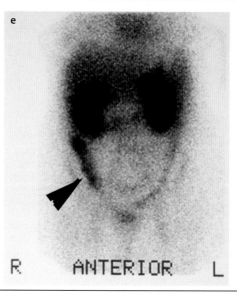
R   ANTERIOR   L

Fig. 9.**37 d** A blood pool scan after administration of technetium-99-labeled red cell in another patient with a less intense bleed shows no abnormality in the first 45 minutes. Kidneys, bladder, liver, spleen, and heart show a homogeneously high radiotracer uptake, as expected. Another scan 20 hours later (**e**) not only indicates the location of the primary bleeding source (arrow) in the cecum but also proves its intraintestinal location because the radiotracer activity is spread out over the colon by the ongoing peristalsis.

Hepatocellular Carcinoma (HCC)

a

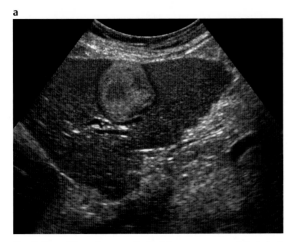

b

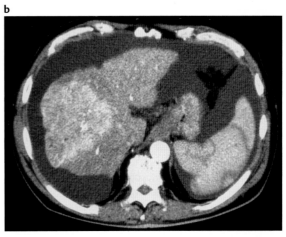

Fig. 9.**49 a** The ultrasound depicts an encapsulated lesion that is partially hyperechoic, partially internally isoechoic compared to surrounding parenchyma. The liver contour is irregular, the liver edge rounded—all of this fits well with a liver cirrhosis that is associated with a higher risk of developing HCC. **b** In this typical case of a hepatocellular carcinoma the liver is diffusely cirrhotic: the parenchyma has a nodular appearance. Ascites is also present already. The early arterial phase after contrast administration (do you see the "tiger pattern" of the spleen?) documents the forceful enhancement of the tumor. (By the way: In which segments according to Couinaud is the tumor located?)

The tumor involves segments VII and VIII.

Cholangiocellular Carcinoma (CCC)

a

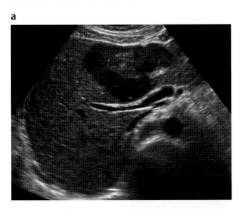

b

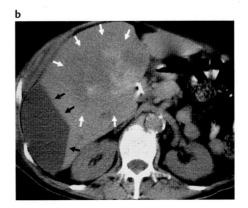

c

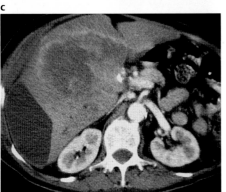

Fig. 9.**50 a** This cholangiocarcinoma is rather hypoechoic along its periphery. Dilated biliary ducts are not present. **b** In another patient the tumor (white arrows) has an irregular margin and is hypodense. In addition there is a subcapsular biloma (biliary retention; black arrows). **c** After contrast the tumor enhances in the periphery in a geographic pattern often seen in CCC.

Diffuse Liver Disease

Checklist: Diffuse Liver Lesion

- Is there alcohol abuse?
- Is the patient overweight?
- Has the patient received chemotherapy?
- Is there a history of chronic hepatitis?
- Is there right cardiac failure?

This Liver Has Done Overtime

Violetta Countess Campari (62) has been examined as part of her follow-up protocol for a previous breast carcinoma. The referring oncologist is naturally interested in whether she has developed any metastases. Giufeng has not found any focal lesions in the liver. She already wants to pass on to the next patient as Gregory comes by and views the images on the monitor with awe. "Just look at that! I need a copy of these," he shouts. "Boy, this is textbook stuff!" Giufeng is taken by surprise; she returns to the scanner and takes another careful look at the images (Fig. 9.**51**).

The Case of Violetta Countess Campari

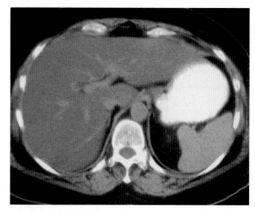

Fig. 9.**51**   Look at this decisive CT scan of Countess Campari. Can you find anything?

→ **What is Your Diagnosis?**

Fatty liver: Another term for this is hepatic steatosis, a frequent incidental finding in liver examinations (Fig. 9.**52a**, **b**). Pathologists see it in approx. 25% of all

Steatosis of the Liver

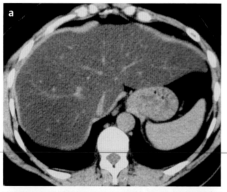

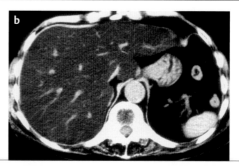

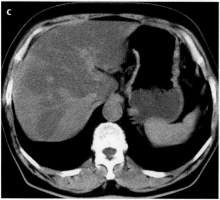

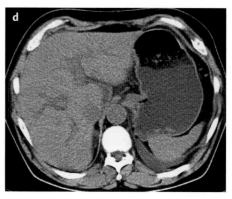

Fig. 9.**52 a**   On noncontrast CT images of the liver the vessels appear brighter than the hepatic parenchyma. Normally it is just the other way round. This is a typical finding in fatty liver. **b** The difference in density naturally becomes even more pronounced after contrast is administered intravenously. If the steatosis is less severe, the vessels may become invisible altogether. **c** This CT-section shows a regional steatosis after chemotherapy. **d** Eight weeks later the liver has returned to its normal homogeneous appearance.

Liver Cirrhosis

a

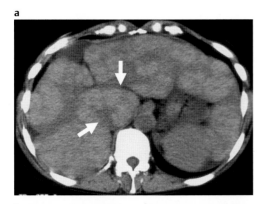

b

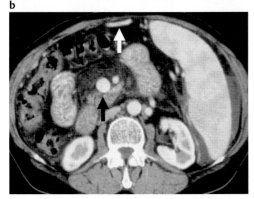

Fig. 9.53 a   In this patient with advanced liver cirrhosis, dense regeneration nodules are detectable even before contrast is administered. The surface of the organ is nodular , the caudate lobe (arrows) is enlarged. **b** If a portal hypertension ensues, the spleen is enlarged, the superior mesenteric vein is often congested (black arrow), and the umbilical vein is recanalized and dilated as part of a collateral system (white arrow), which allows blood to bypass the liver and drain into systemic veins. Note the ascites around the spleen.

otherwise healthy adults. It can develop within a few weeks and can also disappear within such a time frame. In addition to an unhealthy fatty diet and alcohol abuse, diabetes mellitus or chemotherapy can lead to this effect (Fig. 9.**52c**). The steatosis can encompass the whole liver (fatty liver) or remain segmental. If a small part of the liver is spared from the fatty infiltration it can take the appearance of a (pseudo)liver lesion on CT or ultrasound. For obvious reasons, this must be differentiated from focal liver disease such as a primary or secondary tumor. Circumscribed fatty infiltration of the liver parenchyma is often seen adjacent to the falciform ligament. In critical cases, MRI with and without fat saturation or a core biopsy will help differentiate true liver lesions from focal sparing in a patient with otherwise fatty liver.

Liver cirrhosis: Liver cirrhosis manifests itself with a few changes that can be visualized with imaging modalities. The liver volume increases in the early phase, the outer

contour becomes irregular, and regenerative nodules develop (Fig. 9.**53a**). Later the liver may shrink and, as a consequence of progressive fibrosis around the portal vessels and bile ducts and the disorganized regeneration of hepatocytes in nodules, the microcirculation of the liver is gradually destroyed and portal hypertension develops (Fig. 9.**53b**). The consequences are an enlarged spleen, ascites, and increase in the size of collateral veins, which decompress the portal system into the systemic venous circulation, frequently via the veins of the gastric fundus and the esophagus as well as in the retroperitoneum into the left renal vein. These enlarged veins are called varices and bleed easily, a potentially lethal event. The interventional radiologist can create a shortcut from a large portal vein branch into a large hepatic vein within the liver itself by implanting a transjugular intrahepatic portovenous stent-shunt (TIPSS), thus relieving the abnormally high pressure in the portal venous system (see p. 108).

> **!** In a nodular cirrhotic liver, focal lesions such as metastases or hepatocellular carcinomas can be masked and can remain undetected.

Hemochromatosis: Hemochromatosis, an abnormally increased iron deposition within the liver, is easily appreciated even on noncontrast CT because the liver density is diffusely increased in comparison with the spleen and the liver vessels (Fig. 9.**54**). Later a liver cirrhosis develops with all the potential side effects and consequences. The disease occurs in young adults and often necessitates liver transplantation.

→ **Diagnosis:**   Giufeng must confess that she simply overlooked the extensive but homogeneous fatty infiltration of Countess Campari's liver. Gregory knows why: "You probably concentrated too much on the patient's history. There were no metastases and so the examination was all finished for you. Could also have been a simple case of 'satisfaction of search.' You're lucky—in this case it's not a problem. But I definitely need one of the images for my teaching file."

Hemochromatosis

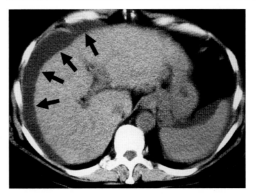

Fig. 9.**54** The density of the liver is increased relative to the density of the spleen. The liver has already developed a cirrhosis, its surface is irregular, and ascites abounds (arrows).

9.8   Diseases of the Extrahepatic Biliary System

Checklist: Diseases of the Extrahepatic Biliary System

- Is there jaundice?
- Is there a history of biliary colic?
- Does the patient have known gallstones?

A Man Sees Yellow

Don Cramp (55) has complained about nonspecific pain in the upper abdomen for two days. His general practitioner has a suspicion that his eyes have turned yellow just a bit. Joey is covering CT today. Mr. Cramp comes straight from the internal medicine clinic and an ultrasound examination to the CT unit. The ultrasound report is handwritten and impossible to decipher. Joey puts it aside to concentrate on the CT examination (Fig. 9.**55**).

The Case of Don Cramp

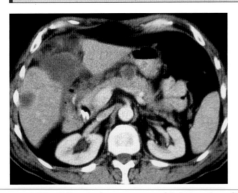

Fig. 9.**55**   What is there to see on this CT section of Mr. Cramp?

➜ What is Your Diagnosis?

Cholecystolithiasis: Gallstones are frequently and definitively diagnosed by ultrasound (Fig. 9.**56a**). Often they are an incidental finding without any symptoms whatsoever. The relevant complications of cholecystolithiasis are:

Acute cholecystitis: This acute inflammation of the gallbladder is frequently the consequence of an obstruction of the cystic duct or the infundibulum of the gallbladder due to a stone. On ultrasound the thickening of the gallbladder wall is typical (Fig. 9.**56a**), and sometimes there is an accompanying inflammatory reaction of the neighboring liver parenchyma (Fig. 9.**56b**). The diagnosis of cholecystitis is made on the basis of the clinical picture, however.

Cholecystolithiasis and Its Consequences

a

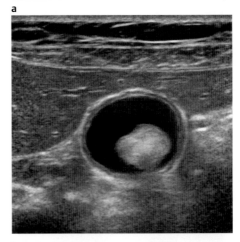

b

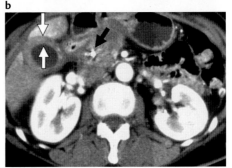

Fig. 9.**56 a**   The stone within the gallbladder is seen well sonographically—the distal acoustic shadow is quite characteristic. The gallbladder wall shows normal thickness. **b** This stone in the common bile duct of another patient (long arrow) has led to a swelling of the gallbladder wall as part of an acute inflammation (cholecystitis, short arrows). The thickness of the bladder wall exceeds the normal value of 1–2 mm.

Stone migration/stone impaction: A migration of a stone into the cystic duct and onward into the common bile duct is always accompanied by colicky pain. If the stone becomes impacted in the infundibulum of the bladder or in the cystic duct, thereby occluding or severely narrowing the common bile duct from outside (Mirizzi syndrome), or if the main choledochal duct is obstructed by stones, bile backs up into the liver; this is also called cholestasis.

Gallbladder carcinoma: A primary adenocarcinoma of the gallbladder can develop in the wall of the gallbladder and its immediate vicinity can be infiltrated by this tumor (Fig. 9.**57**). Risk factors for the development of gallbladder carcinoma are cholecystolithiasis and chronic cholecystitis. One late symptom may be obstructive jaundice. Cholestasis, however, can also have other causes (Fig. 9.**58a**). One possibility is a small cholangiocarcinoma located at the bifurcation of the common hepatic duct (*Klatskin tumor*) that can cause severe cholestasis (Fig. 9.**58b**).

❗ Small tumors can obstruct and dilate the biliary system without themselves being detectable on CT.

Gallbladder Carcinoma

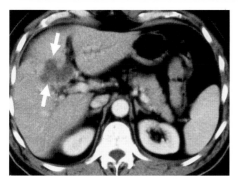

Fig. 9.**57** The tumor is located in the bed of the gallbladder (arrows); it infiltrates the adjacent structures and shows little enhancement after contrast administration.

Biliary Obstruction

a

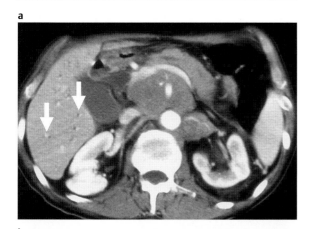

b

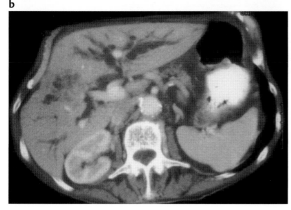

Fig. 9.**58 a** If the dilated biliary ducts are detectable alongside the vessels (arrows) this is called the "shotgun sign." Come back to this image after you have seen the next case to find the cause of the biliary obstruction—or are you smart enough already?

vessels.
biliary obstruction and has already infiltrated the mesenteric
There is a carcinoma of the pancreatic head, which causes the

b In another patient with a Klatskin tumor, the biliary obstruction is even more pronounced. The tumor itself remained beneath the detection threshold of CT.

Caroli Syndrome

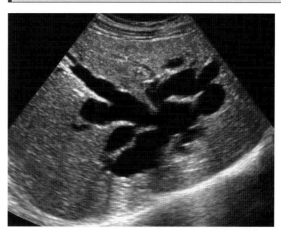

Fig. 9.**59** The extensive dilatation of the bile ducts is well seen. Stones may also be demonstrated with ease.

Caroli syndrome: Caroli syndrome is an extreme and rare form of congenital cavernous ectasia of bile duct dilatations of the biliary system. It is diagnosed very well by ultrasound because the dilatation of the biliary ducts is easily seen (Fig. 9.**59**; see also Fig. 9.**44a**).

→ **Diagnosis:** Joey checks the biliary system and finds it normal in caliber. But the gallbladder bed has a strange appearance. Is this an advanced cholecystitis? And then there is a round lesion close to it in the liver parenchyma! The contour of that lesion is so ill-defined that a cyst seems very unlikely. He adds up all the findings: a carcinoma of the gallbladder with regional metastases in the liver would explain all of it. Giufeng drops by for lunch and agrees—a nice conclusive diagnosis. A week later Mr. Cramp comes back for his staging CT of the chest—a biopsy has confirmed the gallbladder carcinoma.

9.9   Diseases of the Pancreas

Checklist: Diseases of the Pancreas

- Is there a history of alcohol abuse or diabetes?
- Does the patient complain about epigastric pain that radiates to the sides and back like a belt?
- Is there steatorrhea?
- Are the caliber and contour of the pancreas normal?
- Are calcifications present?
- Are the pancreatic ducts dilated or irregular?
- Is there is a definite tissue plane between the pancreas and surrounding structures?

The Case of Timothy Booze

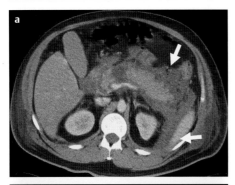

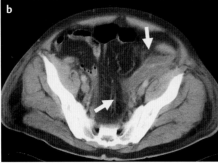

Fig. 9.**60** These are the relevant sections of a CT through Mr. Booze's upper abdomen (**a**) and the pelvis (**b**). Can you think of a diagnosis already?

Disarray of Juices

Timothy Booze (37) is not exactly an uptown boy and life has not been too kind to him. He tends to drown his regular frustrations in alcohol. His fingernails have turned yellow from chain-smoking filterless cigarettes. Yesterday evening he developed constant pain in his upper abdomen. This morning he barely made it to the walk-in clinic of the local city hospital. He simply couldn't take the pain any longer. The physician of the day examines him and then orders a CT to see what's going on in his belly. Hannah is working in the CT unit today and studies the examination. Two of the axial images particularly attract her attention (Fig. 9.**60**).

➜ **What is Your Diagnosis?**

Pancreatitis:

Acute pancreatitis: Acute inflammation of the pancreas is caused by alcohol abuse or blockage of the pancreatic ducts (most commonly by gallstones) in 90% of cases (Fig. 9.**61a**). The extent of the inflammation is best evaluated by CT, but the diagnosis itself is based on the clinical appearance and the laboratory findings—in particular serum amylase and lipase.

Pancreatitis

a Acute pancreatitis

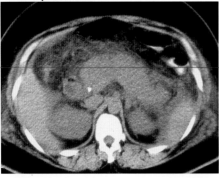

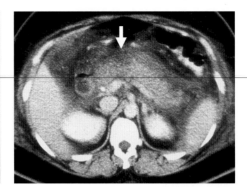

b Chronic pancreatitis

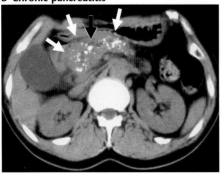

Fig. 9.**61 a** The noncontrast CT scan displaying the corpus and tail of the pancreas demonstrates coexisting swelling and ill-defined margins of the gland (left). Fluid collections extend into the splenic bed. After contrast administration, a perfusion defect in the body of the pancreas is appreciated (right; arrow). This indicates partial organ necrosis. **b** Chronic pancreatitis is characterized by coarse popcorn-like calcifications along the course of the pancreas (white arrows). The pancreatic duct is slightly dilated (black arrow).

Pancreatic Adenoma

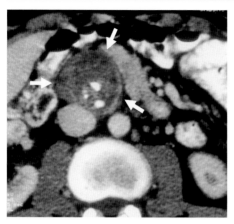

Fig. 9.62   You see here a typical microcystic pancreatic adenoma. The tumor is located anterior to the vena cava and aorta (arrows) and shows characteristic calcifications and small cysts. Histological work-up and verification are necessary in any case.

> ! Not every pancreatitis results in changes of the CT appearance of the gland. Thus pancreatitis cannot be excluded by CT.

Pancreatitis may cause swelling of the gland that may be associated with ill-defined borders. Stranding of the surrounding fat planes develops. The lipolytic and proteolytic pancreatic secretions find their way through the retroperitoneal spaces into and around Gerota's fascia to the kidneys and along the iliopsoas muscle down into the groin. Another commonly affected structure is the mesocolon. Fluid collections, so-called "pseudocysts," can form in and around the pancreas (see also Fig. 7.**11**, p. 108).

> ! The prognosis of the disease correlates with the extent of pancreatic necrosis

Chronic pancreatitis: Chronic pancreatitis is the consequence of recurring bouts of inflammation (Fig. 9.**61b**), frequently in persistent alcohol abuse. Calcifications begin to line the course of the pancreas, the pancreatic ducts (the little side branches in particular) are irregularly dilated, which is easily diagnosed on MRCP.

Pancreatic tumors:

Pancreatic adenoma: A benign adenoma of the pancreas is difficult to differentiate from a pancreatic carcinoma on the basis of imaging alone (Fig. 9.**62**). It should be verified histologically unless there is a very specific history such as Von Hippel–Lindau disease, which is associated with

Pancreatic Carcinoma

a

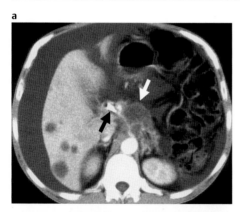

b

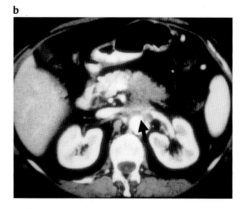

c

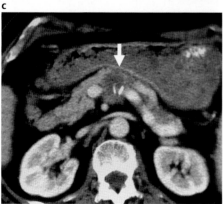

Fig. 9.63 a   This CT section shows an extensive unresectable pancreatic carcinoma. The tumor (white arrow) completely surrounds the celiac trunk. It has caused a biliary obstruction, which has been treated/drained with a biliary stent (black arrow, see the stent tip in the duodenum). Liver metastases and extensive ascites are already present. The reason for the ascites is most likely a peritoneal carcinomatosis. **b** In this patient the cancer infiltrates the duodenum and the para-aortic space (arrow). **c** This tumor alters the organ contour just a little. Only after contrast administration does it become well visible as a low-attenuation lesion surrounded by normally enhancing pancreas (arrow).

multiple pancreatic adenomas. Biopsy is best obtained minimally invasively by ultrasound- or CT-guided percutaneous core needle biopsy or by ultrasound-guided endoscopic biopsy from stomach or duodenal lumen.

Pancreatic carcinoma: Pancreatic carcinoma—when located in the head of the pancreas—becomes symptomatic with painless jaundice in half of cases (Fig. 9.**63a**, **b**). Apart from that the symptoms remain rather nonspecific. Any irregularity of the pancreatic contour is suspicious and should be analyzed with special care (Fig. 9.**63c**). The tumor tends to be hypovascularized in comparison to the surrounding parenchyma. Therefore, multiphasic contrast-enhanced CT or MRI are the best tests to detect its presence. If the celiac vessels, the portal vein and the mesenteric vessels are encased, the tumor becomes unresectable for the surgeon. Therefore the radiologist should carefully examine the relationship of the tumor to the vessels close by and comment on it. Liver metastases are also not infrequent. The detection of a carcinoma within a chronically inflamed organ poses a particular challenge because the pancreatic parenchyma can be scarred from the inflammation and mimic a tumor.

> **!** In the imaging of pancreatic carcinoma, determination of surgical resectability is the primary issue apart from the diagnosis itself.

Islet cell neoplasm: An islet cell tumor, such as an insulinoma or gastrinoma to name the most frequent ones, is normally diagnosed on the basis of the clinical symptoms, which are caused by the hormone production, and with laboratory tests. Imaging is mainly used to localize the tumor preoperatively (Fig. 9.**64**).

→ **Diagnosis:** Hannah has never had any doubt that this must be a case of acute pancreatitis—the clinical history was so obvious. The inflammation is severe in Mr. Booze's case, the fluid collections can be followed all the way into the groin, and a large necrotic defect is present in the body

of the pancreas. Probably pseudocysts will develop in the days to come. Mr. Booze has a few tough weeks ahead of him.

9.10   Diseases of the Peritoneum and Retroperitoneum

> **Checklist:** Diseases of the Peritoneum and Retroperitoneum
>
> • Is the abnormality cystic or solid?
> • Is the abnormality focal (tumorlike) or diffusely infiltrating?

> **Somewhere In Between**
>
> Mary Soames (64) has lost 6 kg within a few weeks. She has not really felt well for more than two months. Joey is the first to have a look at the abdominal CT that was done to find the reason for her weight loss. He notices a lesion in the posterior abdomen that he cannot assign to a specific organ (Fig. 9.**65**). To get to the heart of this he starts with the basics.

→ **What is Your Diagnosis?**

Ascites: Ascites may develop in a number of diseases, *liver cirrhosis* being the most frequent (see Fig. 9.**49b**). Diffuse metastases in the abdomen that sit directly on the peritoneal surfaces also cause ascites (Fig. 9.**66a**). If the peritoneal carcinomatosis is severe, solid tumor nodules and diffuse thickening of the omentum ("omental caking") may be observed (Fig. 9.**66b**, **c**). A paralytic ileus may also ensue (Fig. 9.**66d**).

Islet Cell Tumor

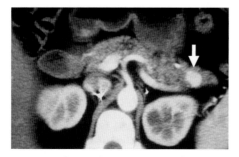

Fig. 9.**64**   This insulinoma (arrow) enhances markedly in the arterial phase of contrast administration. Small tumors can escape detection completely. A nuclear medicine study with radiolabeled octreotide is a very sensitive test to detect even small islet cell tumors. Modern hybrid scanners combine images of the metabolic activity of the tumor with the superb anatomical detail one is acquainted with from CT images.

The Case of Mary Soames

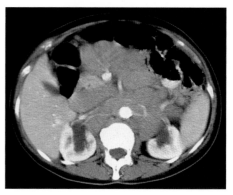

Fig. 9.**65**   Analyze the relevant CT sections of Mrs. Soames. What grabs your attention immediately?

Peritoneal Carcinosis

a

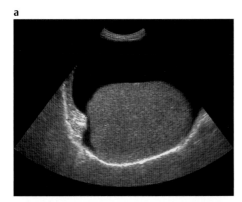

b

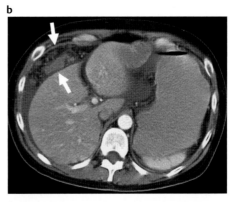

c

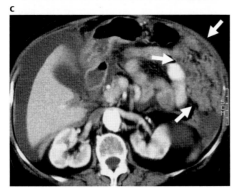

d

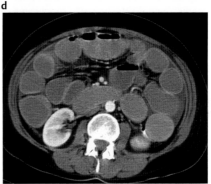

Fig. 9.**66 a** The ultrasound cross-section shows the liver surrounded by ascites. There is a tumor at the underside of the diaphragm. It is a peritoneal metastasis of a pancreatic carcinoma. **b** The CT of another patient shows some tumor nodules in the omentum (arrows) ventral to the liver. **c** The extensive infiltration of the major omentum ("omental caking," arrows) is appreciated on this scan of another patient. **d** In the final stages of extensive peritoneal carcinomatosis a paralytic ileus may develop, which manifests itself in a dilatation of intestinal loops.

> **!** In case of ascites the cause must be found.

Teratoma: A teratoma is an infrequent incidental finding in the abdomen (Fig. 9.**67**). A fatty component and remnants of dental or osseous buds hint strongly at the diagnosis.

Retroperitoneal lymph node enlargement: This is most commonly associated with lymphoma. The nodular structure is typical and they can be discriminated from blood vessels by careful evaluation of successive images and also by contrast administration (Fig. 9.**68**). Some cancers such as testicular cancer can be associated with enlarged lymph nodes in the retroperitoneum next to the large vessels.

Teratoma

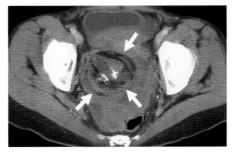

Fig. 9.**67** The fat planes and the calcifications that probably correspond to dental remnants are well appreciated in this case.

Retroperitoneal Lymphoma

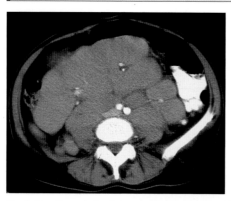

Fig. 9.**68**   The whole abdomen of this patient is filled with en-larged lymph nodes; the mesenteric vessels are surrounded and displaced.

Retroperitoneal fibrosis: This entity is also called Ormond disease (Fig. 9.**69**). It can be induced by medication. Fre-quently, however, the cause remains obscure. Retroperito-neal metastatic disease may look similar; a core needle biopsy may therefore be necessary to verify the histology.

→ **Diagnosis:** Joey has recognized the nodular character of the retroperitoneal mass at once. He considers this to be a lymphoma until proven otherwise. Joey calls up the ward and makes an appointment for a CT-guided biopsy. He hopes, of course, that Dr. Chaban will let him have a go at it. The oncologists are quite happy to get the diagnosis so rapidly and agree to the test.

! Every retroperitoneal tumor needs histological verification.

Retroperitoneal Fibrosis

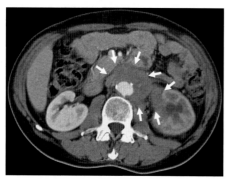

Fig. 9.**69**   The fibrotic tissue in the retroperitoneal space (ar-rows) surrounds the aorta, infiltrates the mesentery, and also involves the renal hilum.

9.11   Gregory's Test

Friday afternoon around 3 p.m., the onrush and ex-citement in the gastrointestinal clinic has died down. McDougal, the technician from Fluoroscopy, has obtained a few of the good old hotdogs from the food shack down-stairs in the lobby. "Watch those breadcrumbs, lads. I don't want them to mess up the developer!" he tells our stu-dents, who are leaning against the x-ray developer unit chewing away quietly. Suddenly the peace is disturbed and backs are straightened. A fair shock of hair appears at the opposite end of the hallway. "It's Blondy the shark," groans Paul. "Quick! Hide the hotdogs!" Giufeng throws him a red-hot angry glance. Gregory strolls over to them and cheerfully hurls a load of x-ray folders on the table in front of the viewbox. "Hi, friends of the opera. Boy, does this smell good. You don't happen to have a spare sausage for this poor fella, have you?" "We're really sorry, Gregory, but there are none left," apologizes Paul with a cold smile. "You can have a bite of mine," Giufeng says into the intense silence. Paul turns pale and Hannah and Ajay fall into a big grin. Greg clears his throat and—very cautiously—bites off a little piece of Giufeng's sausage. "Well, ahem, thanks a lot, Giufeng. Where was I now? Oh yes, well, I have a few cases for you, to get you ready for the weekend as it were. Hey, Paul, how about starting with this one?" "Paul is indisposed," declares Hannah; she pushes Paul back into the second row and positions herself in front of the viewbox. "Show us the beef, Greg!"

Go ahead and try on your own (Fig. 9.**70**)! The last case (Fig. 9.**70n**) is for true intellectuals. You'll find the solutions to the test cases on p. 342.

Test Cases

a This patient has swallowing problems.

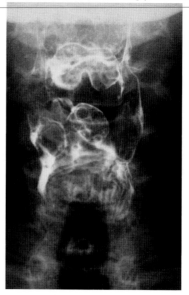

Fig. 9.**70**   ▶

The Case of Joe-James Lee-Chong

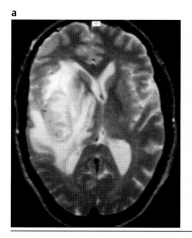

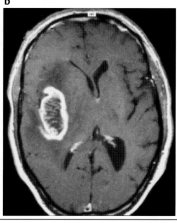

Fig. 11.**12**   Here you see the relevant MRI images of Mr. Lee-Chong. Figure out what kind of MRI sequence images **a** and **b** may be part of.

coronal planes. Now he delves into the complete MRI examination and singles out a representative section (Fig. 11.**12**).

→ What is Your Diagnosis?

Meningioma: Meningiomas are the most frequent intracranial tumors. Their biological behavior is that of a benign tumor, i.e., they do not metastasize. But they can grow over time and press on important neighboring structures in and around the brain and therefore may need to be removed. They originate in the meninges, that is, the periosteum of the skull, the falx cerebri, and the tentorium. Thus they are located extra-axially and are not primary brain tumors in the strict sense. Frequently they involve the skull base. They grow very slowly, often ossify, and expand the neighboring bone and sclerose it. The surrounding brain tissue is rarely edematous. On CT they often appear dense even before contrast is given (Fig. 11.**13**) and they always enhance significantly after intravenous contrast administration. On

MRI meningiomas may be overlooked on noncontrast sequences because they rarely have regressive changes in them and are roughly isointense with brain parenchyma; however, after contrast administration they often show dramatic enhancement (Fig. 11.**14**).

Oligodendroglioma: Oligodendrogliomas constitute about 5% of all true brain tumors of adulthood. They grow slowly, prefer the frontal lobe location, and tend to develop coarse calcifications (Fig. 11.**15**).

Astrocytoma: Astrocytomas (or gliomas) are the most important primary brain tumors. They are classified into four groups (with distinctly different biological behavior and prognosis) that show differences in imaging appearance:

- Grade 1 astrocytomas are also called pilocystic astrocytomas. They occur primarily in children (see Fig. 11.**24**).
- Grade 2 astrocytomas are tumors of early adulthood. They are typically sharply marginated, have little surrounding edema, and enhance only minimally or not

Meningioma on CT

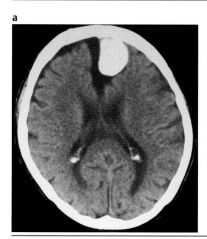

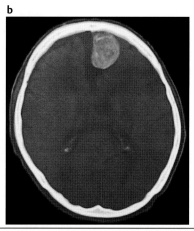

Fig. 11.**13 a**   A noncontrast head CT study clearly depicts the meningioma originating from the falx cerebri. **b** The bone window demonstrates partial calcification of the lesion.

Meningioma on MR Imaging

a

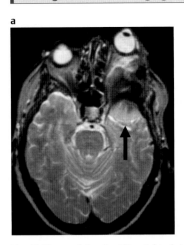

b

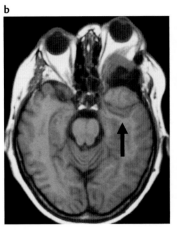

c

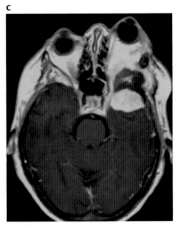

Fig. 11.**14 a and b**   On T2-weighted (**a**) and noncontrast T1-weighted (**b**) MR images you recognize a sphenoid wing meningioma only after a careful analysis of the anatomy. The T2 sequence does not show any associated edema. The soft tissue component is isointense to the cerebral parenchyma (arrow). The adjacent sphenoid wing is expanded and sclerotic. **c** After contrast administration, the situation becomes much clearer: The soft tissue component enhances markedly and is easily differentiated from surrounding normal brain parenchyma. However, the tumor is now almost impossible to distinguish from the orbital fat because no fat-suppression technique was used when this study was acquired!

at all after contrast administration (Fig. 11.**16a**). Morphological differentiation from an infarction is not always possible without a follow-up examination.

- Grade 3 astrocytomas are also called anaplastic astrocytomas. They are tumors of the middle-aged adult. Their margins tend to be diffuse; they are surrounded by considerable edema and accumulate contrast inhomogeneously.
- The grade 4 astrocytoma or glioblastoma multiforme is the most common primary malignant brain tumor. It

predominates in older adults. It is characterized by a pronounced perifocal edema, an intense and frequently serpiginous contrast enhancement, large central necroses, and an unsharp contour (Fig. 11.**16b**). The lesion is difficult to differentiate from an abscess on purely morphological grounds. The tumor has an infiltrative growth pattern and can rarely be resected completely. The part of the tumor that is visible on diagnostic imaging unfortunately represents only the "tip of the iceberg"; at the time of diagnosis, tumor cells have virtually

Oligodendroglioma

a

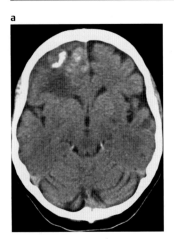

b

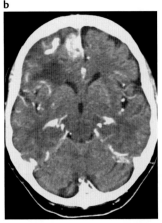

c

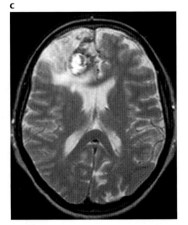

Fig. 11.**15 a**   Noncontrast head CT demonstrates a mass in the right frontal lobe with obvious perifocal edema containing coarse calcifications. **b** After contrast administration, the lesion enhances in an inhomogeneous fashion. This combination of findings is highly suggestive of an oligodendroglioma. **c** The T2-weighted MR image confirms the presence of white-matter edema; the central components of poor signal in the tumor correspond to the calcifications seen on CT.

Astrocytoma

a Astrocytoma grade 2

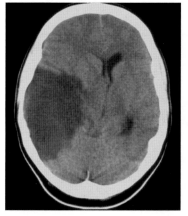 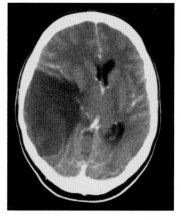

Fig. 11.**16 a** Noncontrast head CT (left) depicts a hypodense, well-demarcated lesion in the right temporal lobe. After contrast administration (right), the tumor, a grade 2 astrocytoma, remains unchanged. A subacute stroke could have a similar appearance. **b** In the T2-weighted sequence (left), edema is seen in the left occipital lobe. After contrast administration, the T1-weighted sequence (right) demonstrates small contrast-enhancing foci, compatible with but not specific for a malignant tumor. This is a grade 4 astrocytoma. Small abscesses, for example, in toxoplasmosis, may look similar.

b Astrocytoma grade 4

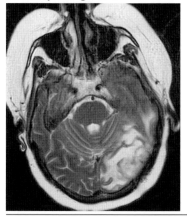 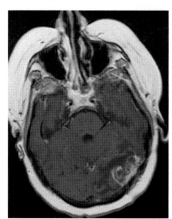

always already spread along white-matter tracts into other parts of the brain, invisible to the radiologist or neurosurgeon.

> ❗ Preoperative imaging of brain tumors requires a complete depiction of their configuration, size, and spatial relationship to important neighboring anatomical structures in three planes with contrast-enhanced T1-weighted sequences.

Hemangioblastoma: Hemangioblastomas occur in middle-aged adults and are preferentially located in the cerebellum. In 15% of cases they are associated with von Hippel–Lindau disease. The typical image appearance is that of a large cyst with a strongly contrast-enhancing mural nodule (Fig. 11.**17**).

Brain metastases: Brain metastases are multifocal in 70% of cases (Fig. 11.**18**). MRI is the most sensitive modality for detection of metastases (Fig. 11.**19**). Metastases are often characterized by extensive perilesional edema and strong contrast enhancement; lung and breast carcinomas are among the most common primary tumors to cause brain metastases.

Hemangioblastoma

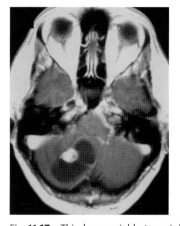

Fig. 11.**17** This hemangioblastoma is located in the right cerebellar hemisphere. The T1-weighted sequence after contrast administration shows the typical appearance of a cyst with a peripheral enhancing nodule.

Brain Metastases

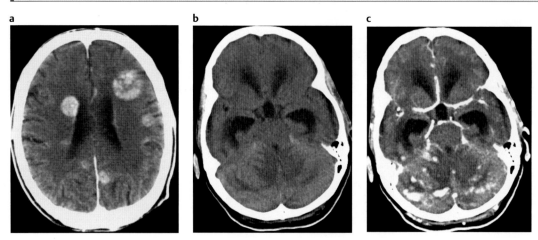

a

b

c

Fig. 11.**18 a**   This postcontrast CT image shows multiple metastases from a bronchial carcinoma. Now the radiation oncologists have to get to work. **b** The exterior CSF space is completely used up in this posterior fossa. A supratentorial obstruction hydrocephalus has developed. The reasons for this are unclear in this precontrast scan. **c** After contrast administration, the metastases in the posterior fossa are delineated with great clarity. The lesions themselves and the surrounding edema led to the obliteration of the exterior CSF spaces.

Detection of Brain Metastases

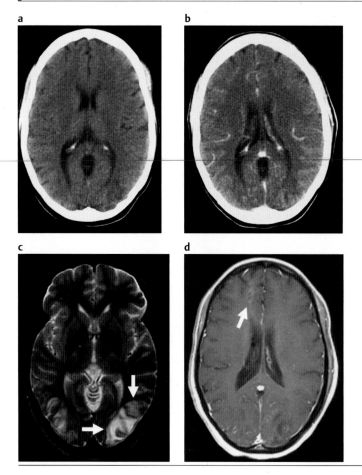

a

b

c

d

Fig. 11.**19**   This image sequence illustrates the differential sensitivity of CT and MRI in diagnosing brain metastases. **a** This noncontrast CT could very well be reported as normal. **b** Even after contrast administration a lesion is difficult to appreciate. **c** It is the T2-weighted MRI that shows the associated edema in both occipital lobes (arrows). **d** The T1-weighted sequence after contrast administration just a little more superiorly suggests a vague contrast accumulation occipitally and another very small metastasis in the right frontal lobe (arrow). These are early brain metastases of a breast carcinoma.

Intracranial Infection

a Tuberculosis

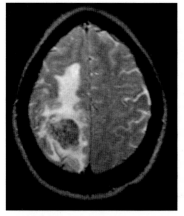
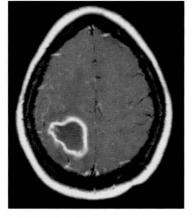

b Toxoplasmosis

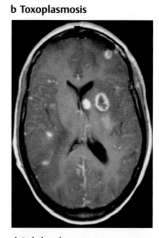

c Invasive aspergillosis

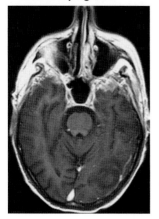
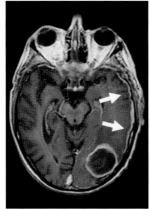

d Subdural empyema

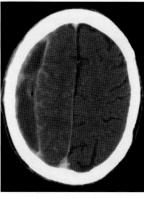

Fig. 11.**20 a** The T2-weighted sequence (left) reveals a tuberculous abscess in the right parietal lobe that is surrounded by extensive edema. In the contrast-enhanced T1-weighted sequence (right), the typical accumulation of contrast in the abscess wall is very well appreciated. **b** Multiple small contrast-enhancing lesions are visible in white matter and subependymally (around the ventricle). Some of them show ringlike structure. This cerebral toxoplasmosis developed in a patient with HIV infection. Based on imaging alone, HIV-associated lymphoma is a possible differential diagnosis. **c** This neutropenic patient with an acute myeloid leukemia has developed a mycotic abscess in the left occipital lobe with no perilesional reaction to speak of even after contrast administration (left). Only two weeks later (right), after the blood marrow has recovered, the patient is able to mount a more vigorous immune response and the same sequence reveals contrast accumulation in the abscess wall as well as along the adjacent meninges (arrows). **d** This chronic subdural hematoma has become infected after a primary and ineffective drainage. After contrast administration, the surrounding leptomeninges enhance significantly.

Brain abscess: A brain abscess develops after the hematogenous spread of septic emboli to the brain (for example, in patients with endocarditis), in immunosuppressed patients, and with direct or venous intracranial spread of bacteria stemming from infected paranasal sinuses (see Fig. 13.**7d**, p. 290) or the mastoid air cells. In an immunocompetent patient, a brain abscess typically shows strong contrast enhancement in the periphery of the lesion and extensive surrounding edema (Fig. 11.**20a**).

Advanced HIV infection, therapeutic immunosuppression after solid organ transplantation, advanced hematological diseases, and aggressive chemotherapy can significantly impair the immune response of a patient and disseminated fungal abscesses may develop (Fig. 11.**20b, c**). These fungal lesions often fail to exhibit the strongly contrast-enhancing abscess membranes that reflect the intact normal immune response in the common bacterial infections. Of course, hematomas can also become superinfected (Fig. 11.**20d**).

Lymphoma: Two percent of all brain tumors are lymphomas. These are particularly frequent in HIV-infected patients. Lymphomas enhance significantly after contrast administration. Morphologically it may be challenging to differentiate them from a glioblastoma or an abscess (Fig. 11.**21**).

Intracranial Lymphoma

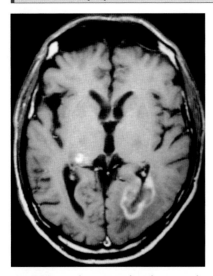

Fig. 11.**21**   In this patient, lymphoma involves the basal ganglia and insinuates itself around the ventricle. Such findings in an HIV patient are difficult to differentiate from toxoplasmosis on morphological grounds. Correlation with laboratory findings helps.

Multiple sclerosis (MS): Multiple sclerosis is a demyelinating disease of early adulthood and of unknown etiology. It may run an acute relapsing or a continuously progressive course. The symptomatology is quite variable, which is why brain tumors must also be excluded as a cause when nonspecific neurological symptoms are encountered. The demyelinated lesions are typically located in the immediate vicinity of the lateral ventricle and are oriented in a centrifugal pattern. In active disease the lesions may accumulate contrast (Fig. 11.**22**). MS is generally diagnosed by CSF analysis.

→ **Diagnosis:** Paul diagnoses a solitary, aggressive, intra-axial primary brain tumor—most likely a glioblastoma. Gregory has to agree: an inflammatory process seems very unlikely on the basis of the patient history. The neurosurgical biopsy performed a few days later unfortunately confirms the suspected tumor type. The Lee-Chongs need a lot of strength now to deal with the dire consequences of this devastating diagnosis.

❗ Brain tumors very rarely metastasize to extracranial locations, but quite a few extracranial tumors metastasize into the head.

Multiple Sclerosis

a

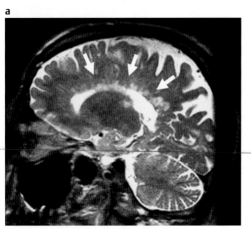

b

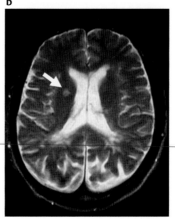

c

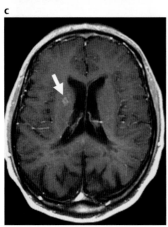

Fig. 11.**22 a**   This parasagittal MR image shows the typical centripetal orientation of the demyelination plaques along the long axis of medullary veins to their best advantage. This phenomenon is sometimes called "Dawson's fingers." **b** The lesions have a high signal in T2-weighted sequences (arrow). **c** In an acute relapse, the lesions tend to accumulate contrast in their periphery (arrow).

The Case of Jerry Flockheart

a   b

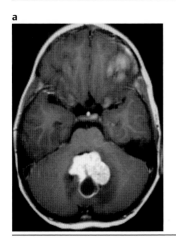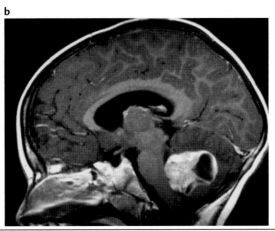

Fig. 11.**23** What comes to your mind when you look at these representative images of Jerry Flockheart's cranial MRI?

Our Child is So Sick

The parents of Jerry Flockheart (8) are extremely worried. The little fellow has repeatedly complained about headaches, cannot walk straight anymore, and has vomited several times during the past week. The pediatrician has immediately requested an MRI. Giufeng and Paul have prepared the frightened boy as well as possible for the examination, especially the long stay in the narrow MR gantry. They want to spare him the general anesthesia that is otherwise necessary. During the examination Jerry's father sits down at the head end of the gantry and talks to him now and then. At last the scan is completed and the first images become available. Jerry has been brave and has kept perfectly still. Both students are eager to view the images on the monitor (Fig. 11.**23**)

→ What is Your Diagnosis?

Pilocytic astrocytoma (see p. 241): Pilocytic astrocytoma, also called grade 1 astrocytoma, is the most frequent brain tumor in childhood. It occurs primarily in the posterior fossa (Fig. 11.**24**) and around the optical chiasm. Frequently the tumor has a cystic component. Its solid parts accumulate contrast intensely.

Medulloblastoma, ependymoma: Medulloblastomas constitute about 20% and ependymomas about 5% of primary brain tumors in children. Both originate in the cerebellum, contain cysts and calcifications, and enhance moderately after contrast administration (Fig. 11.**25**). Both may lead to CSF flow obstruction and thus to a hydrocephalus.

Pontine glioma: This tumor is the third most frequent CNS tumor in childhood (Fig. 11.**26**). It enhances minimally and behaves morphologically like a grade 2 astrocytoma (see p. 241).

Pilocytic Astrocytoma

a   b

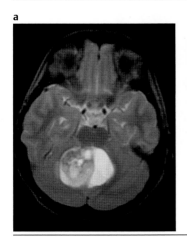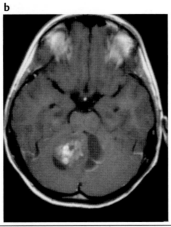

Fig. 11.**24 a** This T2-weighted MR image demonstrates a typical pilocytic astrocytoma. The tumor is partially cystic and lacks surrounding edema. **b** After contrast administration, the solid components enhance significantly.

Medulloblastoma

a

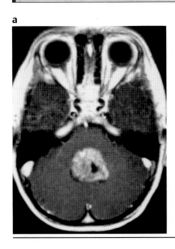

b

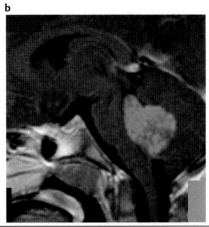

Fig. 11.**25**   The postcontrast axial (**a**) and sagittal (**b**) MR images reveal a mass in or around the fourth ventricle with a small cyst inside. This is a medulloblastoma. Based on its imaging appearance, the differential diagnosis includes an ependymoma.

Pontine Glioma

a

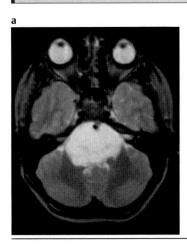

b

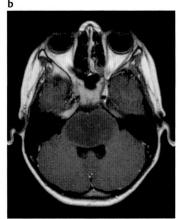

Fig. 11.**26 a**   Massive signal increase and expansion of the pons are very well appreciated on the T2-weighted images. **b** After contrast administration, there is no perceptible enhancement, as is frequently the case in pontine glioma.

Arachnoid cyst: Arachnoid cysts are located extra-axially and as a rule are asymptomatic. They may expand, however, causing headaches in due course. They are preferentially located at the skull base, often in the temporal fossa. In MRI and CT their signal/density follows that of cerebrospinal fluid, with which they are filled (Fig. 11.**27**).

Colloid cyst: This entity is a cystic tumor whose content is rich in protein. It originates in the immediate vicinity of the foramen of Monroe (Fig. 11.**28**). If the tumor blocks the foramen, an obstruction of the physiological CSF circulation results in acute hydrocephalus. This crisis is characterized by a sudden intense headache associated with nausea and emesis. Occasionally syncope ensues. The clinical appearance can be quite characteristic: a young adult suddenly becomes unconscious, falls to the ground, shakes the head and gets up again, becomes unconscious, falls to the ground, shakes the head and gets up again, becomes unconscious ....

Arachnoid Cyst

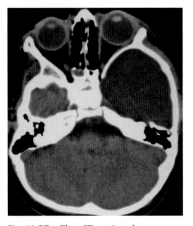

Fig. 11.**27**   The CT section shows a mass of CSF density that has expanded the temporal fossa. This patient suffered from epileptic seizures. Most arachnoid cysts are much smaller and basically represent normal variants.

Colloid Cyst

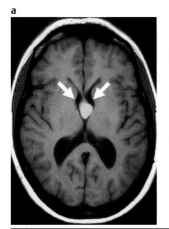
a

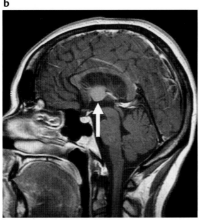
b

Fig. 11.**28 a**   The T1-weighted image beautifully displays this cyst in the area of the foramen of Monroe (arrows) even before contrast administration. It is high in signal because its content is protein rich. **b** This sagittal postcontrast image demonstrates the origin of the cyst (arrow) at the roof of the third ventricle.

Arteriovenous malformation: A congenital vascular malformation may become symptomatic owing to repetitive intraparenchymal and subarachnoidal bleeds. Without therapy the prognosis is dismal. On CT, calcifications within the brain parenchyma point to the diagnosis. MRI shows to advantage the vascular character of the lesion as well as remnants of previous hemorrhages (Fig. 11.**29**). Preferred therapy is minimally invasive occlusion of the lesion by the neurointerventional radiologist (Fig. 11.**30**). This dangerous procedure should only be done by experienced specialists in the field.

→ **Diagnosis:** Giufeng and Paul scratch the back of their heads. This is definitely an infratentorial tumor within or around the fourth ventricle. Medulloblastoma, ependymoma, or a pilocytic astrocytoma? The last is the most probable. A hemangioblastoma would fit morphologically but does not occur in this age group. Gregory comes around and cuts their academic discussion short. "It's gonna have to come out anyway," he says and blows his nose. "For crying out loud, call it a pilo!" Giufeng and Paul are taken aback a little by his cavalier tone—it is a brain tumor in a child, after all. Greg sinks back into his chair: "Listen, folks, for you it is the first pediatric brain tumor. I have been through this a couple of times. You somehow need a little distance from the situation. Otherwise you crack up." He pulls himself up again, adjusts his tie, and walks to the door slowly. "I'm gonna have a word with the parents," he mutters.

Arteriovenous Angioma

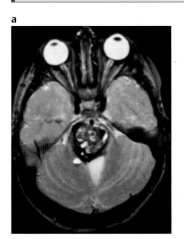
a

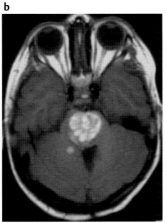
b

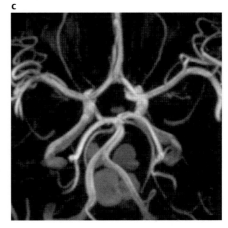
c

Fig. 11.**29 a**   The axial T2-weighted MR section reveals a mass in the pons with very heterogeneous signal. **b** Portions of the tumor also have high signal on the T1-weighted images, indicative of extracellular methemoglobin related to previous hemorrhage. **c** MR angiography (this is an inferior projection of a 3D image) confirms a hypervascular lesion in the pons.

Therapy of an Arteriovenous Angioma

a

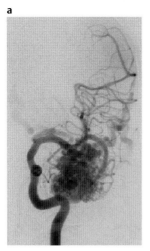

b

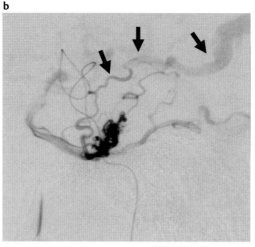

c

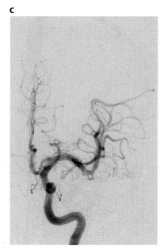

Fig. 11.**30 a** This angiographic image (A-P projection) of another patient shows an extensive vascular malformation in the left temporal region that originates from the middle cerebral artery. **b** Selective angiography with a very fine coaxial catheter shows the angioma and its early venous drainage (arrows) with greater clarity. **c** This angioma was embolized and the normal vascular anatomy was completely reconstituted.

What Should You Pay Attention To in an MR Examination?

The cooperation of the patient is very important in MR imaging because of the long scanning times. In children and uncooperative patients one should make sure ahead of time that they will be able to lie still for the required time and that they will tolerate the unusually loud noises of the gradient coils in the scanner. Individuals who accompany the patient to the examination are permitted to stay in the scanner room but have to follow the same precautionary measures that apply to the patient. Thorough briefing of the patient may save the patient general anesthesia! If general anesthesia is necessary, the whole team should be 100% focused to get all the required information out of the study and to keep the anesthesia time short. And, of course, the lights and the voices in the room should be low.

Perisellar Brain Tumors

Checklist: Perisellar Brain Tumors

- Are there visual disturbances or endocrine symptoms?
- Does the mass originate in the sella or is it extrasellar, compressing the sellar content?
- Is the mass solid or cystic?
- Is the cavernous sinus involved?
- Is the sphenoid sinus normally pneumatized?

The Car Came Out of Nowhere

Cathy Nuremberg (22) has just about recovered from a serious motor vehicle accident that she caused because she ignored someone else's right of way. She feels quite guilty and was relieved when she heard that no one else was seriously hurt. And now she has another problem on top of that: the doctor in the eye clinic whom she consulted merely to get a new pair of ultrachic glasses has sent her for an MRI because something was wrong with her eye examination. The little request note says something about a visual field defect. Paul has talked to Mrs. Nuremberg and is quite eager to see the result of the dedicated sellar MRI (Fig. 11.**31**).

> *Masses in and around the sella can cause endocrine disturbances and characteristic visual field defects.*

→ What is Your Diagnosis?

Tumors:

Pituitary adenoma: Pituitary adenoma is the most frequent sellar or juxtasellar mass. It originates from the anterior pituitary lobe. When a tumor is hormonally active (classic clinical syndromes are acromegaly and Cushing disease), it can be diagnosed early and is frequently very small at the time of diagnosis (microadenoma). A microadenoma does not accumulate contrast as avidly as normal pituitary parenchyma, which is why it appears hypointense in comparison to its surrounding. A hormonally inactive tumor becomes symptomatic as it compresses the neighboring structures (bitemporal hemianopsia, pituitary insuffi-

The Case of Cathy Nuremberg

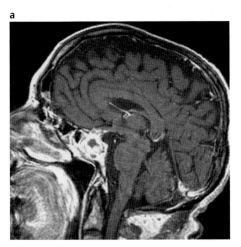
a

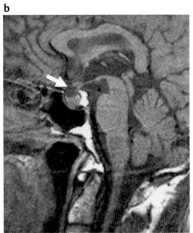
b

Fig. 11.**31 a** Here you see a representative MR section of Cathy Nuremberg's head. Do you notice any abnormalities? **b** Compare her image to this normal sagittal noncontrast MRI section of the pituitary gland. Typically the fine pituitary stalk (arrow) leads to the low-signal-intensity anterior adenohypophysis, which occupies most of the sella, and the smaller high-signal-intensity dorsal neurohypophysis. The brightness of the dorsal pituitary lobe is considered to be due to signal characteristics of its hormone content.

ciency). If the tumor is large it may enhance significantly after contrast administration (Fig. 11.**32**) and invade its vicinity.

> ! After contrast administration, a microadenoma typically appears hypodense in comparison to the surrounding strongly enhancing pituitary gland. A macroadenoma, on the other hand, accumulates contrast rapidly and stands out against the compressed surrounding structures.

Craniopharyngioma: This slow-growing tumor arises from the squamous epithelial remnants of Rathke's pouch in children and young adults. This tumor has cystic, solid, and calcified components as well as a firm capsule (Fig. 11.**33**). From the suprasellar region it can extend into the third ventricle. Compression of perisellar structures may cause bitemporal hemianopia and even pituitary insufficiency may develop.

Miscellaneous perisellar tumors: Metastases to the skull base (Fig. 11.**34a**) as well as regional tumors such as

Pituitary Adenoma

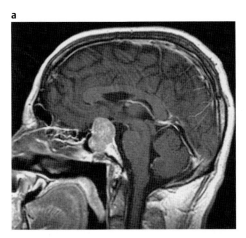
a

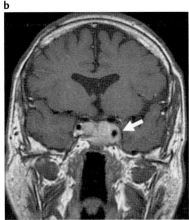
b

Fig. 11.**32 a** Sagittal MRI after contrast administration displays an intensely and homogeneously enhancing tumor that has expanded the sella and presses against the floor of the third ventricle. This is a macroadenoma of the pituitary gland. **b** The coronal MR images document invasion of the cavernous sinus by the macroadenoma and a tumor sleeve extending around the carotid artery (arrow).

Craniopharyngioma

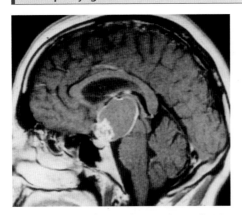

Fig. 11.**33** Sagittal MRI after contrast administration shows a tumor that accumulates contrast intensely in its periphery while its center appears to be cystic. The tumor has invaded the third ventricle. This is a craniopharyngioma.

chordomas of the clivus (Fig. 11.**34b**) or epidermoids (Fig. 11.**34c**) can also lead to compressive symptoms in the perisellar area.

Giant aneurysm: A giant aneurysm can originate anywhere in the circle of Willis and extend cranially, occasionally causing a compression of sellar and/or perisellar components (Fig. 11.**35**).

"Empty sella": The term "empty sella" designates a CSF-filled herniation of the meninges into the sella (Fig. 11.**36**) that can compress, for example, the pituitary gland. A similar situation (and image appearance) may of course develop after sellar surgery.

→ **Diagnosis:** Paul puts two and two together. Mrs. Nuremberg is young and denies any endocrine symptoms. The lesion is primarily cystic and sits in the right location: this should be a craniopharyngioma. Paul is right. The visual field defect is associated with this tumor and its particular location characteristically is a bitemporal hemianopia. In

Other Perisellar Tumors

a Skull base metastasis

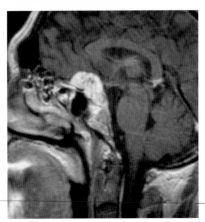

b Chordoma of the clivus

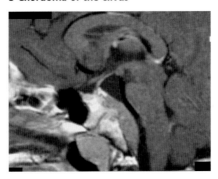

c Epidermoid

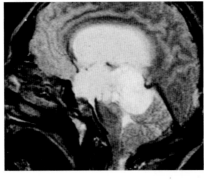

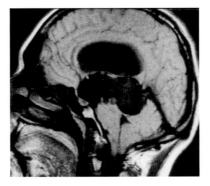

Fig. 11.**34 a** This metastasis from breast cancer is located just anterior to the pituitary. Differentiation from a primary pituitary adenoma is impossible on the basis of imaging alone. Clinical findings and the patient history need to be considered. **b** The clivus just posterior to the sella is expanded and surrounded by a sleeve of strongly enhancing soft tissue. This is

a typical chordoma of the clivus. **c** The cystic epidermoid contains fluid rich in cholesterol that has signal characteristics of CSF on T2-weighted (right) and T1-weighted (left) MR images. This epidermoid has completely obliterated the third ventricle and impinges on the pituitary from a posterior superior direction.

Giant Aneurysm

a   b

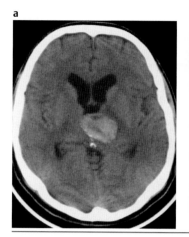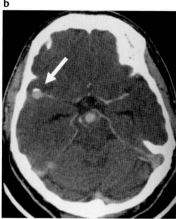

Fig. 11.**35 a** A rounded mass that appears very dense on plain CT impinges upon the third ventricle. **b** Contrast-enhanced CT at a lower level demonstrates not only the lumen of the partially thrombosed giant aneurysm but also an additional aneurysm of the right middle cerebral artery (arrow).

hindsight the accident now also appears in a different light: Mrs. Nuremberg had overlooked a car that came from a side where her visual field is indeed impaired. This is little comfort for the young woman, who now faces cranial surgery. Preoperatively the neurosurgeons want to know about possible invasion of the tumor into the cavernous sinus and get a good idea of the anatomical configuration of this patients' sphenoid sinus, because that is the most practical way to approach and resect the tumor.

Tumors of the Cerebellopontine Angle

Checklist: Tumors of the Cerebellopontine Angle

- Does the mass center within or outside of the porus acusticus?
- Is it cystic or solid?
- Does it merely expand or destroy the bone?

One Ear is Giving Up on Me

Danny Hardware's (54) right ear has been deaf for quite some time. Since he works a pretty noisy steel grinder during the day and likes to spend his evenings playing the drums in his old rock band, he is not really bothered by it. But last week, to his embarrassment, he fell off the stage because of ever increasing dizziness. Now he has had it. The dizziness nags him day and night. A dedicated study of the cerebellopontine angle is performed (Fig. 11.**37**). Pierre, the new third-year student doing a radiology elective, is at Paul's side today. He grabs the images and whips them up on the viewbox before Paul can get going himself. Paul adapts to the situation: "Well now, Pierre, whaddayathink?"

"Empty Sella"

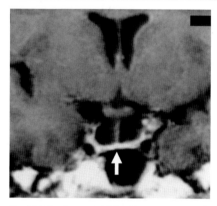

Fig. 11.**36** Coronal MRI after contrast administration illustrates the fine median pituitary stalk and the pituitary gland severely compressed by downward herniation of the meninges (arrow).

The Case of Danny Hardware

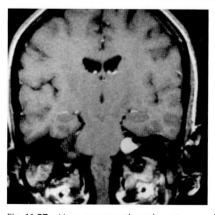

Fig. 11.**37** Here you see the relevant coronal MRI of Danny Hardware's head. Analyze the image. Can you make the diagnosis already?

Acoustic Schwannoma

a   b   c

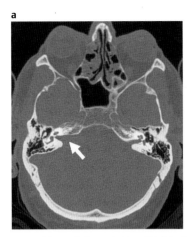
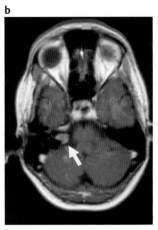
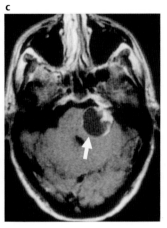

Fig. 11.38 a High-resolution CT of the internal acoustic meatus reveals a funnel-shaped expansion of the right meatus (arrow). **b** The axial T1-weighted MRI after contrast administration documents a small but strongly enhancing tumor at the entry of the internal acoustic meatus (arrow). **c** In another patient, the acoustic schwannoma is a lot larger and partially cystic (arrow).

→ What is Your Diagnosis?

Acoustic schwannoma: The acoustic schwannoma is basically a nerve sheath tumor of the vestibular component of the vestibuloacoustic nerve. It becomes symptomatic with loss of hearing and tinnitus and is also associated with neurofibromatosis type 2. The internal porus acusticus can be expanded over time by the mass (Fig. 11.**38a**). In MRI the intense contrast enhancement of the tumor is very well appreciated (Fig. 11.**38b**). Frequently, cystic components are also observed (Fig. 11.**38c**). Angiographically an acoustic schwannoma usually remains invisible.

Meningioma (see p. 241): This tumor frequently arises from the skull base (Fig. 11.**39**). It does not expand the acoustic porus and appears very vascular on catheter-based angiography.

Glomus jugulare tumor: The glomus jugulare tumor arises from the paraganglionic tissue around the skull base and may erode the tip of the petrous bone (Fig. 11.**40a**, **b**). Patients tend to hear a systolic murmur because the tumor is very vascular. The therapy of choice is neurosurgical, but preoperative embolization is often requested to limit intraoperative blood loss (Fig. 11.**40c**, **d**).

→ Diagnosis:
Pierre is fired with ambition. Frantically he leafs through the large book on neuro-MRI that he has found in one of the drawers. After a few minutes he looks up: "Textbook example of an acoustic schwannoma!" he declares triumphantly with his elegant French accent. "Right you are," growls Paul. Gregory stops by on his way to the neurointerventional suite: "Hey, a typical janitor's lesion!" Pierre is puzzled and for an explanation turns to Paul, who gives him a secretive glance: "Gregory thinks that this a lesion so easy to see that even the cleaning lady can diagnose it. 'Janitor' means 'concierge,' Pierre. Gregory

picked that up when he was in New England for, oh let's see, Greg, was it three or four weeks that you 'worked' in Boston?" he asks Gregory slyly. Greg ignores Paul and hurries on to his original destination. Pierre hasn't lost the big grin on his face: "A 'istological diagnosis is a 'istological diagnosis," he says, unperturbed.

> ❗ B.i.Bs—people who have "Been in Boston"—are quite frequent in academic institutions around the world: some of them identify themselves to their peers by wearing bowties. If you want to please them, ask them about the "when," the "where," the "with whom." Remain wry when inquiring about the "how long" as it touches the private sphere in some. The question "what really came out of it" should be reserved for folks with stable friendships.

Meningioma of the Cerebellopontine Angle

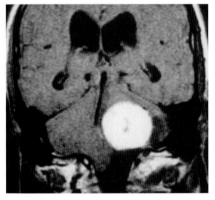

Fig. 11.39 This large tumor considerably enhances with contrast. It does not reach the internal acoustic meatus, in contrast to the typical acoustic schwannoma. This turned out to be a meningioma of the cerebellopontine angle.

Congenital Malformations of the Brain

a Meningocele

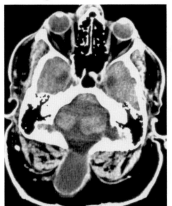

b Dandy–Walker complex

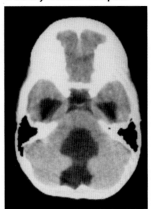

c Arnold–Chiari malformation

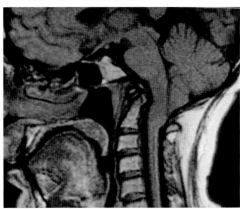

d Agenesis of the corpus callosum

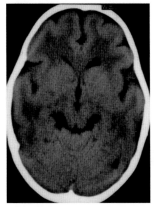

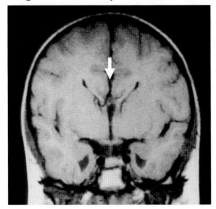

e Pachygyria

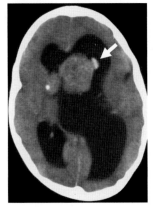

f Tuberous sclerosis

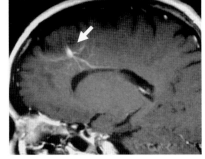

g Venous angioma

Fig. 11.**46 a**   This meningocele presents itself as a dorsal out-pouching of the dura through an osseous defect. The dural pouch is filled with CSF. **b** On this axial CT image the vermis is missing, the fourth ventricle is enlarged, and the temporal horns are dilated considerably, indicative of hydrocephalus. This is a patient with Dandy–Walker complex. **c** Descent of cerebellum and brainstem into the spinal canal is characteristic of the Arnold–Chiari malformation. There is also an associated malformation of the osseous craniocervical junction zone. **d** The corpus callosum is missing completely (arrow, left image) on this coronal MR image (compare the normal anatomy in Fig. 11.**32b**). Agenesis of the corpus callosum leads to a club-shaped dilata-tion of the posterior horns of the lateral ventricles (right image). **e** This 1-year-old, severely retarded child has extremely thick-ened and coarse-appearing gyri. This configuration is termed pa-chygyria. Compare to the normal gyri in Fig. 11.**1a**. The child also suffered from corpus callosum agenesis that caused the club-shaped dilatation of the posterior horns. **f** Tuberous sclerosis is characterized by the formation of tubers (nodules) alongside the ventricular wall (subependymally), which may calcify (ar-row). **g** This median sagittal MR image, which was obtained after contrast administration, displays an atypically thick centripetal vein (arrow). This is a textbook case of a venous angioma.

▶

Congenital Malformations of the Brain

h Sturge–Weber syndrome

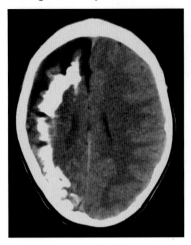
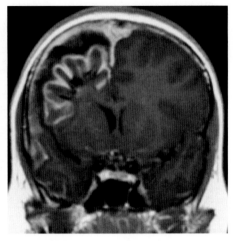

Fig. 11.**46h** In this patient with a Sturge–Weber angiomatosis, the cranial CT reveals extensive calcification of the gray–white matter junctional zone (left), which can sometimes even be appreciated on plain radiography of the skull. The angiomatous region accumulates contrast avidly, as seen on this coronal MR image after gadolinium administration (right). The calcified portion appears as a signal void.

Who Are the Persons behind These Names?

Walter E. Dandy was a neurosurgeon in Baltimore in the first half of the 20th century. He was an assistant to Harvey Williams Cushing and the first to develop a method to look inside the living brain: pneumencephalography. **Arthur E. Walker** was a younger colleague of his.

Julius Arnold and **Hans Chiari** were pathologists in the late 19th century, the former in Heidelberg, the latter first in Prague and then in Strasbourg.

Anomalies of the corpus callosum: Agenesis of the corpus callosum is often associated with other complex brain malformations (Fig. 11.**46d, e**). It can be complete or partial.

Pachygyria: Disturbed migration of the neuronal cells during the embryonal period can interfere with the orderly formation of the brain cortex. This is the case, for example, in pachygyria (Fig. 11.**46e**) where the cortical gyri are thickened and abnormally smooth.

Tuberous sclerosis: This inherited autosomal-dominant disease is associated with intellectual retardation and a facial skin efflorescence called adenoma sebaceum. Subependymal hamartomas are found in the brain parenchyma, which typically calcify partially (Fig. 11.**46f**).

Angioma:
Venous angioma: A venous angioma represents an abnormally prominent vein draining normal functional brain tissue and is not normally associated with any other developmental deficits or symptoms. As a rule these lesions are normal variants without any therapeutic relevance (Fig. 11.**46g**) but they must not be mistaken for an arteriovenous malformation of the brain because their removal leads to venous infarction of the parenchyma drained by this vessel.

Arteriovenous angioma: For details on this entity see above (p. 249).

Sturge–Weber syndrome: This autosomal congenital dominant disease may also occur de novo. Patients may have a cutaneous vascular nevus ("port wine stain"), seen usually along the distribution of the trigeminal nerve, and are mentally retarded. CT or MRI demonstrates an ipsilateral angioma in the parieto-occipital region, which is regularly calcified. The hemisphere is atrophic at the same time (Fig. 11.**46h**).

→ **Diagnosis:** Giufeng and Paul are absolutely convinced that this is a case of Sturge–Weber syndrome. Gregory gives them a big smile: "That is what the anesthesiologist said half an hour ago. Had you been here earlier and looked at the little boy before the study you would have noticed the port wine stain in his face. It is a nice case for us—unfortunately not so for the boy and his parents."

! Congenital brain malformations can be very complex. These patients belong in experienced neuropediatric centers where sound genetic counseling is also available.

11.6   Spinal Cord Tumors

Checklist: Spinal Cord Tumors

- Is there paraparesis?
- Is the spinal cord of normal caliber and of normal signal on T2-weigthed images?
- Is the spinal canal of normal caliber?

If masses are present in the spinal canal

- Is the mass intradural or extradural, intramedullary or extramedullary?
- Is it solid, cystic?
- Is there evidence for peripheral enhancement?
- Radicular symptoms
- Is there any malalignment of the spinal column?
- How wide is the osseous spinal canal? How wide are the intervertebral foramina?
- How extensive is the degeneration of the intervertebral disks, the intervertebral, uncovertebral, and facet joints?

When Both Legs Fail

Ann Ray (45) is brought to the MRI unit on a Sunday afternoon on a stretcher. During the past week she has felt an increasing lower limb weakness. This weekend her legs quit on her altogether. Her desperate husband and the two adolescent kids had called the on-call general practitioner, who immediately had her transferred to the hospital. The neurologist on duty diagnosed an acute paraplegia and asked for an immediate MRI (Fig. 11.**47**). Giufeng and Paul know that this is a classic indication for an emergency MRI—day or night. After the obligatory sagittal scans of the whole lumbar spine, the suspicious area is also examined with axial scans.

→ **What is Your Diagnosis?**

Massive intervertebral disk prolapse: Massive prolapse of a disk can lead to acute paraplegia (Fig. 11.**48**).

Extradural spinal tumor: Typical extradural spinal tumors are multiple myeloma (Fig. 11.**49a**) and lymphoma. Masses originating in parenchymal organs may also invade the spinal canal by direct extension (Fig. 11.**49b**).

Intradural spinal tumor:

Intradural extramedullary spinal tumor: The most frequent intradural *extramedullary* spinal solid tumor is the spinal meningioma. It is a slow-growing tumor that may also expand the spinal canal (Fig. 11.**50a**; see also p. 241). Metastases—often spread via the CSF—also settle in the thecal sac (Fig. 11.**50b**). They are a feared complication, particularly in pediatric tumors of the posterior fossa.

Intramedullary spinal tumor: intramedullary spinal masses tend to be primary CNS-type tumors such as astrocytomas and ependymomas. Metastases are also seen (Fig. 11.**50c**).

Spondylodiskitis: Bacterial spondylodiskitis may be associated with an epidural abscess and can impinge on the thecal sac, resulting in acute paraplegia (see Fig. 8.**41**, p. 143). The involvement of the intervertebral space is characteristic, with a loss of diskal height, loss of vertebral end plate distinction, and strong accumulation of contrast in the periphery of the disk.

Spinal trauma and preexisting spinal canal stenosis: In a stenotic spinal canal even minor trauma may induce major cord damage. This can be due to sudden compression of the whole myelon (Fig. 11.**51a**) or the focal compression of the anterior spinal artery (Fig. 11.**51b**).

The Case of Ann Ray

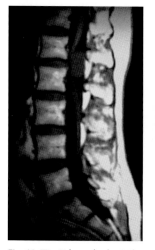
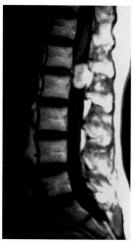

Fig. 11.**47**   Take a look at these representative MR images of Ann Ray. Do you have a suspicion what this could be?

Intervertebral Disk Prolapse

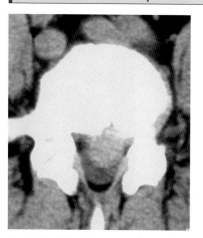

Fig. 11.**48**   The CT section obtained parallel to the vertebral end plates shows severe compression of the thecal sac by soft tissue isodense to intervertebral disk substance. This is a massively prolapsed disk.

Extradural Spinal Tumor

a Plasmacytoma

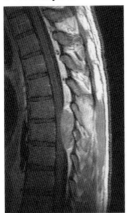

b Pancoast tumor

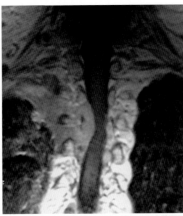

Fig. 11.**49 a** The spinal cord on this sagittal T1-weighted contrast-enhanced MR image is compressed considerably by the soft tissue component of a plasmacytoma. Plasmacytoma frequently causes destruction of the cancellous and cortical bone. **b** The coronary T1-weighted MRI section after contrast administration reveals a Pancoast tumor, a mass originating in the pulmonary apex that may invade the spinal canal through the neuroforamina and subsequently may cause spinal cord compression. Cranially it involves the brachial plexus and can present with Horner syndrome.

Intradural Spinal Tumor

a Spinal meningioma

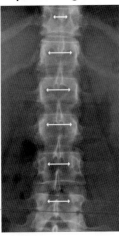

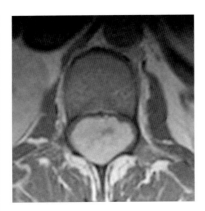

Fig. 11.**50 a** This spinal meningioma is even detectable on the lumbar radiograph (left) because its slow growth has forced the pedicles apart (arrows). The axial T1-weighted MR image obtained after contrast administration (right) displays the avidly enhancing tumor, which has expanded the spinal canal. **b** A number of smaller and one larger metastases of an esophageal carcinoma are seen here studding the spinal cord. The primary tumor has directly invaded the spinal canal at a higher level. **c** After contrast administration, the intra-axial spinal metastasis of a breast carcinoma is very well appreciated.

b Thecal metastatic disease

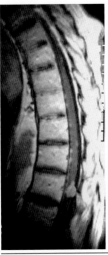

c Metastatic disease involving the spinal cord

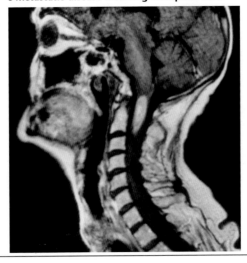

Test Cases

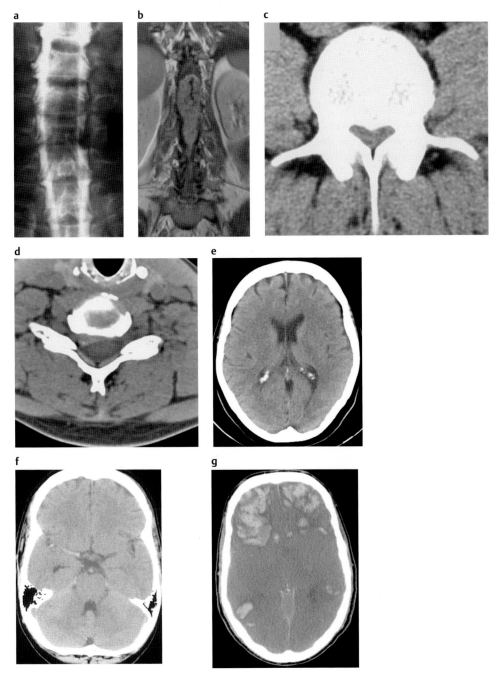

Fig. 11.**57 a–g**   All histories are withheld.

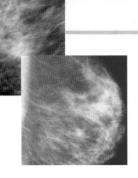

12 Breast

The radiological examination of the female breast (mammography) assumes a very special status within the spectrum of all imaging modalities, for several reasons. First of all, it is a pure soft tissue examination with which ultrafine calcifications are supposed to be detected. For that reason it is performed with a much lower exposure voltage than normal in projection radiography (25–32 kVp) (see p. 34).

> **!** With this technology carcinomas can be found that are only a few millimeters in size. Nowhere else in the body can current radiology hope to achieve anything like that.

Secondly, the contact between the radiologist and the patient is particularly close—something that is not the rule in other radiology subspecialties (with the exception of interventional radiology). The time of the examination is often a period of intense psychological stress for the women involved. Within a few minutes a recently palpated breast lump might turn out to be a harmless cyst or a potentially lethal carcinoma with all its implications for the private and professional future of the patient. The resulting turmoil of emotions does not leave the diagnostician unaffected. A clear decision cannot always be reached right away; uncertainty must be carefully considered and explained by the radiologist, who needs to make very specific recommendations for further diagnostic work-up at the conclusion of the encounter with the patient.

Eventually, however, and this is something to rub in real deep, mammography is a modality that can lower breast cancer mortality by up to 40% if done technically well by expert mammographers in the context of a well-organized population-based breast screening program. No other imaging modality even comes close to that kind of extraordinary impact on women's health! Ultrasound and MRI of the breast are secondary but essential auxiliary modalities for evaluation of the breast (Table 12.**1**).

Table 12.1 Suggestions for diagnostic modalities in breast imaging[1]

Clinical problem	Investigation	Comment
Mammographic screening in asymptomatic patients[2]		
Screening <40 years	Mammography	Not indicated because there is no proven benefit to screening of women <40 years old who are not at increased risk of breast cancer. Breast cancer is uncommon under the age of 35 and the sensitivity of mammography for detection of malignancy can be reduced in younger patients owing to dense breast parenchyma.
Screening 40–49 years	Mammography	Women seeking screening at this age should be made aware of the risks and benefits. While cancers can be diagnosed by screening, total benefit to the population of this age group is limited.
	US	Only as special adjunct to mammography in women with dense breasts and those with implants.
Screening 50–64 years	Mammography	Decreased mortality results from regular population-based and quality-controlled certified screening in this age group.
	US	Only as a special adjunct to mammography in women with dense breasts and those with implants.
Screening 65+ years	Mammography	Screening by invitation in some programs until 70 years. Self-referral required in some programs.
	US	Useful adjunct to mammography in women with dense breasts and those with implants.

▶

Table 12.**1 Suggestions for diagnostic modalities in breast imaging**[1] (Continued)

Clinical problem	Investigation	Comment
Family history of breast cancer	Mammography	Evidence of benefit is emerging for women at significantly increased risk in their 40s and appears to outweigh the harm of screening. Screening should only be undertaken after genetic risk assessments and appropriate counseling as to the risks and unproven benefits. Consensus is that screening of women <50 years old with a family history should only be undertaken when the lifetime risk of breast cancer is greater than twice the average. Further guidelines for mammographic and other forms of screening in these women remain under review.
	US	Useful adjunct to mammography in women with dense breasts and those with implants.
Women <50 years having or being considered for hormone replacement therapy (HRT)	Mammography	HRT has been shown to increase density and benign changes in the breast. There is a related drop in sensitivity and specificity and an increased recall rate in screening of such breasts. There is no evidence to support performance of routine mammography prior to starting HRT. Women on HRT 50 years old and over can be appropriately monitored within a regular breast screening program.
	US	Only as a special adjunct to mammography in women with dense breasts and those with implants.
Augmentation mammoplasty (50 years and over)	Mammography, US	As part of the regular breast screening program: mammography is best performed at a static unit as there may be a need for extra (implant displacement) views and US.
Symptomatic patients		
Clinical suspicion of carcinoma	Mammography	Referral to a breast clinic should precede any radiological investigation. Mammography ± US should be used in the context of triple assessment—clinical examination, imaging, and cytology/biopsy.
	US	The modality of choice for women <35 years old. Should be performed at specialist breast clinic.
	MRI	Breast MRI should be considered after histological proof of cancer to exclude multifocality or multicentricity and if disagreement arises between imaging and pathology results.
? Carcinoma recurrence (posttherapy)	Mammography	For detection.
	US	For detection and image-guided biopsy.
	MRI	In ambivalent cases at least 6 months after surgery or 12 months after radiotherapy.
Generalized lumpiness, generalized breast pain or tenderness, or long-standing nipple retraction	—	In the absence of other signs suggestive of malignancy, imaging is unlikely to influence management. Focal, rather than generalized pain may warrant investigation.
Cyclical painful breasts (mastalgia)	—	In the absence of other clinical signs suggestive of malignancy and localized pain, investigation is unlikely to influence management.
Augmentation mammoplasty (clinical suspicion of carcinoma, rupture)	US, MRI	The assessment of integrity of breast implants and potentially co-existing palpable masses requires specialist skills and facilities. MRI is the most comprehensive study.

▶

Table 12.**1 Suggestions for diagnostic modalities in breast imaging**[1] (Continued)

Clinical problem	Investigation	Comment
Paget disease of the nipple	Mammography	Will show abnormality in 50% of women. Helpful to determine the possibility of image-guided biopsy. When invasive disease is confirmed, it influences surgical management of the axilla.
Breast inflammation	US	Can distinguish between an abscess requiring drainage and diffuse inflammation, and can guide aspiration when appropriate.
	Mammography	May be of value where malignancy is possible.

[1] Modified after: RCR Working Party. *Making the best use of a Department of Clinical Radiology. Guidelines For Doctors*, 5th ed. London: The Royal College of Radiologists, 2003.
[2] In many countries quality-assured population based mammographic breast screening is not yet in place.
MRI, magnetic resonance imaging; US, ultrasound.

Is Breast Screening Worthwhile?

Ten of 100 women eventually get breast cancer; three of those die of the disease. Population-based quality-controlled screening (as performed in Sweden, the Netherlands, Australia, the United Kingdom, to name just a few) saves the life of one of these three women. One percent of all women are thus kept from dying from breast cancer. To reach this result, the Dutch health system spends about 1% of its total health budget. Just imagine if the residual 99% of the budget had a similar effect!

12.1   How Do You Analyze a Mammogram?

Always view a mammogram under optimal lighting conditions, that is, with a bright viewbox, well collimated, with a magnifying glass at hand, a hot or bright light on your side, and all of this in a room with low ambient light. To do a bilateral comparison, always put both sides on the viewbox facing each other. Make sure you have a look at previous films, which should also be mounted on the viewbox. If old mammograms exist but are not available to you at the time of image interpretation, perform a preliminary interpretation, request the prior mammograms, and review the images again when they become available. At that time, an addendum to the report should be made. Only image analysis under such strict conditions yields the maximum diagnostic results that we owe our patients.

! Mammography calls for: bright viewbox, bright light, bright brain.

How Do You Evaluate the Image Quality?

The optical density of the film is optimal if you can appreciate the skin contour well with the hot light. The glandular parenchyma should be penetrated to the extent that vessels are discernible even in the densest areas of the breast. Principally the breast images should be as symmetric as possible. Digital mammography systems allow adjustment of some image parameters by the radiologist, which can compensate to a certain degree for suboptimal exposure while interpreting the radiograph. However, this option does not replace careful radiographic technique. The positioning of the breast by the mammography technologist should be such that:

- The mamilla is always imaged as integral part of the skin contour and is seen in profile on the craniocaudal view
- The fatty tissue dorsal to the glandular parenchyma and/ or the pectoral muscle are—if barely—visible on the craniocaudal view
- On the oblique projection the contour of the pectoral muscle runs from the approximate middle of the upper film edge to the approximate middle of the dorsal film edge.

! In mammography, highly motivated, exquisitely trained, and communicative technologists are crucial.

What Do You Have to Pay Attention to in Image Analysis?

First compare the **distribution of the glandular parenchyma** of both breasts: it should be distributed almost symmetrically (Fig. 12.**1a**). Breasts are not always of the same size, however!

When **stellate lesions** are seen (Fig. 12.**1b, c**), try to determine whether they are due to the superimposition of normal parenchymal structures or whether the architecture of the breast is truly disturbed, that is, distorted or scirrhous. Is the stellate figure visible on the second projection? Sometimes a magnified coned-down view is needed to differentiate a real stellate lesion from a summation phenomenon. Spot compression views can also be very useful in this situation: a radiolucent compression paddle is applied to the area overlying the observed stellate lesion. The added focal pressure causes the various layers of normal breast tissue to spread out, while a stellate

Mammogram: Normal Findings

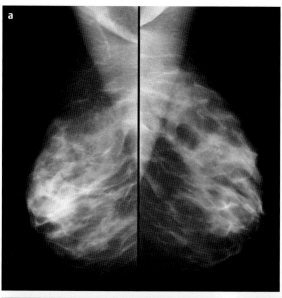

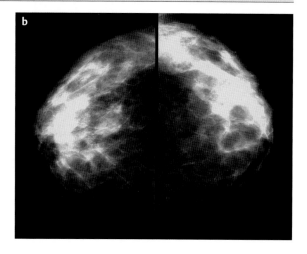

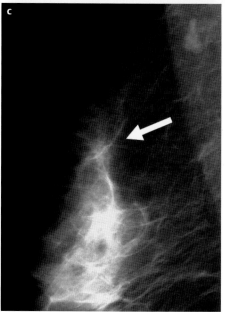

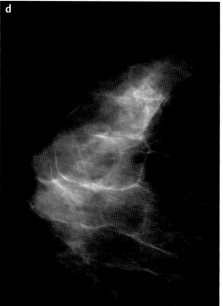

Fig. 12.**1 a** You see the normal medial oblique view of both breasts (note the contour of the pectoral muscle coursing down to the middle of the posterior image margin). The lobulated appearing parenchyma is distributed almost symmetrically in both breasts. **b** On this craniocaudal view the fat tissue posterior to the glandular parenchyma is well appreciated. **c** This oblique view shows a stellate figure (arrow) in the axillary tail of the breast. **d** The structure is invisible on the craniocaudal view. It was due to a superimposition of multiple different normal structures.

cancer will not spread and may in fact become more conspicuous as the superimposed tissue is moved out of the way. Is there a soft tissue mass in the center of the star? Are there any calcifications visible inside?

If there is a **circumscribed soft tissue mass** in the breast, examine its contour with care. Does it have sharp borders all the way around? Do you perhaps see a halo—a narrow rim of decreased density—around the mass? Or do finger-like extensions of the mass seem to infiltrate the neigh-boring tissue? Are there any calcifications associated with the mass?

Finally, the mammograms are searched with a magnifying glass and the skin contour is assessed with a hot light. Again, are there **calcifications** detectable? If yes, are they large and coarse or fine, linear, or branching? Do they follow the normal course of vessels or do they align themselves to the glandular duct system? Magnification views facilitate the analysis of suspicious calcifications.

In a symptomatic patient, a palpable lesion or a positive mammographic finding will be further assessed by an ultrasound examination for further characterization.

Ready for Your First Case? Let's Go!

The mother of Hannah's best and long-time girlfriend has recently learned that she has breast cancer. Hannah has experienced the woman's and the family's constant worry during her visits to the hospital and thus has a very personal interest. She has looked forward to her stay in the breast clinic to learn more about this dreadful disease. She also very much enjoys the contact with the patients, which is much more intense than elsewhere in the radiology department. Dr. Skywang receives her warmly and promises to give her a good introduction into the matter.

The Case of Meg Dyan

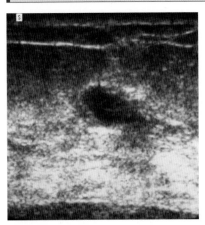

Fig. 12.**2**   This is the relevant ultrasound image of the lesion in Mrs. Dyan's breast.

12.2   Tumorlike Lesions and Tumors of the Breast

Checklist: Breast Tumors

- Are both breasts depicted symmetrically?
- Is the entire breast parenchyma included on the image?
- Are there any masses?
- How do they relate to their neighborhood?
- Do they alter the parenchymal architecture?
- Are microcalcifications detectable?

Horror at Dawn

Meg Dyan (26) is horrified: on Saturday morning, while taking a shower, she has felt a lump in her left breast that she believes was definitely not there before. Her breasts always feel a little lumpy and shortly before her menstrual period they tend to be swollen and painful to touch. But now this! The whole weekend was a mess, trying to get help and information on what this could be. An internet search freaked her out even more. First thing on Monday she got herself an emergency appointment in the breast clinic after talking to on the phone to a trusted colleague and her gynecologist. The mammography technologist sends her directly to the radiologist of the day. Dr. Skywang and Hannah listen carefully to her story, ask about occurrence of breast cancers in her family, and then physically examine her breasts. There is a palpable lump, no doubt about it, about 1.5 cm in size. It is mobile relative to the chest wall. The overlying skin is soft and unremarkable. Hannah scans both breasts carefully with the ultrasound probe under Skywang's supervision and then concentrates on the lump in the left breast (Fig. 12.**2**).

Fibroadenoma

a

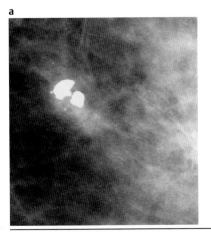

b

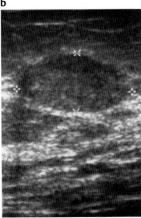

Fig. 12.**3 a**   These coarse calcifications are a typical mammographic finding associated with a fibroadenoma. They are reminiscent of popcorn. The soft tissue mass of the actual adenoma is also visible. **b** Sonographically, a fibroadenoma typically displays a homogeneous internal echo and a regular and smooth border. The echo shadow is minimal, just barely different from the surrounding glandular parenchyma.

No Reason to Panic!

The normal structure of the glandular breast can be so irregular that separate lumps are felt although they represent nothing but variations of the normal parenchyma. This is particularly so shortly before the menstrual period, when the breasts also tend to be rather dense. For that reason any imaging should be performed in the second week of the menstrual cycle.

→ What is Your Diagnosis?

Fibroadenoma: This is a benign tumor of the breast that develops in younger women and then remains in place for a while and often involutes later in life, especially after menopause. In older women, new fibroadenomas are a rarity and are always very suspect. On physical examination, the fibroadenoma is usually a very mobile lesion. As it may grow rapidly and occasionally reaches a spectacular size, patients are often frightened. The mammogram displays the fibroadenoma as an oval and smoothly marginated mass, frequently speckled with coarse calcifications that may remind you of popcorn (Fig. 12.**3a**). Sonographically the appearance of a fibroadenoma is compatible with a solid mass that shows a rather homogeneous internal echo without any dorsal echo shadowing and also a smooth contour (Fig. 12.**3b**). If the appearance of the lesion is not that clear-cut or if there is suspicion otherwise, an ultrasound-guided core needle biopsy is rapidly performed, which usually ends the diagnostic uncertainty.

Cysts of the Breast

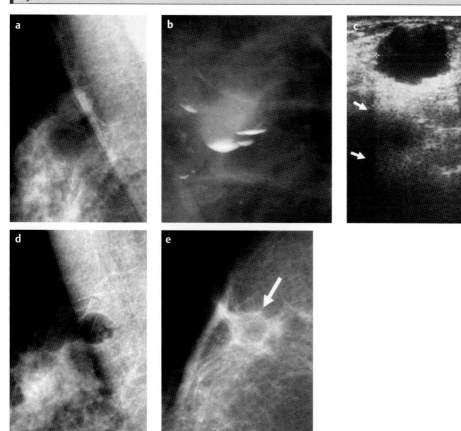

Fig. 12.**4 a**   This cyst projecting over the contour of the pectoral muscle has the typical appearance of a benign lesion: a well-defined and smooth margin along the entire circumference. Could this also be a fibroadenoma? Sure. Can breast cancer be excluded? Not based on the mammogram alone. **b** This lateral magnified view of a breast shows a lamination in some cysts, which are partially filled with milk of calcium—the so-called "teacup" phenomenon. This appearance is pathognomonic for cysts. **c** The ultrasound appearance of cysts is straightforward: there is no internal echo and an increased through-transmission of sound, which causes a segmental hyperechogenicity of the tissue distal to the cyst (arrows). **d** If the cyst has been punctured and evacuated, air is frequently injected into it again. This is done for two reasons: On the one hand, a subsequent mammogram can now image the cyst wall and any tissue previously masked by the cyst content because of potentially equal radiographic density. This is particularly important in large cysts. On the other hand, it is hoped that the air instillation will support the shrinking of the cyst and prevent recurrence. **e** This patient had a breast carcinoma removed two years ago. The patient history makes an oil cyst the most likely diagnosis for this lesion in the tumor bed. The lesion is of fat density and shows a thin capsule (arrow). A lipoma of the breast could also look like this.

Cyst: A cyst often has its origin in dilated glandular ducts or lobules. It can gain size quickly, can become inflamed, and also—but very rarely—contain a cancer. Mammographically it appears in most instances as a well-marginated rounded mass (Fig. 12.**4a**). The cysts may contain "milk of calcium," which causes a characteristic interface between the cyst fluid and small calcific particles layering along the dependent portion of the cyst: this is best observed on mammograms taken with a horizontal beam. This so-called "tea-cup" phenomenon is seen on strictly lateral projections (Fig. 12.**4b**). Occasionally the cyst wall may calcify. On ultrasound a clear-cut cyst shows no internal echogenicity at all and a strong through-transmission of sound (a sector of higher echogenicity directly distal to the cyst; Fig. 12.**4c**). Absolute proof, of course, is provided by the ultrasound-guided puncture and aspiration of the cyst fluid. If any blood residua are perceived within the aspirated fluid, it should be sent to the pathologist for cytological analysis. In older women and in otherwise very dense breasts, the cyst fluid should be replaced by air before the mammography is repeated. On this immediate follow-up mammogram the cyst wall and the immediate neighborhood of the cyst are scrutinized again with special care (Fig. 12.**4d**).

An *oil cyst* is a remnant of an injury to the breast that has caused a hematoma and some focal fatty tissue necrosis. The patient history is, of course, the clearest hint at the true nature of the process. On the mammogram the oil cyst appears as a round mass of fatty density (Fig. 12.**4e**). Sonographically it cannot be distinguished from a simple cyst.

➜ **Diagnosis:** The ultrasound examination has been the definitive modality in Mrs. Dyan's case. Hannah is abso-

Relief

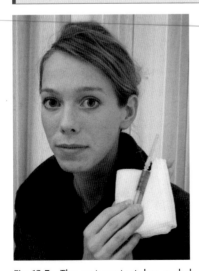

Fig. 12.**5**   The cyst content has a dark coloring, much like Coca Cola. From the look in Mrs. Dyan's eyes you can tell she's been through 2 days of worry and feels a great relief after the diagnosis and aspiration of this benign cyst.

The Case of Nastassja Rimzky I

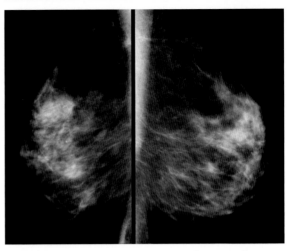

Fig. 12.**6**   These are the mammograms of Mrs. Rimzky.

lutely certain: the mass in Mrs. Dyan's breast is definitely a cyst that has acutely increased in size. A number of other smaller cysts are spread over the rest of the parenchyma. When she tells the patient the good news, Mrs. Dyan takes

Hematoma in the Breast

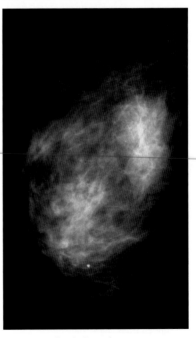

Fig. 12.**7**   This lady underwent a vacuum core biopsy for a suspect breast lesion two days prior to this follow-up mammogram. A rather large hematoma has developed close to the chest wall. Patient history is the key in this case. But beware! Not every injury to the breast is remembered or admitted to. The reverse is also true: if a lump is discovered in the breast, minor injuries are often blamed as the cause. This may be an unnecessary reminder, but patient psychology plays an important role in medicine.

a deep breath and turns her head sideways. As she turns her head back a little later and looks Hannah straight in the face, her eyes are filled with tears. Hannah also feels choked up a bit and smiles warmly to reassure her. The cyst is punctured under ultrasound guidance, and the fluid is evacuated and sent to the cytology laboratory just to be absolutely sure (Fig. 12.**5**). Back in the waiting room, Mrs. Dyan embraces her colleague who has accompanied her.

Tell Me the Truth, Doc!

Nastassja Rimzky (35) has been sent for mammography by her gynecologist. During a routine examination, this physician has palpated a lump in her right breast and sent her for a diagnostic mammogram to further work it up. Mrs. Rimzky had discontinued her breast self-examinations a long time ago. It made her too nervous, she says. She is quite tense now. There is no family history of breast cancer, but her family is rather small. She finds breast compression during mammography quite painful. Hannah studies the films with great care. In the right breast she finds a suspicious mass (Fig. 12.**6**).

→ What is Your Diagnosis?

Fibroadenoma, cyst: These have been discussed above (see p. 273) and may occur in any developed breast.

Scar, hematoma: A scar or a hematoma, either posttraumatic or postoperative, can also have the mammographic appearance of a soft tissue mass (Fig. 12.**7**).

Invasive breast carcinoma: An invasive breast carcinoma can have a variety of appearances. If it has a shaggy or ill-defined border (Fig. 12.**8a**) or if it significantly disturbs the surrounding parenchymal architecture of the breast, this diagnosis is more likely. But breast cancer can also reside inside the parenchyma without any visible involvement of the immediate vicinity; its contour may be sharp and smooth (Fig. 12.**8b**). On ultrasound, acoustic shadowing and an irregular margin are the most frequent findings (Fig. 12.**8c**).

Intramammary lymph nodes: These are particularly frequent in the lateral quadrants of the breast. Mammographically they may be centrally lucent; their contour is lobulated and a little dent may be visible that corresponds to the hilum of the lymph node (Fig. 12.**9**).

Invasive Breast Carcinoma

a

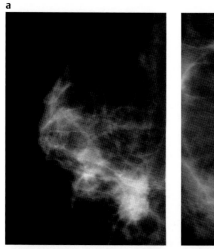 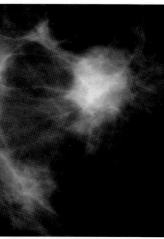

Fig. 12.**8 a** This large lesion (left) has changed the architecture of the neighboring breast tissue. The magnified view in another projection (right) displays the scirrhous extensions of the tumor into the glandular parenchyma. **b** This tumor does not visibly invade the surrounding tissue. Mammographically it could also be a cyst or a fibroadenoma. An ultrasound examination should definitely be performed for further characterization. **c** The ultrasound examination yields crucial additional information: There is definite distal echo shadowing. Cysts fall off the list of differential diagnoses. A core needle biopsy is performed right away under ultrasound guidance. The histological result was an invasive ductal carcinoma.

b

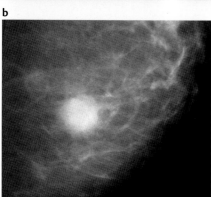

c

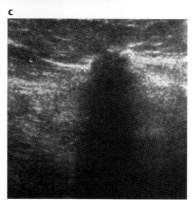

Intramammary Lymph Nodes

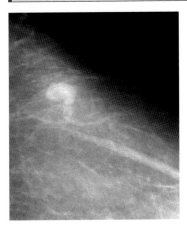

Fig. 12.**9** Lymph nodes typically show a little hilar retraction and a fine lobulation.

→ **Diagnosis:** After some consideration Hannah has little doubt that this lesion is a breast cancer. On the magnified views she has also detected a little calcification, which is the case in up to 40% of all carcinomas (Fig. 12.**10a**). Dr. Skywang asks her to perform an ultrasound of the lesion, which also points towards a malignant character of the lesion (Fig. 12.**10b**). Dr. Skywang advises the patient to have an ultrasound-guided core needle biopsy done. Mrs. Rimzky agrees right away. The final result is available two days later: it is an invasive breast cancer. MRI of both breasts is then performed, which demonstrates several other lesions in close vicinity to the dominant lesion (Fig. 12.**10c**).

> ❗ In more than 40% of mastectomy specimens, pathologists find additional foci of cancer that went undetected by mammography and/or ultrasound. Contrast-enhanced magnetic resonance tomography of the breast can find many of these lesions with great accuracy and reliability.

Mrs. Rimzky undergoes surgery only a few days later. Instead of the initially planned quadrantectomy, a complete mastectomy and axillary lymph node dissection is done. Fortunately the lymph nodes prove to be unaffected.

That Tiny Bit of Calcium

Dorothy Lamour (45) has dropped by the breast clinic to get herself "screened." After being told that the clinic is not part of a breast screening scheme, she pauses for a while, then complains about lumps she has felt in both breasts recently. On clinical examination, Hannah confirms the lumpy consistency of both breasts but cannot find any dominant lesion. Skywang repeats the examination and comes to the same conclusion. Mrs. Lamour does not know of any breast cancer in her family. Mammograms are done and put on the

The Case of Nastassja Rimzky II

a

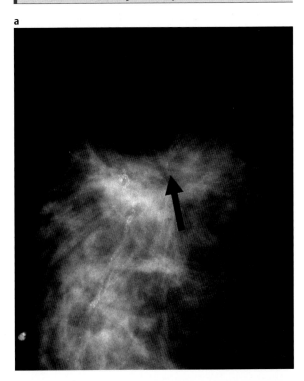

b

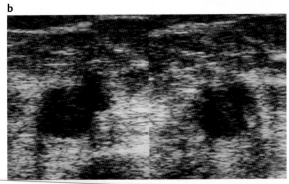

c

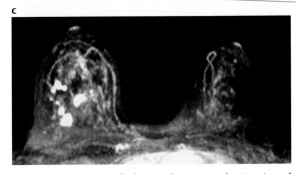

Fig. 12.**10 a** The magnified view documents the invasion of the surrounding tissue by the cancer a little better. There are fine irregular calcifications in the center of the lesion (arrow). **b** Sonographically, Hannah sees an irregularly marginated, partially hypoechoic mass. This is definitely not a cyst. The minimally increased through-transmission does not change her opinion at all. **c** The MRI examination verifies the lesion and finds additional tumors in the same breast.

13 Face and Neck Imaging

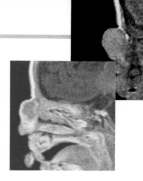

Ear, nose, and throat (ENT) specialists and oral and maxillofacial surgeons consult with radiologists on a regular basis. The ophthalmologists come less often. Classical problems are inflammation of the paranasal sinuses, the dental status, or the localization of metallic foreign bodies in the eye (Table 13.**1**). Any other face, head, and neck imaging problems tend to get very interesting fast. Frequently the neurologists and the neurosurgeons are also involved. Often confirmation of a clinically suspected diagnosis or the further characterization of a lesion or tumor before aggressive therapy is the objective. Facial fractures will be dealt with in Chapter 14 on "Trauma."

Table 13.1 Suggestions for diagnostic modalities in face and neck imaging[1]

Clinical problem	Investigation	Comment
Disease of the nose, the sinuses, the ear, and the salivary system		
Congenital disorder	MRI/CT	Definitive examination for all malformations. CT may be needed to define bone and skull base abnormalities. Sedation or general anesthesia may be necessary for young children.
Sinusitis	XR	Acute sinusitis can be diagnosed clinically. If symptoms persist >10 days, XR or limited sinus CT is indicated. Findings are often nonspecific and encountered in asymptomatic individuals.
	CT	If maximal medical treatment fails, if complications arise (e.g., orbital cellulitis), if malignancy is suspected and surgery is anticipated.
Middle or inner ear symptoms (including vertigo)	CT	Evaluation of symptoms requires ENT, neurological, or neurosurgical expertise.
Salivary gland mass	US	Initial method of choice. Highly sensitive and specific. Can be combined with biopsy.
Diseases of the neck		
Mass of unknown origin	US	First-line investigation for characterization. Can be combined with biopsy.
	MRI/CT	If the full extent of the lesion is not determined in US, for identifying other lesions and staging.
Congenital disorder	See above.	See above.
Diseases of the TMJ and the teeth		
TMJ dysfunction	XR	For documentation of osseous degenerative change.
	MRI	Definitive investigation.
Dental status	XR	To find or exclude dental foci, particularly before immunosuppressive therapy.

A-P, anterior–posterior; CT, computed tomography; ENT, ear, nose, and throat; MRI, magnetic resonance imaging; TMJ, temporomandibular joint; US, ultrasound; XR, radiography.

▶

Table 13.1 Suggestions for diagnostic modalities in face and neck imaging[1] (Continued)

Clinical problem	Investigation	Comment
Diseases of the eye		
Orbital lesion	MRI	Investigation of choice. Beware of metallic foreign bodies.
	US	Consider for intraocular lesions.
	CT	To evaluate the osseous structures and the nasolacrimal duct.
Orbital trauma	CT	When orbital trauma is combined with major facial trauma. Additional 3D reconstructions are very helpful.
Orbital foreign body	XR	Single soft-exposure lateral XR can exclude a metallic foreign body. Additional A-P XR before MRI is considered.
	CT	Required by some specialists if a metallic foreign body is found by XR.
	US	If a foreign body is radiolucent or XR is difficult.
Acute visual loss	MRI/CT	MRI is preferable for suspected lesions of the optic chiasm.
	Angiography	Specialist referral is indicated.

[1] Modified after: RCR Working Party. *Making the best use of a Department of Clinical Radiology. Guidelines For Doctors*, 5th ed. London: The Royal College of Radiologists, 2003.
A-P, anterior–posterior; CT, computed tomography; ENT, ear, nose, and throat; MRI, magnetic resonance imaging; TMJ, temporomandibular joint; US, ultrasound; XR, radiography.

13.1   Diseases of the Nose and Sinuses

Checklist: Diseases of the Nose and Sinuses

Congenital lesions
- Is there are a communication to the subarachnoid space or the brain?

Paranasal sinuses
- Are the sinuses pneumatized normally?
- Are they normally radiolucent? Have they lost volume? Or is there an air–fluid interface?
- Are the bony structures destroyed or displaced?
- What previous surgical procedures have been performed?

That Little Nasal Hump

Agostino Martinez (3) has been brought by his worried parents. He is going to be operated on for a little bulge at the base of his nose that has been present since birth. The surgeons want to know the precise extent of the tumor before they resect it and have therefore requested MRI. Giufeng got the word of this interesting case from Greg, who is all exited about it. She actually manages to be the first to view the images as they pop on the monitor one by one (Fig. 13.**1**). Greg has also told her that it is the extremely complex embryological development of the facial bone with all its pitfalls that makes this examination necessary. Normal fusions, for example, may be delayed or omitted (see Fig. 3.**3**,

The Case of Agostino Martinez

a
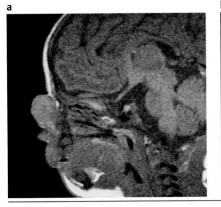

b
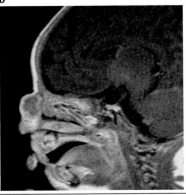

Fig. 13.**1 a** This T1-weighted sagittal MR image shows a lobulated tumor at the base of the nose. **b** After contrast administration, the periphery of the lesion enhances markedly. A communication to the subarachnoid space was not seen on this or on other images in this study.

p. 9) or tissue may be left behind or misdirected on its path of migration. Congenital midline lesions of the face can extend deep into the cranium and ultimately even extend to the subarachnoid space or the brain. Ill-informed surgical procedures may result in serious complications such as cerebrospinal fluid (CSF) leak or meningitis.

Giufeng is mulling over what exactly the problem is with little Agostino and reviews the scan again.

➔ What is Your Diagnosis?

Nasofrontal encephalocele: An encephalocele is a protuberance of the dural sac that contains CSF and brain tissue. It can be located anywhere along the neuroaxis posteriorly (Fig. 13.**2**) as well as anteriorly. If it contains no brain tissue, it is also called a meningocele.

Dermoid: A dermoid consists of ectodermal tissue (epidermal and dermal elements) left behind during an embryological migration process. Its facial variety is found at the base of the nasal ridge and expands the bone there (Fig. 13.**3**). It can also be a component of a nasal CSF fistula.

Nasal glioma: The nasal glioma consists of sequestered brain tissue at the base of the nose (Fig. 13.**4**). It may have a fibrous connection to the subarachnoid space but lacks a communication to the CSF space.

➔ Diagnosis: Giufeng has looked for the relevant finding. There is no apparent communication between the tumor and the CSF space. A defect in the bone is not seen.

Meningocele

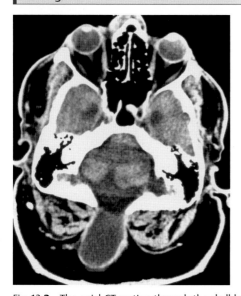

Fig. 13.**2** The axial CT section through the skull base demonstrates a posterior osseous defect through which a dural pouch extends into the subcutaneous tissue. This does not contain any brain tissue.

Agostino's small bulge can be resected in a cosmetically optimal fashion. It is most likely a benign nasal glioma that has no malignant potential and does not tend to recur. Greg, who had been held back by a conversation with the chairman, reviews the case himself and agrees with her conclusions. The Martinez family can calm down again. Pathological examination after resection confirmed the presence of brain tissue in this lesion.

Dermoid

a

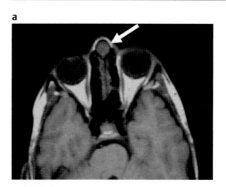

b

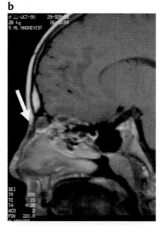

c

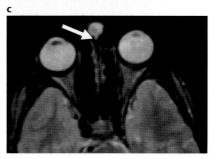

Fig. 13.**3 a** The axial T1-weighted MR image through the nasal base depicts a small tumor (arrow) in the nasal ridge surrounded by signal-free bone. **b** On the sagittal image obtained after contrast administration, there is a suggestion of a cutaneous fistulous tract (arrow) but no evidence for communication with the CSF space. **c** The T2-weighted axial image shows a small dorsal dimple of the tumor (arrow), indicating a possible communication with the intracranial space. Histological examination was compatible with a dermoid.

Nasal Glioma

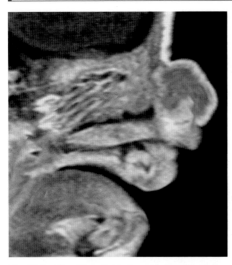

Fig. 13.**4** The T1-weighted sagittal section after contrast administration demonstrates a tumor at the nasal base. A tract to the CSF space is not present. This is a nasal glioma.

A Problem of the Grottos

Sid Cavern (54) has been sent to the radiology department by his doctor to get some sinus radiographs done. The clinician has treated him for a sinusitis for a little while and is worried now because the clinical symptoms have not changed at all despite prolonged therapy. Paul and Hannah are covering the bone unit today. Having gathered a little experience with these patients, they know that two types of radiographs are needed for the proper evaluation of the paranasal sinus: the Waters view (Fig. 13.**5a**) to see the frontal, ethmoidal, and sphenoid sinuses well and the Caldwell view (Fig. 13.**5b**) for the important maxillary sinus. The two interns analyze the radiographs of Mr. Cavern (Fig. 13.**6**). Alternatively, the paranasal sinus can be evaluated with a limited coronal CT. No intravenous contrast administration is needed for this test and a few representative cuts provide a good overview and can exclude a significant inflammatory abnormality. However, in the case of Mr. Cavern, the plain films are well executed and nicely display the pathological finding.

Technique of Sinus Radiography (Caldwell and Waters Views)

a

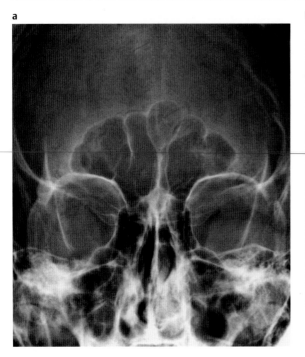

b

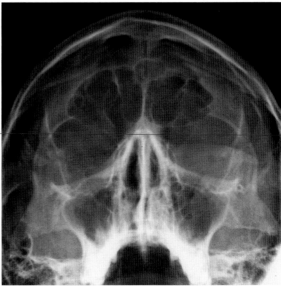

Fig. 13.**5 a** The Caldwell view is obtained by placing the nose and forehead of the patient against the x-ray cassette and by tilting the tube caudally. The image depicts the frontal, ethmoidal, and sphenoid sinuses. The overlying petrosal bone masks the maxillary sinus. By the way, you can see the superior orbital fissure and the round foramen beautifully on this projection. Do you remember which structures run through these openings? **b**

The Waters view is obtained with the chin raised and placed on the x-ray cassette and with the nose 1–1.5 cm off the plate while the x-ray beam stands perpendicular to the cassette. In this projection the frontal and maxillary sinuses as well as the nasal cavity are well appreciated. In this patient there is a cutaneous swelling on the left due to trauma.

The Case of Sid Cavern

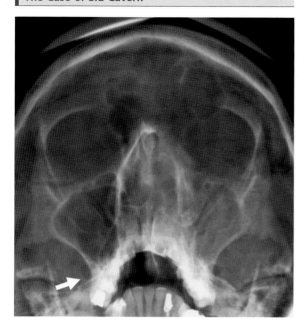

Fig. 13.**6** There is loss of normal radiolucency of the left maxillary sinus. The nasal cavity also appears to be too dense. Is it also expanded? Just to bug you—the oval foramen is well visible on the right side (arrow). The small foramen spinosum immediately lateral to it makes it easy to differentiate from other openings. Which nerve runs through this foramen? Which CSF-filled structure lies directly behind it?

Of course, it is the mandibular division of the trigeminal nerve. And the trigeminal or gasserian ganglion lies behind it.

→ What is Your Diagnosis?

Sinusitis:

Acute sinusitis: Acute sinusitis may go along with a collection of infected secretions in the sinus that can obliterate the sinus completely or partially—an air–fluid level may be visible on the sinus radiographs (Fig. 13.**7a**). Acute sinusitis is mostly viral in nature, but a dental cause must always be considered. If the dental abnormality is not treated or if the drainage of the paranasal sinuses is hampered—owing to stenosed ostia or chronically swollen mucous membranes—conservative therapy may fail. To evaluate which surgical procedure is best suited, a dedicated CT of the paranasal sinuses is necessary because it depicts the osseous septae and the soft tissues with superb clarity. If the sinusitis is left untreated or therapy is unsuccessful, extension into the facial soft tissues (Fig. 13.**7b**) is possible. If the infection reaches the orbit (Fig. 13.**7c**), damage to the optical nerve or the eye bulb may result. If the infection perforates into the cranial vault, the consequences may be fatal (Fig. 13.**7d**). Septic cavernous sinus thrombosis is another feared complication of any serious and long-standing infection in the nasal/paranasal tissues.

Chronic sinusitis: Chronic sinusitis is the end result of recurring or therapy-refractory sinus infections (Fig. 13.**8**). If the perisinusoidal bone is sclerosed and the sinus itself has lost volume, this diagnosis can be made on the basis of imaging.

Acute Sinusitis and Its Complications

a Acute maxillary sinusitis

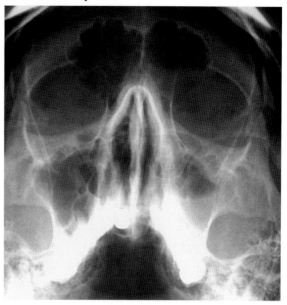

b Perforation into the facial soft tissues

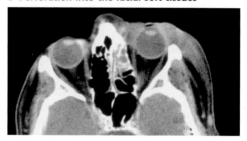

c Perforation into the orbit

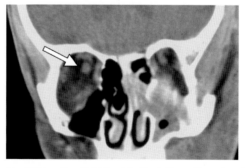

Fig. 13.**7 a** The fluid level in the left maxillary sinus indicates sinusitis if the clinical symptoms fit. A fracture of the maxilla could, of course, also produce such a fluid level when bleeding into the sinus occurs. **b** The axial CT image through the orbits (note the eye lenses) demonstrates an infiltration of the left periorbital soft tissues as a consequence of a treatment failure in maxillary sinusitis. Nicely depicted are the medial and lateral ocular muscles as well as the course of the optic nerve on the right. **c** This coronal CT image through the posterior orbit—note the optic nerve (arrow) and the orbital muscles on the right—documents the extension of acute maxillary sinusitis into the orbit.

▶

d Perforation into the intracranial vault

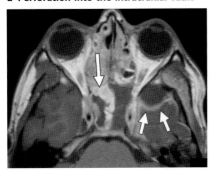
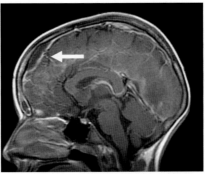

Fig. 13.**7 d** The axial T1-weighted MR image (left) obtained after contrast administration (the content of the eye bulb is dark) shows fluid retention in both sphenoid sinuses with marked mucosal enhancement particularly in the right sinus (long arrow). There is an additional fluid pocket in the temporal fossa (short arrows) that is surrounded by enhancing, swollen meninges. This is a potentially lethal epidural abscess associated with meningitis as a consequence of sinusitis! Note another frontal epidural abscess on the image on the right (arrow).

Benign tumor:

Retention cyst: A retention cyst is a fluid-filled, slowly expansile mass arising from the paranasal mucous membranes that can be found in up to 10% of all adults (Fig. 13.**9a**). Most retention cysts remain clinically silent. They can occasionally erode bone. The cysts may grow out of the maxillary sinus through the ostiomeatal complex and become clinically apparent as choanal polyps.
Osteoma: This benign bone tumor tends to occur in the frontal sinus (Fig. 13.**9b**). The high density of the round or lobulated tumor on the radiograph makes this an easy and definite diagnosis.
Juvenile angiofibroma: Male adolescents may develop a juvenile angiofibroma (Fig. 13.**9c**). This arises in the pterygopalatine fossa and extends into the nasopharynx and can obliterate the sinus. Surgeons prefer embolization of this very vascular tumor prior to resection.

Malignant tumor: If conservative therapy fails or if there is radiographic evidence for osseous destruction (Fig. 13.**10a**), malignant processes need to be considered. To properly evaluate the extent of the tumor, the potential infiltration of vessels, nerves, muscles, and parotid glands as well as the lymph node status for subsequent therapy, MRI is the modality of choice (Fig. 13.**10b**). CT (with 3D reconstructions) is excellent for assessment of osseous structures and operative planning but lacks the superior contrast resolution for soft tissue structures that MRI has to offer.

→ **Diagnosis:** Hannah thinks that chronic sinusitis is the most likely diagnosis. Paul is bothered by the fact that Mr. Cavern has never had problems with his sinuses in the past. They are still discussing as Gregory happens to drop by on his way to the neurointervention suite. He observes that the nasal septum is destroyed and is also alerted by clinical history and the age of the patient:

"This is an aggressive process until proven otherwise, kiddos. Think cancer!" Hannah reluctantly agrees—she simply did not analyze the image with sufficient care. At a second glance it seems so obvious. This won't happen to her again. The histological diagnosis a week later comes back from the laboratory as squamous cell carcinoma.

> Four eyes see more than two. To ask someone with more experience for help is not a sign of weakness … on the contrary it is quite smart. For experienced radiologists it is an honor to help the neophyte—they tend to feel tickled—and you as the neophyte profit from it. But be warned: Radiology is a complex field. "Old hands" may also miss a thing or two—and they know it.

| Chronic Sinusitis

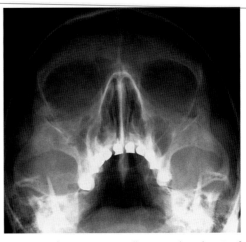

Fig. 13.**8** This Waters view illustrates the sclerosis of the bone and volume loss in both maxillary sinuses in a patient with chronic sinusitis. The left frontal sinus is opacified; the right one is not seen at all.

Benign Tumor

a Retention cyst

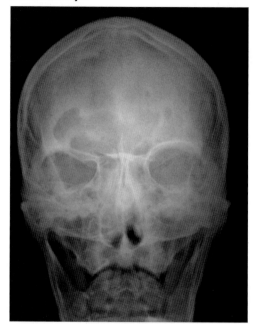

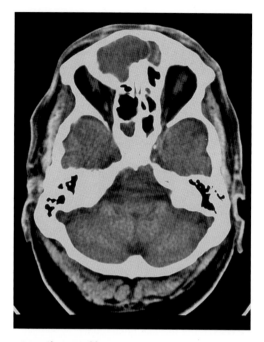

b Osteoma

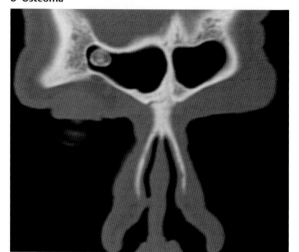

c Juvenile angiofibroma

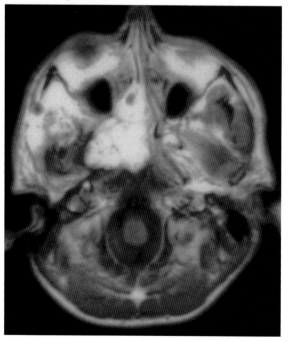

Fig. 13.**9 a**   The anterior-posterior radiograph of the skull (left) documents an expansion of the right frontal sinus with sclerotic margins. The orbital roof is depressed; the left frontal sinus is obliterated. The axial CT image (right) confirms expansion of the right frontal sinus and shows an impressive deviation of the septum to the left. The cause of this is a retention cyst. **b** A coronal CT section displays a round body of osseous density and structure in the frontal sinus, probably extending from the roof of the sinus. It is a typical osteoma. **c** The axial T1-weighted MR image obtained after contrast administration documents a large, nodular mass in the dorsal roof of the nasopharynx. This appearance, together with the clinical findings, is compatible with the diagnosis of a juvenile angiofibroma.

Malignant Tumor

a
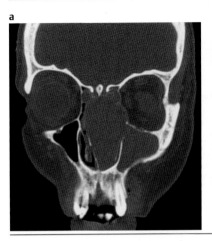

b
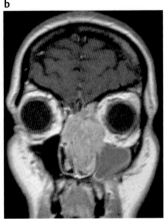

Fig. 13.**10 a** The left maxillary sinus and the nasal cavity are obliterated; the osseous nasal septum, the left sided conchae, and the medial orbital wall (also called lamina papyracea) are destroyed on this coronal CT image viewed in bone window settings. **b** On this coronal MR image after contrast administration, a homogeneously enhancing mass in the nasal cavity and its extension into the frontal sinus are shown. The maxillary sinus was, in retrospect, opacified secondarily to retention of fluid. Are you looking at a T1- or a T2-weighted sequence?

13.2   Disease of the Ears

Checklist: Ears

• Is the mastoid sufficiently pneumatized?
• Are the cells of the mastoid obliterated?

Lucky Song

Carlos Antenna (32) has been fighting a middle ear infection for a couple of weeks. He suffers from pain and his hearing has decreased. He was a bit late to visit his ENT specialist because he has been traveling much lately for professional reasons. He has not really been taking his expensive antibiotics, either, because he left the package at home. Now another spike of fever has forced him to see his doctor again. The colleague immediately referred him to radiology for a radiograph. Hannah has a real close look at the Schüller view (Fig. 13.**11**).

Do You Know about the Schüller Projection?

When performing a Schüller projection, the central x-ray beam (an imaginary line running from the focus on the x-ray anode to the center of the image) is in line with the external opening of the auditory canal of the imaged side. The extent of pneumatization of the mastoid, the distribution and degree of aeration of the mastoid air cells, and the contour of the porus acusticus can be evaluated very well. Dedicated thin-section temporal bone CT is the study of choice for complex problems.

The Case of Carlos Antenna

a
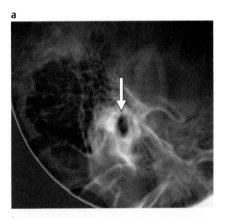

b
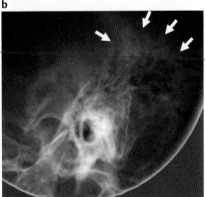

Fig. 13.**11** **a** On the symptom-free side, the mastoid air cells are pneumatized normally posterior and superior to the prominent porus acusticus (arrow), which is surrounded by dense bone. Directly anterior to the porus, the mandibular condyle is seen in its articular niche. The faint arching structure a little above and anterior to the temporomandibular joint is the auricle, which is bent forward for this examination. **b** On the symptomatic side, the upper part of the mastoid is attenuated, which indicates a filling of the air cells with reactive secretions or pus (arrows).

Air in the Mastoid?

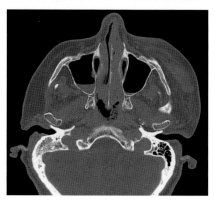

Fig. 13.**12** This patient shows a significantly decreased pneumatization of the mastoid air cells on the right side. Middle-ear infections are much more frequent in this setting. The fluid levels in both maxillary sinuses in this patient were due to trauma.

→ **Diagnosis:** The radiological findings in Mr. Antenna's radiograph confirm the clinical impression of a mastoiditis as consequence of a prolonged middle ear infection. Because of the long duration and Mr. Antenna's fever spikes, the decision is made to perform MRI to exclude extension of the process into the cranial vault. Mr. Antenna finally comes to terms with the gravity of the situation and is quite relieved when the MRI turns out to be normal. He promises to closely follow his doctor's advice in the future. Hannah remembers patients with similar problems she has seen in the weeks gone by. She recalls a CT of another patient that showed significantly reduced pneumatization of the mastoid air cells (Fig. 13.**12**) due to recurrent past ear infections in younger years. She also reminds herself of patients in whom the diagnosis was made by MRI (Fig. 13.**13a**) and where events took a dramatic turn for the worse (Fig. 13.**13b**).

13.3 Diseases of the Temporomandibular Joint

Checklist: Temporomandibular Joint (TMJ)

- What is the relative position of the dorsal disk to the mandibular condyle?
- Does it glide along during mouth opening?
- Is the appearance of the mandibular condyle symmetric?

Chewing and Problem Solving

Isabella Nutcracker (41) is passing through a very exciting phase in her life as an engineer. During her nerve-wracking work in the Sydney cross-city tunnel project she has now developed an excruciating pain in her right facial half. She feels a click when opening her mouth. The head and neck surgeon has sent her for a dedicated functional MRI of the temporomandibular joint to establish the cause of her suffering. Giufeng covers the MRI unit today and is—as usual—very well prepared for the examination.

 What Does Giufeng Know about the TMJ?
She knows that the joint consists of two distinct compartments that are divided by a disk with a dumbbell-like configuration. The disk is suspended by ventral and dorsal ligaments and translates the force from the mandibular condyle to the articular tubercle of the temporal bone. As the mouth is opened, the condyle slides out of the mandibular fossa underneath the articular tubercle. If the mouth is closed, the dorsal part of the disk stands in the 12-o'clock position

Complications of Otitis Media

a Mastoiditis

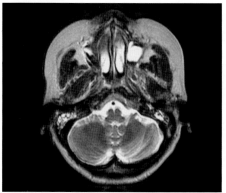

b Brain abscess

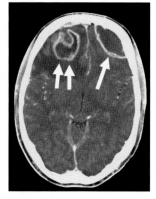

Fig. 13.**13 a** The axial T2-weighted MRI section through the mastoid shows fluid on both sides. This is indicative of mastoiditis. The patient also presented with the symptoms of middle-ear infection. As an unrelated finding the study shows a reten-tion cyst in the left maxillary sinus. **b** In another patient the middle-ear infection has perforated into the cranial vault. An acute and potentially lethal epidural (long arrow) and even an intracerebral abscess (short arrows) have resulted.

relative to the mandibular condyle (**a**); as the mouth is opened it moves to the top of the condyle (**b**). The mandibular condyle may be hypoplastic, the joint may show degeneration. Bear in mind the enormous forces that the small temporomandibular joint must withstand—that explains why this joint is so prone to developing problems.

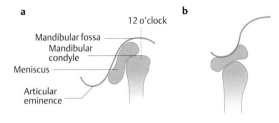

a   b

12 o'clock

Mandibular fossa
Mandibular
condyle
Meniscus
Articular
eminence

Giufeng reviews Mrs. Nutcracker's MRI looking separately at each side with the mouth opened and closed (Fig. 13.**14**).

→ **What is Your Diagnosis?**

Luxation: In *fixed luxation* the disk remains anterior to the mandibular condyle no matter whether the mouth is open or closed, and it is frequently compressed (Fig. 13.**15a**). There are also patients with *intermittent luxation* in whom the disk slides into its normal position when the mouth is opened (Fig. 13.**15b**).

→ **Diagnosis:** The findings are clear in our engineer's case. Both mandibular condyles show a normal configuration. Giufeng diagnoses a fixed luxation of the disk on the right side. She could not find an abnormality on the left. Now the head and neck surgeons must do what they can to give the tunnel project a real shove.

13.4   Injuries and Diseases of the Orbit

Checklist: Injuries and Diseases of the Orbit

Injuries
- Are there intraorbital metallic foreign bodies?
- Are the osseous orbital structures intact?

Masses
- In which compartment (bulb, orbit, skull base, pre-septal or postseptal space) is the mass located?
- Does the mass displace or infiltrate the neighborhood?
- Is there a known primary malignancy?

| **The Case of Isabella Nutcracker** |

a   b

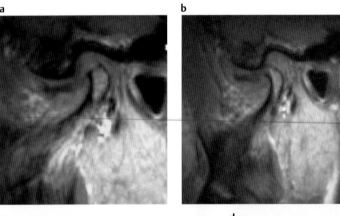

Fig. 13.**14** The images of this study are aligned parasagittally at a slight angle in order to optimally demonstrate the function of the temporomandibular joint. The ventral side is on the left of the image. Images **a** and **b** depict the right joint, **c** and **d** the left joint. First localize the mandibular condyle, then identify its slip track along the articular tubercle, and finally find the low-signal disk. The upper part of the images shows the temporal lobe, the lower posterior part the pneumatized and therefore almost signal-free mastoid.

c   d

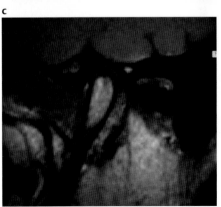
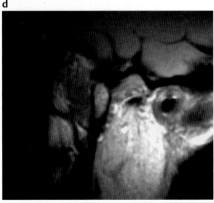

Dislocation

a Fixed dislocation

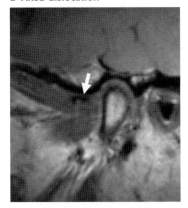
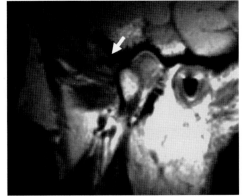

b Reducible dislocation

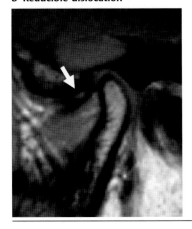
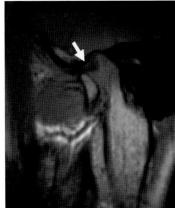

Fig. 13.**15 a**   This disk (arrow) is identified ventral to the mandibular condyle no matter whether the condyle is in the mandibular fossa when the mouth is closed (left) or whether it sits under the articular tubercle when the mouth is open (right). **b** This disk (arrow) is seen anterior to the mandibular condyle (at about 10 o'clock) when the mouth is closed (left). It is subluxed anteriorly. As the mouth opens (right) it assumes its normal translational position between the mandibular condyle—which has now moved ventrally—and the articular tubercle.

Teamwork

Alfried von Trupp und Stahlbach (56) is well known in the world of abstract art for his large, sophisticated stainless-steel sculptures. While he was putting the finishing touches to his latest project "Grand Onlooker" with an angle grinder, his protective goggles fell off and a metallic splinter flew into his eye. The ophthalmologist on call was unable to determine the precise location of the splinter during the ocular examination. His chairman—a great lover of the arts himself—was called but also failed to see the foreign body clearly enough. Joey reviews the orbital radiographs on which the little metal chip is identified very well (Fig. 13.**16a**). MRI is clearly not the modality of choice to establish the precise location of a metallic foreign body—that much he knows. The metallic fragment would be dislodged by the strong magnetic field and further harm would come to the eye. The CT of the orbit (Fig. 13.**16b**) displays the foreign body quite well, despite the artifacts, but the eye surgeons feel that its location relative to the lens and the bulbar axis is still not clear enough for a straightforward atraumatic removal. They ask for a radiograph according to *Comberg*, which is a dedicated examination developed specifically for the purpose of localizing intrabulbar metallic foreign bodies. Now it's Mrs. Koch's turn: she is the most veteran and experienced x-ray technician and she performs the study meticulously under the eager eyes of the whole team (Fig. 13.**16c**). Joey lends her a hand. Have a look at the radiograph. Can you indicate the exact location of the foreign body on the schematic drawing (Fig. 13.**16d**)?

! An experienced, dyed in the wool, motivated x-ray technician is a true treasure. If you show your appreciation of and interest in their work they will support you in your work, too.

That "Evil" Stare

Loretta Hotblood (45) has developed the "evil stare" as she calls it herself. She has noticed that her eyes protrude from the orbit, more so on the right than on the left. In addition, she has difficulties closing her eyelids, which is why her eyes have a tendency to feel dry. Apart from the reactions of other people on the bus and at

The Case of Alfried von Trupp und Stahlbach

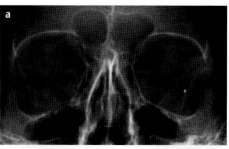

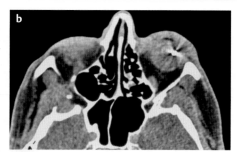

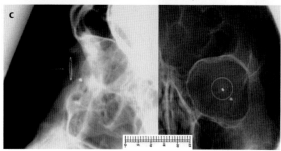

Fig. 13.**16 a**   The radiograph of the orbit clearly shows a foreign body in the left eye. If visible during the clinical ophthalmological examination, it can be removed without further imaging. **b** The axial CT through the orbit also demonstrates the foreign body; however, its precise location relative to the lens and the anterior chamber of the eye remains unclear. **c** The Comberg set aligns itself to the axis of the lens. The foreign body can now be localized relative to the lens axis and the metal ring in two projections.

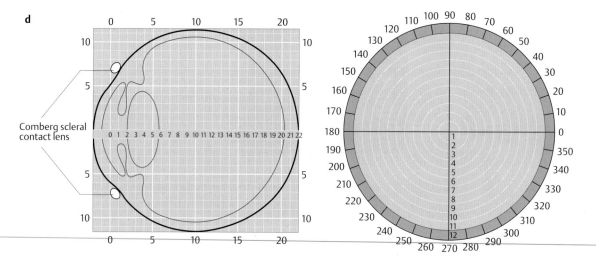

d The metal ring of the Comberg set is indicated in the drawing on the left. The axis of the Comberg set corresponds to the center of the circle on the right drawing. Now go ahead and sketch the foreign body into the diagram.

work, she is bothered particularly by increasing double vision. Her visual acuity has also dwindled. The endocrinologist has diagnosed an endocrine orbitopathy, but conventional therapy has so far not led to any substantial improvement. For that reason, additional radiation therapy is being contemplated. Before this procedure, MRI is indicated to verify the diagnosis, to exclude other causes of exophthalmos, to rule out a potential compression of the optical nerve, and to document the pretreatment status. Paul and Joey cover the examination and analyze the images (Fig. 13.**17**). They know they have to carefully exclude the presence of a number of tumors that may cause exophthalmos.

→ **What is Your Diagnosis?**

Endocrine ophthalmopathy: In endocrine orbitopathy (or Graves disease) the orbital muscles enlarge. The volume of the intraorbital fat increases as well (Fig. 13.**18**).

Things You Can Learn from Graves

Graves was the Irish doctor who first described endocrine ophthalmopathy in 1835 and also one of the first bedside teachers. He was an extraordinary man, his linguistic talents being so extreme that he was taken in custody as a **German** spy in Austria for two weeks when traveling there without proper identification. On another journey, in the Mediterranean, he

The Case of Loretta Hotblood

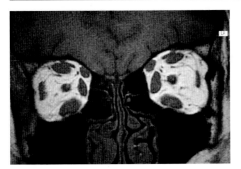

Fig. 13.**17** This MRI sequence with enhancement of the orbital fat depicts a coronal image directly posterior to the eyeball.

Endocrine Ophthalmopathy

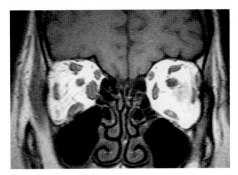

Fig. 13.**18** The coronal T1-weighted MR image through the orbit demonstrates very well the centrally located optic nerve and the enlarged ocular muscles on the left—a typical finding in endocrine ophthalmopathy.

saved a ship and its rebellious crew by taking over command during a storm. The ship suffered a leak, the pumps broke down, and the crew attempted to abandon ship. Graves destroyed the only lifeboat with an axe and repaired the pumps with leather from his own shoes, and all aboard survived. No doubt you know institutions that could do with formidable men like that today.

Carotidocavernous fistula: An exophthalmos may also be caused by a carotidocavernous fistula (Fig. 13.**19a**). This

entity is a posttraumatic or an idiopathic communication between the carotid artery and the venous cavernous sinus that may have a direct mass effect on the retrobulbar orbit and cause locoregional venous hypertension. Prominent filling of the conjunctival vessels and a vascular bruit detectable by auscultation with a stethoscope are pathognomonic. Interventional radiologists have the opportunity to solve this problem with bravery. After documen-

Carotidocavernous Fistula

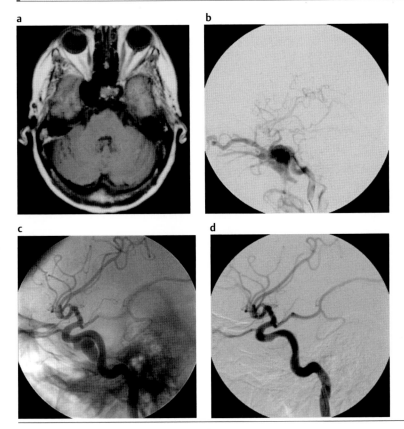

Fig. 13.**19a** This T1-weighted MR image of the skull base displays a large signal-free structure posterior to the right orbit. It is a large vessel segment that certainly does not belong there. **b** A subtraction angiography is performed by administering contrast via a catheter into the right common carotid artery—you can see the catheter tip—and subtracting the precontrast image from the postcontrast images. An enormous dilatation of an artery in the cavernous sinus with early venous drainage is documented. This is indicative of a carotidocavernous fistula. **c** To close the fistula, it is filled with detachable balloons. The rest of the vascular lumen will hopefully thrombose later, but the early venous drainage has already stopped. **d** After the intervention, the subtraction shows a normalized vascular flow.

Meningioma

a

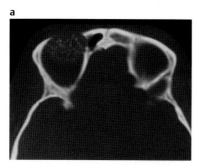

b

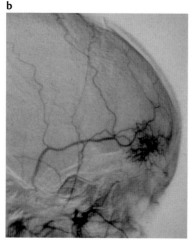

Fig. 13.**20 a**   Review of this head CT in bone windows shows a bizarre calcification below the orbital roof. This is suggestive of a meningioma because these tumors tend to calcify in such a fashion. **b** Angiography reveals the typical spoke-wheel-type vascular pattern of a meningioma.

tation of the large-caliber fistula (Fig. 13.**19b**), detachable balloons can be introduced through a catheter (Fig. 13.**19**c), filled in situ, and left behind, occluding the fistula.

Meningioma: This benign tumor originates from the meninges and is often found adjacent to the sphenoid bone or the orbital roof. It frequently calcifies (Fig. 13.**20a**) and enhances strongly after contrast administration in a typical

Lymphoma of the Skull Base

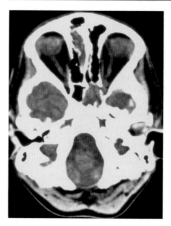

Fig. 13.**21**   This patient complained of an acute decrease of visual acuity on the left. The axial CT section displays the tumor, which extends from the sphenoid sinus into the left orbit and (on other slices) into the optic canal.

spoke-wheel fashion (Fig. 13.**20b**). If surgical removal is contemplated, a preoperative embolization of the richly vascularized tumor by the interventional radiologist is often requested—this time of course not with balloons but with coils or small particles that get caught in the capillaries of the tumor.

Metastases/lymphoma: Metastatic disease and lymphoma must always be considered in the differential diagnosis (Fig. 13.**21**). They often display infiltrative and destructive growth. In Mrs. Hotblood's case, breast carcinoma would be the most likely primary tumor.

Osteopetrosis: Osseous expansion of the orbit and the sphenoid bone may also cause a protrusion of the eye bulb. This is seen with osteopetrosis (or "marble bone disease" [Fig. 8.**30c**, p. 137; see also Fig. 8.**30c**, p. 137)] and Camurati–Engelmann disease (see Fig. 8.**30d**, p. 137), where the bones become denser and enlarge over time. Both diseases are normally diagnosed during childhood. The cranial foramina become progressively narrowed, often resulting in cranial nerve palsy. Involvement of the optic nerve is particularly precarious and is not uncommon.

Osteopetrosis

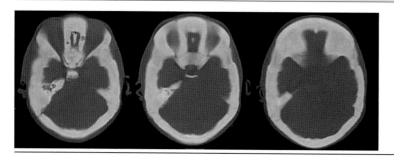

Fig. 13.**22**   The bone windows of this cranial CT show an enormous increase in density and volume of the bone. It is obvious that the osseous foramina will eventually be so narrow that compression of the respective central nerves is inevitable and that the eyeball will be forced out of the orbit.

Plexiform Neurofibroma

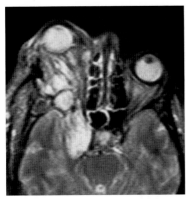

Fig. 13.**23** The axial T2-weighted MR image demonstrates a large mass at the skull base that has invaded and filled up most of the orbit. It presents with a high signal and a nodular structure—a typical pattern for a plexiform neurofibroma.

Plexiform neurofibroma: Finally, a plexiform neurofibroma of the orbit is one of the hallmarks of neurofibromatosis (Fig. 13.23). It manifests during late childhood and frequently also involves the eyelids and the other neighboring soft tissues.

→ **Diagnosis:** On the basis of clinical history and the MR images, Paul and Joey favor typical endocrine ophthalmopathy as the diagnosis. They are right. Radiation therapy may start now.

13.5 Diseases of the Neck

Checklist: Neck Masses

- Is the tumor solid or cystic (centrally necrotic)?
- Is the tumor solitary?
- Does its location correspond to the typical lymph node sites?
- Which anatomical structure does it originate from?

One Swelling Too Many

Sylvester Mascarpone (35) has recently noted a swelling on the right side of his rather muscular neck. The swelling does not hurt, but the cosmetic asymmetry bothers him quite a bit. He smokes a Havana cigar every evening while sitting in front of the fireplace, which is a habit his friends at the gym like to tease him about. Joey helps him to find a comfortable position inside the MRI gantry. Mr. Mascarpone has been a little claustrophobic since he was trapped for three hours in a defective metal costume during filming of his last blockbuster film. Joey explains the course of the examination to him once again, slowly administers half an ampule of diazepam intravenously, and puts a light, bright cloth over the patient's eyes. He also sits down at the other end of the MRI gantry to remain close to the patient. Afterwards, Paul and Joey look at the images together (Fig. 13.**24**). They discuss the potential diagnoses.

→ **What is Your Diagnosis?**

Malignant tumor: In smokers, malignant tumors of the face and neck are frequent (Fig. 13.**25a**). Often they are diagnosed by the patient or clinically before any abnormality can be verified with imaging modalities. This

The Case of Sylvester Mascarpone

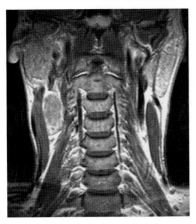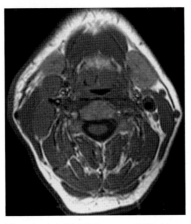

Fig. 13.**24** These are the relevant coronal (**a**) and axial (**b**) MR images of Mr. Mascarpone. Do you see an abnormality?

Malignant Tumor of the Head and Neck

a

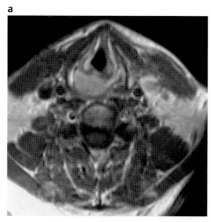

b

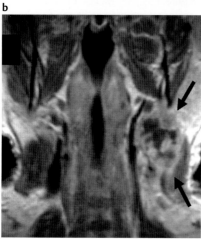

Fig. 13.**25 a**   Contrast-enhanced axial T1-weighted MR imaging shows the approximate level of the vocal cords. The enhancing mass posterior to the airway causes an obvious asymmetry—an essential radiological observation in the complex head and neck area. This proved to be a carcinoma of the hypopharynx. **b** The enlargement and peripheral irregular contrast enhancement of a left sided regional lymph node (arrows) lateral to the signal void of the carotid artery on this T1-weighted image proves the regional lymphatic spread. For your orientation: in the middle of the image you see the airway; cranially on both sides at a distance the relatively signal-free mandibular bone with the masseter muscle lateral and the pterygoid muscle medial to it.

is particularly true for tumors of the oral cavity. Parotid tumors are also often first noticed by the patients themselves. Histopathological examination is required in most cases before a treatment decision can be made; biopsy is facilitated by ultrasound guidance in deep lesions. MRI is the most comprehensive modality to evaluate the local extent and regional lymph node involvement (Fig. 13.**25b**) in patients with head and neck cancer.

Lymph node enlargement: Lymphadenopathy may be due to lymphoma, metastatic disease, or reactive inflammation, for example, in tuberculosis. An ultrasound examination (Fig. 13.**26a**) with subsequent removal of a tissue core

by needle biopsy helps obtain a tissue diagnosis. If lymphoma is diagnosed, staging is best complemented by CT (Fig. 13.**26b**).

Cervical cysts: Congenital malformations such as lateral or median cervical cyst can cause swelling in the cervical region. The *lateral cervical cysts* or *branchial cleft cysts* (Fig. 13.**27**) are remnants of the embryonal set of gills. They are located lateral to the jugular vein and dorsal to the submandibular salivary gland. They often become clinically apparent when an acute inflammation develops inside. A fistulous connection of the cysts to the skin surface may form and prompt a search for the underlying etiology. *Median cervical cysts* originate from remnants of the thyroglossal duct, particularly at the base of the tongue. Clinically the tumor is soft and elastic and moves during swallowing.

Paraganglioma or glomus tumor: Any pulsatile mass of the neck is diagnosed and treated with special caution. A premature core needle biopsy may result in severe hemorrhage. Paragangliomas arise from extra-adrenal

Lymphadenopathy in the Head and Neck Region

a

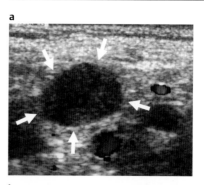

b

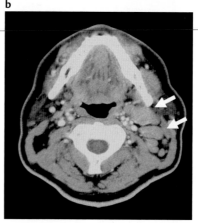

Fig. 13.**26 a**   Ultrasound shows a significantly enlarged lymph node (arrows) in the direct vicinity of the jugular vein. The Doppler signal helps distinguish vessels inside the node and in its neighborhood. This patient had a lymphoma. **b** The CT demonstrates the whole extent of the lymphatic spread dorsal to the mandibular angle (arrows). Multiple nodes of different size are seen. CT of chest and abdomen was subsequently performed for complete staging.

Lateral Cervical Cyst

a

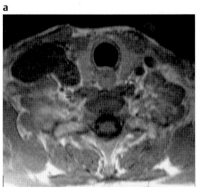

b

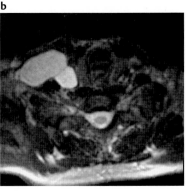

Fig. 13.**27 a**   The axial T1-weighted MR image displays a lesion in the right anterolateral cervical soft issues, nearly homogeneous and low in signal. **b** The T2-weighted, fat-saturated image confirms the cystic character of the mass (fat saturation is incomplete in the posterior subcutaneous fat for technical reasons).

Paraganglioma

a

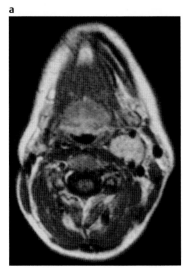

b

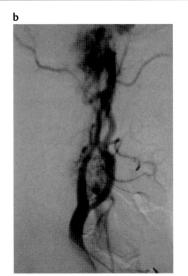

c

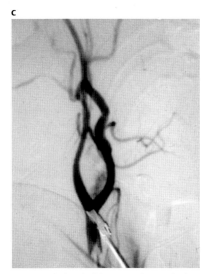

Fig. 13.**28 a**   A strongly contrast-enhancing mass in the left carotid bifurcation is visible in this axial MRI section of the tongue base. **b** Selective angiography with the catheter tip in the left common carotid artery documents several well-vascularized tumors at the bifurcation and the skull base. **c** After embolization with small particles via a branch of the external carotid artery, the vascular blush is gone and chances for a safer and effective curative surgical procedure are greatly improved.

portions of the sympathetic nervous system. They can arise at different levels along the cervical vascular bundle. In Mr. Mascarpone's case a paraganglioma of the carotid bulb would need to be considered. Cervical paragangliomas are typically located at the carotid bifurcation and enhance intensely after contrast administration (Fig. 13.**28a**). Because the lesion is very vascular, a preoperative embolization via the branches of the external carotid artery is often requested by the surgeons (Fig. 13.**28b, c**).

Arteriovenous fistula: Aneurysms or an arteriovenous fistula can also cause a pulsatile mass or bruit anywhere in the body. If the fistula has a large caliber, the arteriovenous shunt volume may induce high-output cardiac failure. The documentation of an arteriovenous fistula (Fig. 13.**29a, b**) and frequently also its therapy—embolization with balloons or metallic coils (Fig. 13.**29c**)—is performed by the radiologist.

→ **Diagnosis:** Joey and Paul have made up their minds. This is definitely a lateral cervical cyst in a typical location. The patient is visibly relieved by the good news. His sedation makes it necessary to keep him in the unit him for a little while before his driver can take him back to the Park Hyatt in his turbo-charged Humvee. The head and neck surgeons will take care of him in due course.

Arteriovenous Fistula

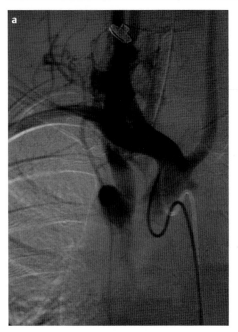
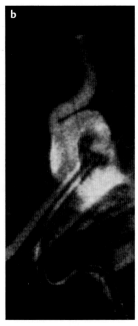
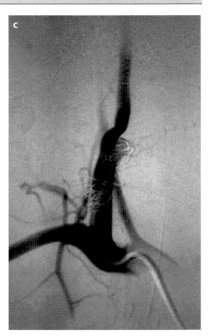

Fig. 13.**29 a**   Angiography with the catheter tip in the brachio-cephalic artery illustrates the immediate venous shunting into the azygos vein system (at the orifice into the vena cava, the contrasts medium is diluted). The first segment of the vertebral artery is significantly dilated by the increased blood flow; its caliber resembles that of a large carotid artery. **b** Selective angiography using an individually angulated projection and with a catheter in the vertebral artery orifice depicts the arteriovenous fistula to its best advantage. The vessel running cranially is the normal segment of the vertebral artery. **c** After embolization of the fistula with metallic coils, normal anatomical blood flow is restored.

13.6   The Teeth You Need

Hank Colgait (35) has been sent by an oromaxillofacial surgeon. Lately he has felt a painful swelling in his left mandibular angle during eating. The colleague has asked for an orthopantomograph (OPG). Orthopantomography is a dedicated and technically sophisticated tomographic technique in which tube and film cassette rotate around the head of the patient. Greg reviews the film (Fig. 13.**30**) and asks our students to have a good look themselves. This patient, he says, has a whole number of diagnoses. Apart from a maxillary fracture about 20 years ago and the loss of several teeth in the course of time he also has:
- A granuloma of the dental radix
- One impacted and another normal "wisdom tooth"

- One intact and one amputated dental bridge and
- The reason for Mr. Colgait's pain

Our students grab the form and assign their observations to the respective teeth. Do you want to have a go at it also?

Maxilla	18 17 16 15 14 13 12 11	21 22 23 24 25 26 27 28
Mandible	48 47 46 45 44 43 42 41	31 32 33 34 35 36 37 38
	Right	Left

Have you sorted it out? The correct answers are found on p. 342.

Table 14.1 **Suggestions for diagnostic modalities in trauma imaging**[1] (Continued)

Clinical problem	Investigation	Comment
Very high risk of intracranial injury ■ Deteriorating consciousness or neurological signs (e.g., pupil changes) ■ Confusion or coma persistent despite resuscitation ■ Tense fontanelle or sutural diastasis ■ Open or penetrating injury ■ Depressed or compound fracture ■ Fracture of skull base	CT (immediately!)	**Urgent neurosurgical and anesthetic referral indicated,** which must be sought in parallel with imaging.
Thoracic and lumbar spine		
No pain, no neurological deficit	No imaging	Physical examination is reliable in this region. When the patient is awake, alert, and asymptomatic, the probability of injury is low.
Pain, no neurological deficit or patient not able to be evaluated	XR painful area	A low threshold for XR when there is pain/tenderness, a significant fall, a high impact MVA, other spinal fracture present, or if it is not possible to clinically evaluate the patient.
	CT/MRI	CT or MRI if XR suggests instability or posterior element fractures or leaves information to be desired.
Neurological deficit ± pain	XR	For initial assessment.
	MRI	Whole-spine MRI is the best method of demonstrating ligamentous injuries, intrinsic cord damage, cord compression, cauda equina injuries, and vertebral fractures at multiple levels.
	CT	Best for detailed analysis of bone injury. Multiplanar and 3D reconstructions are obligatory. Often used in the context of dedicated "trauma spiral" CT encompassing chest and abdomen.
Pelvis and sacrum		
Fall with inability to bear weight	XR pelvis plus lateral hip	Physical examination may be unreliable. Check for femoral neck fractures, which may not show on initial XR, even with good lateral views.
	CT, MRI, bone scan	Useful in selected cases when XR is normal or equivocal.
Urethral bleeding and pelvic injury	Retrograde urethrogram	To show urethral integrity, leak, rupture. Consider cystogram or delayed postcontrast CT if urethra is normal and there is suspicion of bladder leak.
Trauma to coccyx or coccydynia	XR coccyx	Not indicated routinely as normal appearances are often misleading and findings do not alter management.
Upper limb		
Shoulder injury	XR shoulder	Some dislocations present subtle findings. As a minimum, orthogonal views are required.
	US, CT, MRI	Have a role in soft tissue injury
Elbow injury	XR elbow	To show an effusion. Routine follow-up XRs not indicated in "effusion, no obvious fracture."
	CT, MRI	In complex injuries and ambivalent XR.

CSF, cerebrospinal fluid; CT, computed tomography; CTA, CT angiography; CXR, chest radiograph(y); FB, foreign body; MRI, magnetic resonance imaging; MVA, motor vehicle accident; NM, nuclear medicine; US, ultrasound; XR, radiography

Table 14.1 Suggestions for diagnostic modalities in trauma imaging[1] (Continued)

Clinical problem	Investigation	Comment
Wrist injury	XR	Four-view series is needed where scaphoid fracture is suspected.
	MRI, NM, CT	If clinical doubts persist, MRI, NM, or CT are reliable, MRI being the most specific. There is increasing use of MRI as the only examination in complex injuries.
Lower limb		
Knee injury (fall/blunt trauma)	XR	Not indicated routinely, especially where physical signs of injury are minimal. Inability to bear weight or pronounced bony tenderness, particularly at patella and head of fibula, merit radiography.
Ankle injury	XR	Not indicated routinely. Features that justify XR include: the elderly patient, malleolar tenderness, marked soft tissue swelling, and inability to bear weight.
Foot injury	XR	Not indicated routinely, unless there is true bony tenderness or ongoing inability to bear weight. Even then the demonstration of a fracture rarely influences management. Only rarely are XRs of foot and ankle indicated together; both will not be done without good reason. Clinical abnormalities are usually confined to foot or ankle. If XRs are not taken, advise return in one week if symptoms persist. CT is indicated for complex midfoot or hindfoot injuries.
? Stress fracture	XR	Indicated, although often unrewarding.
	NM or MRI	Provide a means of early detection as well as a visual account of the biomechanical properties of the bone.

[1]Modified after: RCR Working Party. *Making the best use of a Department of Clinical Radiology. Guidelines For Doctors*, 5th ed. London: The Royal College of Radiologists, 2003.
CSF, cerebrospinal fluid; CT, computed tomography; CTA, CT angiography; CXR, chest radiograph(y); FB, foreign body; MRI, magnetic resonance imaging; MVA, motor vehicle accident; NM, nuclear medicine; US, ultrasound; XR, radiography

→ Abdominal Ultrasound

Checklist: Abdominal Ultrasound in Polytrauma

- Is there any free fluid in the abdomen? Is there any fluid in the pleural spaces, in the pericardium?
- Are any parenchymal organs visibly injured?
- Is there fluid detectable around the aorta?

Giufeng starts to scan sagittally from the right side of the patient and follows the liver edge to the front, thus displaying Morrison's pouch, the recess between the liver and the right kidney (Fig. 14.1a).

! A sign of a significant visceral organ injury, free fluid in the abdomen is best visualized in Morrison's pouch.

Giufeng cannot find any free fluid and reports this to the keeper of the minutes protocolling all events in the resuscitation room, including the exact time of the US examination. A follow-up ultrasound just 30 minutes later—after circulatory stabilization of the patient (see also Fig. 14.31b)—may show an entirely different situation. Rapidly she scans the liver, both kidneys, the spleen, and the aorta for abnormalities and then checks the pleural space on both sides as well as the pericardium (Fig. 14.1b) for fluid. She pushes the ultrasound unit back into the corner.

→ Radiograph of the Chest

By now the first radiograph of the chest appears on the viewbox (Fig. 14.2). Giufeng's heart races, her mouth is dry. She takes a deep breath and tries to be systematic in her analysis despite all the adrenaline rush of the situation.

Patient A: Ultrasound

a, b Abdomen

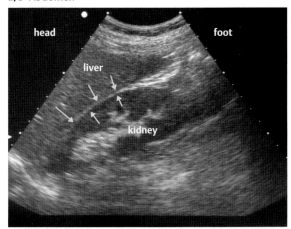

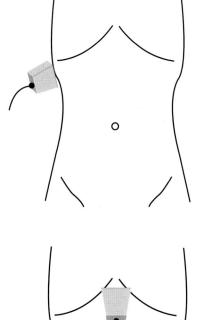

c, d Heart

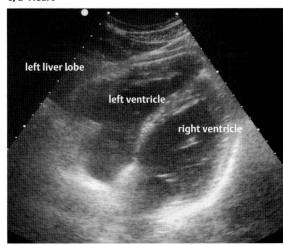

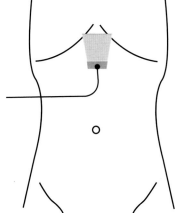

Fig. 14.**1 a** View of the Morrison's pouch. The fine peritoneal recess between liver and right kidney (arrows) is Morrison's pouch. This is where free fluid collects early and where it cannot be mistaken for fluid in any hollow organ. **b** The US probe is located in the superior lateral abdominal wall (sagittal section).

c View of the heart. Do you see the interventricular septum and both cardiac ventricles? Fluid in the pericardium would manifest itself as a dark stripe between the liver and the heart. **d** The ultrasound probe is positioned just inferior to the xiphoid process and is tilted cranially.

Checklist: **Radiograph of the Chest in Polytrauma**

- Is the endotracheal tube well positioned?
- Is there a pneumothorax or even a tension pneumothorax?
- Are central venous lines correctly placed?
- Are there rib fractures, particularly in the region overlying the spleen?
- Is there a pulmonary edema, a lung contusion?
- Is the mediastinum widened? Beware: Patient positioning!
- Is the diaphragm intact?

Is the endotracheal tube correctly positioned? Your first concern must be the endotracheal (ET) tube. Its tip should

ideally be 1.5 cm above the tracheal bifurcation. If it is placed lower, movements of the patient may lead to selective intubation of a main bronchus with a consecutive reduced aeration or even collapse of the contralateral side. Volume loss ensues and eventually displaces the mediastinum to the contralateral side (Fig. 14.**3**). In order not to injure the vocal cords, the tube cuff should be located well inferior to them, around the level of the 5th cervical vertebral body. Are you sure the tube is inside the trachea? A lot of air in the stomach may indicate incorrect intubation of the esophagus, either presently or in the immediate past (Fig. 14.**3**). The anesthesiologist must be alerted to the fact at once and perform clinical examination including auscultation to check ET tube position!

Patient A: Radiograph of the Chest

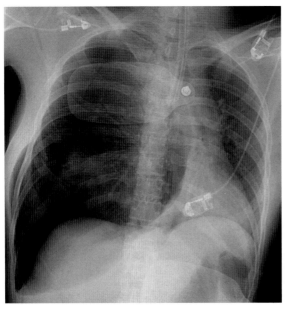

Fig. 14.**2** This is the chest radiograph of patient A. Do you see any abnormality? Use the checklist for your image analysis.

Is there a pneumothorax? The second major thing to consider is the potential complications of the vascular access. If the large internal jugular or subclavian veins are punctured, the lung apex is particularly at risk, especially if several attempts are necessary before venous access can

be established. Is there evidence for a pneumothorax (Fig. 14.**4a**, **b**)? In supine portable CXRs the air in the pleural space moves anteriorly. A fine rim of decreased attenuation along the heart and diaphragm contour may be the only indication of a pneumothorax. There is another sign to look for, however.

> **!** The deep pleural recesses are only reached and unfolded by free air in the pleural space (Fig. 14.**4c**). This is the rather specific "deep sulcus sign" of a pneumothorax.

If there is a tension pneumothorax (Fig. 14.**4d**) that causes a mediastinal shift to the contralateral side, the ventilation of the contralateral lung and the venous backflow into the chest are impaired. Rapid relief of the increased pressure in the pleural space is crucial.

Catheters, textile folds, rib margins, the medial contours of the scapulae, and skin folds (Fig. 14.**4e**) can simulate a pneumothorax because they may look like the outline of the visceral pleura.

> **!** Check for crossing anatomical structures: any "pleural line" that is crossed by pulmonary vessels on their way to the periphery cannot be the pleural outline in pneumothorax.

Are the central venous lines correctly placed? Subclavian or jugular venous lines should harmonically follow the course of the vena cava (Fig. 14.**5a**) and not reach the level of the tricuspid valve (Fig. 14.**5b**) in order to avoid catheter-induced arrhythmias. A catheter to measure the central pulmonary pressure (Swan–Ganz catheter) is advanced through the right heart into the pulmonary

Where is the Tube?

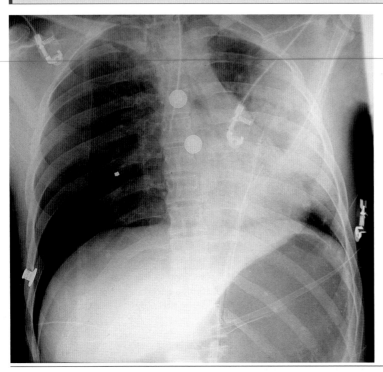

Fig. 14.**3** The tip of the tube is located in the right mainstem bronchus! The left lung is increased in density owing to atelectasis and has lost volume; the mediastinum is displaced to the left. The stomach is significantly overdistended as a consequence of a previous esophageal intubation, which has since been corrected. During the accident or during intubation, the patient has aspirated a dental filling. There is another extremely important finding visible on this radiograph. Do you see it?

Yes, of course, there is a tension pneumothorax on the right. The metal gadgets are ECG electrodes. The fine lines superimposed over the upper abdomen are textile folds.

Pneumothorax

a Pneumothorax

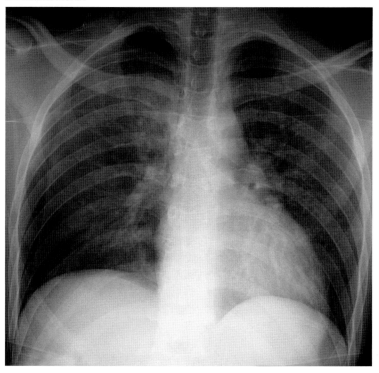

b Apical pneumothorax

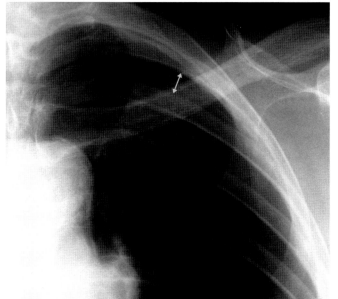

c "Deep sulcus sign"

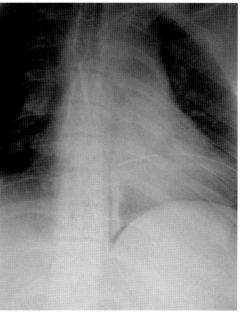

Fig. 14.**4 a** The pleural margin appears as a fine line running along the right thoracic wall that is not traversed by any vessels. A tension pneumothorax is not yet present. To prevent its development, an intrathoracic tube may need to be inserted. **b** In another patient, only a fine line is visible apically between the third and fourth ribs dorsally (arrow). If you are not absolutely sure, you can have the radiograph repeated in expiration. This technique often makes the air-filled pleural space wider and better visible. **c** Paravertebrally on the left you see the pointed deep pleural recess, also called "deep sulcus sign." The partially airless left lower lobe is seen reaching into it but not filling it. A chest tube has already been inserted in this patient.

▶

Pneumothorax

d Tension pneumothorax

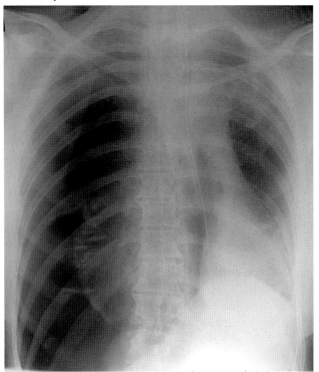

e Wrong diagnosis

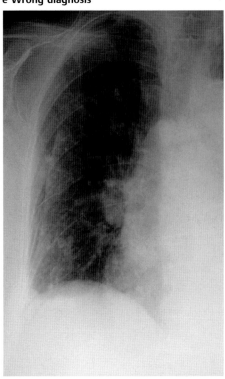

Fig. 14.**4 d** Vascular markings are lacking in the periphery of the right hemithorax (compare to the left hemithorax). The visceral pleura and with it the collapsed lung are appreciated with ease. The right hemidiaphragm is severely depressed, while the mediastinum is displaced to the contralateral side (note the course of the nasogastric tube within the esophagus). Subcutaneous emphysema is present in the right cervical region. The parietal pleura was probably injured during a vascular puncture. Immediate intervention is necessary! **e** In this radiograph a rather dense line is visible that is traversed by the pulmonary vasculature—it thus cannot be a pneumothorax. The line is paralleled by a dense stripe of attenuation a few centimeters wide: you are looking at a skin fold. Remember: These bedside patients are resting on the film cassette and not everyone is as well built as you are.

artery. For certain measurements the catheter is wedged into a more peripheral pulmonary arterial vessel and temporarily a small balloon is inflated at its tip. The balloon should be deflated at all other times.

Are there rib fractures, particularly overlying the spleen? The presence of a rib fracture or even serial rib fractures (Fig. 14.**6**) in the left lower hemithorax greatly increases the probability of a coexisting splenic injury. Rib fractures may cause a pneumothorax, even a tension pneumothorax (see above). Is there evidence for a hemothorax? Circumscribed consolidations in the lung at this stage tend to be due to lung contusions (Fig. 14.**6**).

Is there pulmonary edema? Are there lung contusions? Perihilar symmetric patchy opacities and ill-defined blood vessels indicate *pulmonary edema* if (very important!) the radiograph is performed with sufficient inspiration (Fig. 14.**7**). Causes may include an overly aggressive fluid resuscitation during the initial emergency care. In elderly patients a cardiac decompensation can also be induced by the trauma itself.

If—particularly in the presence of rib fractures—circumscribed consolidations are detectable in the lung of a freshly traumatized person, *lung contusions* are the most likely cause (Fig. 14.**6**). They consist of pulmonary hemorrhages that tend to clear within a few days. The injuries to the lung can, however, also lead to tears of the pulmonary parenchyma, so-called lung lacerations (Fig. 14.**6**). Opacities in dependent lung areas may also be due to atelectasis or aspiration.

Is the mediastinum widened? The mediastinum is always wider in the recumbent than in the upright patient. The diaphragm pushes upward, especially in the fatter individual, and compresses the mediastinum. In addition the venous backflow is increased, which also adds to the mediastinal volume. Any rotation of the patient around the longitudinal axis also makes the mediastinum appear wider. For that reason it is crucial that the patient is positioned straight for the radiograph; this is not always trivial in an emergency room or intensive care setting. Assessing the relative position of the spinous processes between the medial edges of the two clavicles (ideally centered)

Central Venous Catheter

a

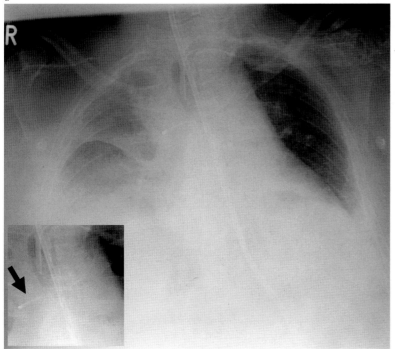

b

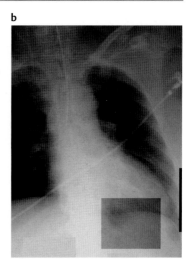

Fig. 14.**5 a** A central venous catheter has been introduced via the left jugular vein and has then deviated into the azygos vein, where its tip appears to have a very high density. It is, however, imaged orthogonally or "down the barrel."

b On this radiograph you can follow the central venous catheter through the right atrium into the apex of the heart (see window). Does anything else strike you?

The tube is positioned too low!

Serial Rib Fractures

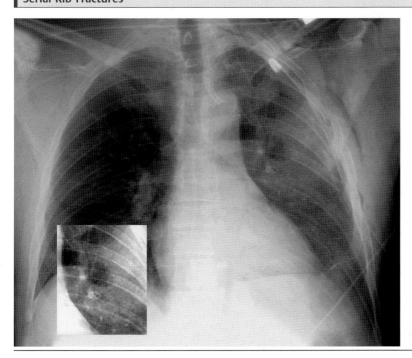

Fig. 14.**6** This patient suffered from serial rib fractures (ribs 3–6 on the left). A pneumothorax has already been taken care of with an intrathoracic chest tube in drainage. The lung in the vicinity of the fracture is considerably increased in density: The alveoli are filled with blood, which is why the bronchi are beautifully visible as black stripes, so-called "positive air bronchograms" in a patient with a lung contusion. Within this zone there is a circumscribed area of increased lucency (see also the inset)—this is a pulmonary tear. The pulmonary hemorrhage clears within a few days. The pulmonary tear may take months to heal.

Pulmonary Edema

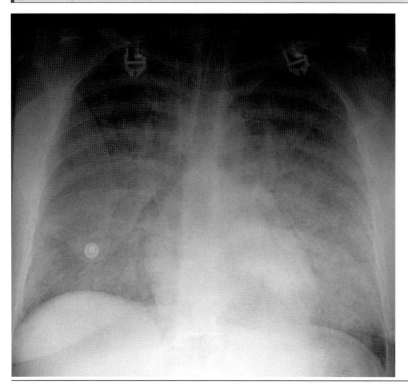

Fig. 14.**7** Severe alveolar edema is characterized by positive air bronchograms and perihilar symmetrical opacities. The distribution of the consolidations resembles the outline of a butterfly in flight (or even a less popular creature), which is why perihilar alveolar lung edema is often labeled as "butterfly edema" or "batwing edema." This patient underwent vigorous fluid resuscitation and defibrillation (you can see the large transparent electrode of the defibrillator superimposed on the right chest) and developed pulmonary edema in this context.

Pneumomediastinum

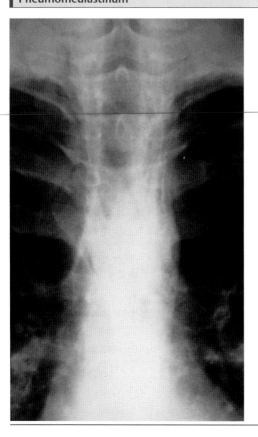

Fig. 14.**8** This view of the upper mediastinum shows some fine, dark stripes parallel to the trachea and the large mediastinal vessels, for example, the brachiocephalic trunk. There must be air in the mediastinum. Have a close look!

Rupture of the Diaphragm

a

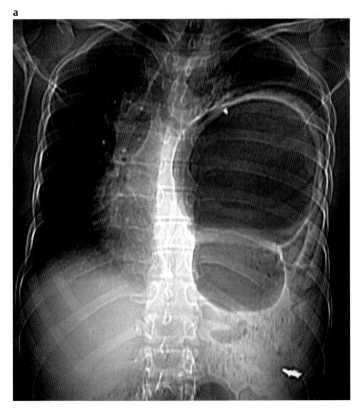

b

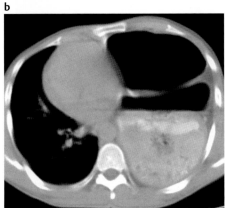

Fig. 14.**9 a**   The hemidiaphragm on the left is obliterated. Parts of the colon and the stomach have prolapsed into the chest. **b** CT confirms the finding. The stomach is located high in the left hemithorax.

helps to determine the degree of rotation of the patient around the body axis. If the rotation is taken into consideration and the mediastinum still appears to be abnormally wide, a contrast-enhanced CT of the chest should be done—particularly in those patients with high-speed motor vehicle accident (MVA) trauma or some other deceleration trauma. This is to exclude any treatable injuries to the large vessels, especially traumatic aortic dissection or aneurysm formation. Blood in the mediastinum seen on CT can be an indirect hint. If there is a pneumomediastinum (Fig. 14.**8**), a tracheal or bronchial tear should be considered.

Is the diaphragm intact? If the outline of the diaphragm is invisible or if there are bowel loops seen inside the thorax (Fig. 14.**9a**), a CT (Fig. 14.**9b**) should be done to assess the presence of a rupture and look for associated injuries. Most diaphragmatic ruptures occur on the left side because on the right the diaphragm is protected by the sturdy liver.

Giufeng calls the diagnoses out loud for the taker of the minutes to jot down: "Tube malpositioned in the right main bronchus, severe tension pneumothorax on the right, serial rib fractures on the right (4th–8th ribs); volume loss of the left lung; mediastinal shift to the left." The defibrillation electrode is still fixed to the chest.

What Pathology Do You Find Here?

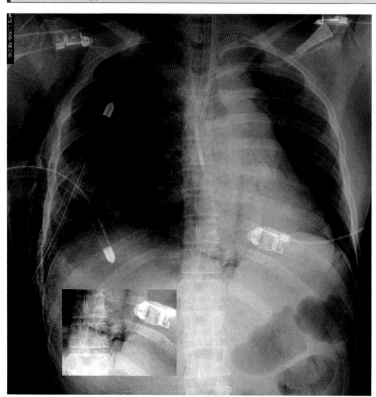

Fig. 14.**10**

There is a "deep sulcus"(see inset) next to the spine on the left. If you look closer, you will find a fine line along the accentuated heart contour. This patient also has a pneumothorax on the left! The tube position must be corrected and another chest drain must be inserted on the left.

The reasons for the prior cardiac arrest are evident now: only the side with the tension pneumothorax was being ventilated.

The trauma surgeons had already suspected the tension pneumothorax on clinical grounds and had inserted two chest drains on the right after a first quick glance at the CXR. They had also ordered a follow-up radiograph imme-

diately after first CXR was out and before Giufeng was finished with her analysis. Giufeng realizes at once that the drains have not had quite the intended effect: the mediastinum is still displaced to the left because it was apparently mainly the right main bronchus intubation that had caused the decreased aeration and the ensuing atelectasis of the left lung. Fortunately, the anesthesiologist listened to Giufeng and corrected the tube position right after Giufeng had called the incorrect tube position. But Giufeng now recognizes another important finding (Fig. 14.**10**). Any idea what it might be?

→ Lateral Radiograph of the Cervical Spine

By now the lateral radiograph of the cervical spine is ready for inspection. The trauma surgeons and the anesthesiologist want to know how careful they have to be during repositioning of the patient and whether the stiff collar can be taken off. The radiograph of the cervical spine is always difficult to evaluate and any mistakes can be fatal.

Patient A: The First Radiograph of the Cervical Spine

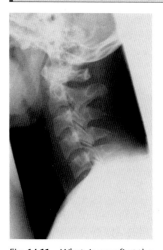

Fig. 14.**11**   What is your first thought when you see this image? What are the consequences?

! Twenty percent of all polytraumatized patients have an injury of the cervical spine, a dislocation injury (particularly in deceleration trauma), or a compression injury due to extreme axial loading forces impacting vertebral bodies in the longitudinal direction. It is therefore crucial to check the cervical spine with great care. Definition, outline of all vertebral bodies, and posterior elements and their alignment must be smooth and harmonic!

Auxiliary Lines for the Evaluation of the Cervical Spine

a 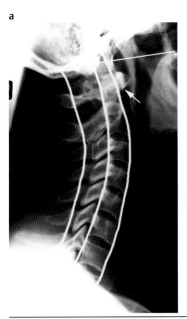   b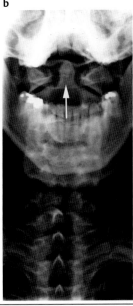

Fig. 14.**12 a**   The auxiliary lines for the evaluation of the configuration of the lateral cervical spine run (from anterior to posterior) along the anterior edges of the vertebral bodies, along the posterior edges of the vertebral bodies, and along the anterior contour of the posterior vertebral arches. Another auxiliary line—the Chamberlain auxiliary line—courses from the hard palate to the occiput. The apex of the dens should not traverse it. Another important point is the atlantodental distance (arrow)—it may not exceed 4 mm. Finally, the prevertebral soft tissue rim above the level of the esophageal inlet (about C4/5) may not exceed 7 mm in adults. **b** In the anterior–posterior projection, imagine lines along the spinous processes (do not get thrown off by bifid processes!) and the intervertebral joints. The well-centered position of the dens axis (arrow) relative to the atlanto-occipital joints and to the C1–C2 intervertebral joints is checked with care. (But beware: Is the patient positioned straight?)

Checklist: **Radiograph of the Cervical Spine in Polytrauma**

- Are all cervical vertebral bodies visualized? (Find a strong person to pull down the shoulders or have oblique views performed!)
- Are all auxiliary contour lines well seen and normal in appearance?
- Is the dens axis centered?
- Do the prevertebral soft tissues appear normal?
- Any residual doubts? Get a CT!

Giufeng is quite relieved that Gregory has come to her help. Both delve into the radiograph (Fig. 14.**11**). First they make sure the whole cervical spine is documented; then they look at the configuration of the spine (normal lordosis?) and the harmonic course of the auxiliary lines along the anterior and posterior edges of the cervical bodies, the posterior margin of the spinal canal (on the lateral projection), and the spinous processes (on the lateral and anterior–posterior projection) (Fig. 14.**12**). They study the intervertebral joints, the intervertebral disk spaces, the vertebral body configurations, and the prevertebral soft tissue stripe. Is the dens axis well centered on the A-P projection?

Giufeng and Gregory know that the occipitocervical junction zone down to C2/C3 shows some peculiarities in trauma (Fig. 14.**13**).

Occipitocervical junction injuries down to C2/C3:
Jefferson fracture: The Jefferson fracture is a typical compression fracture due to axial loading (for example, a head-first dive into shallow waters). The anterior and posterior arch of C1 is split (Fig. 14.**14a**), which causes a

dangerous instability. On the dedicated view of the dens or in a coronal CT reconstruction (Fig. 14.**14b**), the C1 joint facets of the C1/C2 segment are displaced laterally.
Dens fracture: The dens fracture is the most frequent traumatic lesion of the upper cervical spine. It is classified according to Anderson into fractures of the top of the dens (Anderson I, probably stable), the base of the dens (Anderson II, probably unstable, Fig. 14.**15a**, **b**), and the body of the axis vertebra (Anderson III, mostly stable, Fig. 14.**15c**).

Fractures of the Upper Cervical Spine

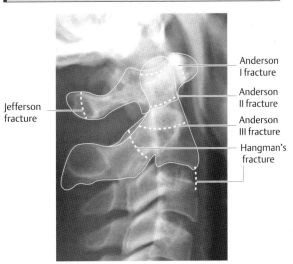

Jefferson fracture

Anderson I fracture
Anderson II fracture
Anderson III fracture
Hangman's fracture

Fig. 14.**13**   Illustrated are the most important fractures of the upper cervical spine.

Jefferson Fracture

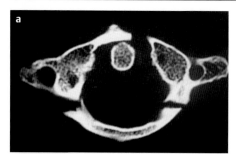

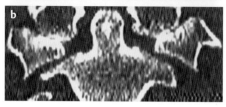

Fig. 14.**14 a**   This CT image shows a fracture of the anterior and posterior arches of the atlas ring. It is quite obvious that this fracture is frequently unstable. The dens axis has completely lost its osseous fixation. **b** The lateral migration of the joint facets is best documented by this CT image, which was reconstructed in a plane that shows the abnormality to better advantage. The transverse ligament that normally holds the dens in place must also be torn.

Traumatic spondylolisthesis: The second most frequent fracture is the traumatic spondylolisthesis of C2, also called "hangman's fracture" because it is caused by a sudden hyperextension such as occurs during hanging (Fig. 14.**16**). Depending on the force of the hyperextension,

Traumatic Spondylolisthesis

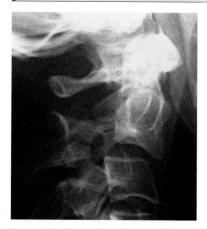

Fig. 14.**16**   This patient hit the dashboard of his car in a motor vehicle accident. He did not have his seatbelt fastened nor was an airbag installed in his car. The resulting hyperextension has broken his C2 vertebral arch and torn the ligamentary apparatus between C2 and C3. This fracture is evidently unstable.

the arch of C2 breaks bilaterally (type 1, potentially unstable). If the ligaments and the disk of the articular segment C2/C3 rupture partially (type 2) or completely (type 3), a higher degree of instability results.

> ! The dens fracture is the most common, the traumatic spondylolisthesis is the second most common, and the atlas fracture is the third most common fracture of the upper cervical spine.

Dens Fracture

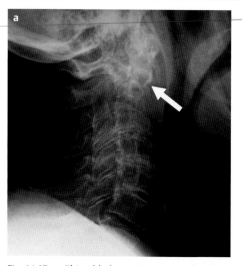

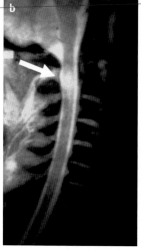

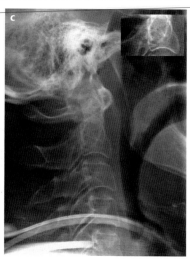

Fig. 14.**15 a**   This elderly patient—note the degeneration of the intervertebral spaces—has a fracture of the base of the dens (arrow) classified as Anderson II. **b** An MRI examination of a similar fracture in a different patient illustrates the potential consequence of the resulting osseous instability.

The T2-weighted, sagittal section documents a signal increase (arrow) along the course of the spinal cord. This signal indicates a contusion of the spinal cord. **c** This patient has an Anderson III fracture (see inset).

Ligamentary Injury of the Cervical Spine

a

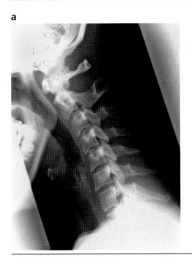

b

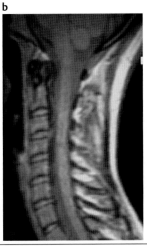

Fig. 14.**17 a** This patient suffered a whiplash trauma during a motor vehicle collision. The radiograph in flexion shows a subtle kink at the level C3/C4. **b** The MR image confirms the disk prolapse at this level.

Ligamentous injuries: Primary ligamentous injuries are of great relevance for any future rehabilitation. They are diagnosed after primary emergency care has been concluded using function studies (Fig. 14.**17a**) and MRI (Fig. 14.**17b**).

Spinal column injuries caudal to C3: Giufeng realizes that the so-called "normal spine" begins at C3. Starting at that level the spinal injuries are categorized as:

- Compression fractures (type A)
- Flexion–distraction fractures (type B)
- Torsion injuries (type C)

The involvement of the posterior edge of the vertebral body is, of course, essential because it indicates a potential hazard to the spinal canal. Fractures of the lower cervical spine mostly evolve in flexion–distraction movement patterns (type B). Any restriction of the spinal column flexibility, such as seen in ankylosing spondylitis (Fig. 14.**18a**) or Forrestier disease (Fig. 14.**18b**), increases the risk of unstable fractures even after minor trauma.

While Giufeng is still busy studying the radiograph, Greg has already ordered a repeat study: C6 and C7 are not depicted at all. The new radiograph is performed as an oblique view because, even with two strong trauma surgeons pulling the patient's shoulders footward, the cervicothoracic transition zone could not be adequately imaged on the lateral projection. The new finding scares the living daylight out of Giufeng (Fig. 14.**19**). There is a considerable misalignment between C6 and C7: the ligaments of this section must be torn completely. This is a typical torsion injury (C-class spinal injury). The instability can cause a paraplegia. Extreme caution and the stabilization of the cervical spine are warranted.

Preexisting Spinal Problems That Increase Trauma Risk

a Ankylosing spondylitis

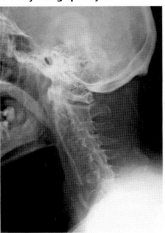

b Forestier disease

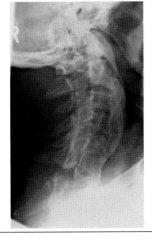

Fig. 14.**18 a** In ankylosing spondylitis, also called Bechterew disease, slowly progressive ossification of the complete ligamentous apparatus of the spinal column occurs. You have already seen the prototypical appearance of the "bamboo spine" in Fig. 8.**44b**, p. 146. Note the fracture at the C6/7 level after a minor trauma in this patient. **b** In Forestier disease only the anterior longitudinal ligament of the spinal column ossifies, but the effect is the same: the spine loses all its elasticity. Every motion that results in any significant axial loading force on the spine constitutes a considerable fracture risk for these patients. Minor trauma has led to a fracture of the C7 in this case.

Patient A: The Additional Projections of the Cervical Spine

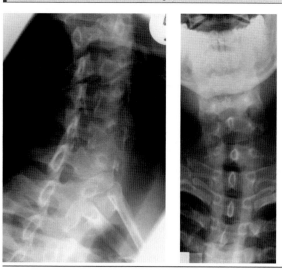

Fig. 14.**19**   Here you see important additional views of the cervical spine in an oblique (**a**) and a posterior–anterior (**b**) projection. Now the pathology should be clear!

Patient A: Cranial CT

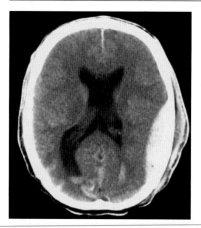

Fig. 14.**20**   Analyze the cranial CT of patient A. Can you already call the diagnoses? All of them?

→ Cranial CT

After successful circulatory stabilization by the anesthesiologists, patient A is brought to the CT suite. Paul has been waiting for him. The severity of the trauma and the unclear neurological status of the respirated and deeply sedated patient necessitate a head CT. The risk of an intracranial injury is quite high. Cautiously, the patient is moved over onto the CT table. While the anesthesiologists monitor the patient, Paul sits down in front of the CT workstation and analyzes the study as the images appear on the screen one by one (Fig. 14.**20**). Can you help him? What is the right diagnosis? Before you start, have a look at representative sections of a normal head CT (Fig. 14.**21**).

Generalized cerebral edema: A generalized lethal edema (Fig. 14.**22**) can develop as a consequence of a severe head trauma. The resulting impaction of the brainstem against edges of the foramen magnum or clivus may compromise the vascular supply of the brain. Secondary infarction can

Normal Findings in a Cranial CT

a   b

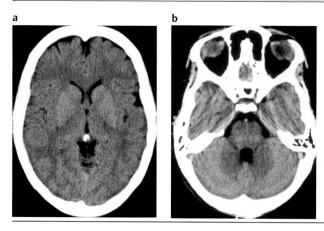

Fig. 14.**21 a**   This is a normal CT of a 50-year-old. The inner and outer CSF spaces are well appreciated. Gray and white matter are easily differentiated from each other and are of normal density. **b** The basal and posterior fossa cisterns are also well seen.

Generalized Brain Edema Due to Head Trauma

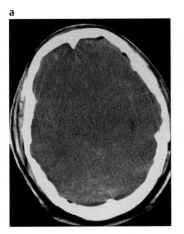 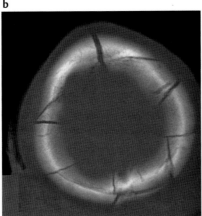 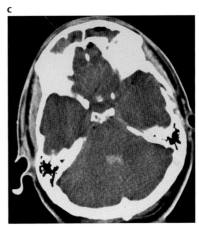

Fig. 14.**22** This 40-year-old patient was hit by a wooden plank falling from a building. The pupils had already become unreactive to light in the ambulance helicopter. **a** In comparison to the normal CT (see Fig. 14.**21a**), the inner and outer CSF spaces are completely obliterated and differentiation between the gray and white matter is impossible. The sylvian fissure and the frontal sulci are outlined with dense material (blood). The midline is not displaced, however. These findings are compatible with severe generalized brain edema and subarachnoid hemorrhages. **b** A more cranial CT section in a bone window shows the reason for the extensive changes: a burst fracture of the skull. As the cranial vault does not permit sufficient expansion of an edematous brain, the intracranial pressure consequently increases. In less severe states of edema, a conservative antiedematous therapy or a wide surgical fenestration of the skull may be successful—in this patient any help comes too late. **c** A CT image at the level of the posterior fossa demonstrates a complete lack of external CSF space. The fourth ventricle is filled with blood (compare Fig. 14.**21b**). This patient was later transferred to the intensive care ward for the determination of brain death (24-hour flatline EEG, neurological examination). Hopefully, organ donation is an option in this case to help someone else in need.

develop, resulting in death or permanent brain damage. A similar diffuse edema may be the sequel of a longer-lasting brain hypoxia, for example, in prolonged shock, drowning, suffocation, or strangulation (Fig. 14.**23**). The consequences are identical.

Epidural hematoma: An epidural hematoma (Fig. 14.**24**) carries a high risk for the patient. It is often an arterial, fracture-induced bleed. It fills the space between the skull bone and its periostium, the dura mater. This space is, of course, limited by the cranial sutures where the periosteum is tightly fixed. Any blood in this space will elevate the dura, assuming the shape of an expanding cushion. Relatively little blood can thus result in quite a pulsating space-occupying lesion affecting the adjacent brain like a "steam hammer." This development can be very swift and is naturally accelerated by a successful circulatory stabilization. Immediate neurosurgical intervention is life-saving!

Subdural hematoma: A subdural hematoma (Fig. 14.**25a**), induced by tearing of bridging veins, can spread relatively freely underneath the dura mater (from the viewpoint of the neurosurgeon opening the skull)—subdurally. The bony sutures do not hinder the spread. Frequently, however, an *acute subdural hematoma* goes along with brain contusions that significantly worsen the prognosis. Considerably better are the chances of patients in whom a *subacute subdural hemorrhage* manifests itself only after an interval free of neurological symptoms. The longer

Generalized Brain Edema Due to Strangulation

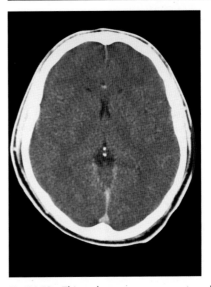

Fig. 14.**23** This unhappy young man strangled himself in an effort to commit suicide. The hypoxia has led to a generalized edema. There are no hemorrhages to note on the precontrast image (not shown). The normal bright structure in the midline is the falx cerebri. The contrast-enhanced CT shows the superior sagittal venous sinus dorsally. The bright spots ventrally in the midline are the anterior cerebral arteries; the very dense midline spots a little dorsal to the center are typical calcifications in the pineal gland.

Epidural Hematoma

a

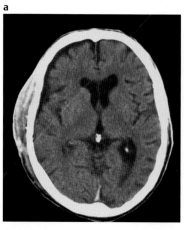

b

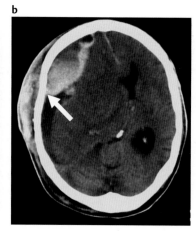

c

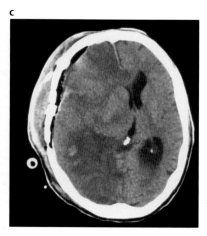

d

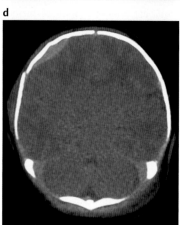

Fig. 14.**24 a**   The initial CT was performed immediately after the polytraumatized patient had reached the emergency unit. There is a considerable right-sided scalp hematoma. There is no evidence for cerebral edema; the midline structures are not shifted. **b** A few hours later, the patient has become comatose. Repeat study reveals a typical epidural hematoma in the right frontal region. The bleed does not traverse the coronal suture (arrow) posteriorly. The brain surface appears considerably indented ("steamhammer effect"). The midline is now shifted to the left by more than 1.5 cm. Not only the brain but also the supplying cerebral arteries are displaced and consequently squeezed against the falx cerebri and the tentorium. Immediate relief by craniotomy is needed to save this patient. **c** The follow-up study after the craniotomy documents the detrimental consequences of the midline shift. The vascular territories of the anterior and posterior cerebral artery as well as parts of the territory of the medial cerebral artery on the right are swollen and decreased in density—all of this is indicative of brain infarction. Parietally on the right there is an additional brain hemorrhage—due either to a traumatic contusion or to a hemorrhagic infarction. There is some residual postsurgical air seen in the epidural space. The midline shift has decreased only minimally—by now it is caused by the pronounced edema of the right hemisphere. **d** In this neonate who fell off the table during a diaper change, a right frontal epidural hematoma is accompanied by severe global edema.

Subdural Hematoma

a

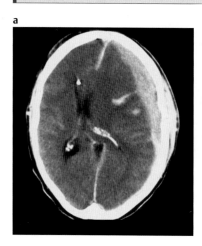

b

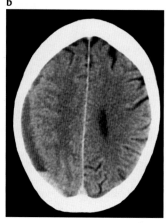

Fig. 14.**25 a**   This patient was involved in a high-speed motor vehicle accident and suffered a head trauma. As a consequence, a large subdural hematoma developed on the left that spread over the surface of the brain and led to a substantial midline shift. The brain contusion has resulted in an intraparenchymal hemorrhage, which is seen frontally on the left. Faint subarachnoid blood is seen bilaterally (see Fig. 14.**27** for comparison). Immediate neurosurgical intervention is also necessary in this patient. **b** This woman complained about a continuing headache since she hit her head against a low ceiling in her basement. The cranial CT shows a right-sided chronic subdural hematoma that has a fluid–fluid level (serum above and the erythrocytes in the dependent part of the hematoma) and very little resulting mass effect.

Intracranial Hematoma

a

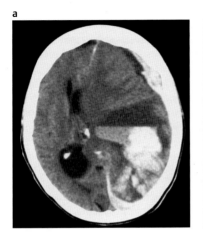

b

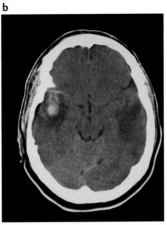

Fig. 14.**26 a** There is a small left-sided sub-dural hematoma and severe hemorrhage into the brain parenchyma in the occipito-parietal region in this patient. The hemor-rhage shows layering. The additive mass ef-fect of both disease processes increases the intracranial pressure and causes severe mid-line shift, which is probably also the reason for the obstructive hydrocephalus of the right lateral ventricle. The right posterior horn of the lateral ventricle is grossly dilated. The on-going CSF production further contributes to the intracranial pressure increase. Surgical de-compression of the ventricular system is cru-cial to give the patient a chance of survival. **b** In another patient, a deceleration trauma has led to a brain contusion temporally on the right (and a fracture, not visible in this window setting) with an associated contre-coup tem-porally on the left.

this interval, the better the chances of survival. Both the acute and the subacute subdural hematoma may be trea-ted by neurosurgical drainage through one or several burr holes in the skull or openly with craniotomy and eva-cuation. The *chronic subdural hematoma* (Fig. 14.**25b**) may not become symptomatic until weeks after the under-lying marginal trauma. If necessary, it is also flushed and drained via a burr hole.

Intracranial hematoma: An intracranial hematoma (Fig. 14.**26a**) can also occur as a sequel of a severe brain contusion. It may be relieved surgically. In deceleration trauma, "coup" and "contre-coup" lesions may be seen (for the few non-francophiles: punch and counter-punch). These consist of hemorrhages in opposing regions of the brain (Fig. 14.**26b**). In addition, smaller *subarachnoid he-*

morrhages—detectable as fine bright lines or dots within the sulci—can occur as a collateral injury (Fig. 14.27). Subarachnoid hemorrhages (SAH) in the absence of sig-nificant trauma are most often caused by rupture of a pre-existing aneurysm and resulting hemorrhage (see p. 235, Chapter 11).

Paul's head is spinning, but finally he makes up his mind: there is a classic epidural hematoma along the left super-ior convexity of the brain. The scalp in this area is swollen as consequence of a direct trauma. The sulci are swollen and the white-matter/gray-matter distinction is de-creased, both findings indicating locoregional cerebral edema. Occipitally on the right the sulci are filled with blood. This is a subarachnoid hemorrhage as part of a "contre-coup" phenomenon. The ventricular system is

Intracranial Hematoma with Subarachnoid Hemorrhage

a

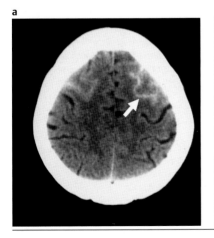

b

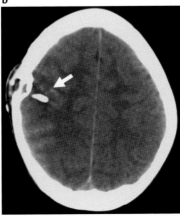

Fig. 14.**27 a** Here you see a small subar-achnoid hemorrhage (SAH, arrow) that was associated with an occipital brain contusion a few centimeters lower. Note the filling of the sulcus with dense blood. **b** A punch with an iron rod caused this depressed fracture of the skull on the right side. Amazingly, a subtle SAH (ar-row) is the only resulting intracranial ab-normality.

dilated considerably, which must be due to an obstruction of the CSF drainage. The reason for this remains obscure for Paul, but Gregory comes in time and solves the puzzle: he points out the blood in the right posterior horn of the lateral ventricle, where a small fluid–fluid interface with the CSF is present. Somewhere there must be a parenchymal bleed that has ruptured into the ventricular system. The tiniest blood clot from this source can obstruct the aqueduct connecting the third and fourth ventricles and thus lead to hydrocephalus requiring surgical ventriculostomy. Patient A is transferred immediately to the neurosurgical OR.

Patient B

Meanwhile, another heavily traumatized patient (B, name unknown, male, about 45 years old) is rushed into the CT scanner.

What Must Paul Consider in Deceleration Trauma?

Paul knows that aortic injuries are one major problem after high-speed motor vehicle accidents and other deceleration traumas. A rupture of the aortic wall is only survived if the adventitia, the outer wall of the aorta, remains intact. The aortic arch is held in place by the outflows of the cervical vessels and the ligamentum arteriosum (the remnant of the fetal ductus arteriosus of Botalli, which runs between the superior surface of the origin of the left pulmonary artery and the inferior surface of the arch of the aorta; It passes superolaterally from inferior to superior attachments, the latter is about the level of the origin of the left subclavian artery from the aorta). Ninety percent of all aortic ruptures originate directly distal to the ligamentum arteriosum. They may be associated with a dissection.

Radiograph and CT of the chest: A CXR that was performed in another primary care hospital shows a mediastinal widening (Fig. 14.**28a**). As a consequence, the otherwise stable patient was transferred immediately. Paul initiates a dissection protocol type chest CT pre and post contrast administration (Fig. 14.**28b**).

Checklist: Chest CT in Polytrauma

- Is there hemorrhage in the mediastinum?
- Are all large vessels normal?
- Is there air present in the mediastinum?
- Is there fluid in the pericardium?

Aortic injury: An *incomplete aortic rupture* (Fig. 14.**29a**)— the complete rupture is not survived—fortunately causes a detectable mediastinal widening in about 80% of cases. In up to 50% of cases a simultaneous hemothorax is seen. The aortic rupture is best appreciated by rapid spiral CT, where the aorta can be reconstructed in three dimensions or in fine two-dimensional slices. If this technology is not available, catheter-based transfemoral aortography needs be performed. A pseudoaneurysm (Fig. 14.**29b–d**) is the natural sequel of an untreated incomplete aortic rupture. *Aortic dissection* (Fig. 14.**29e**, see also p. 79) is frequently associated.

Cardiac injury: A cardiac injury is also possible in deceleration trauma. Hemorrhage into the pericardium, leading to tamponade, is the most frequent injury requiring surgical intervention. Penetrating trauma, for example, a stab wound (Fig. 14.**29f**) or a gunshot injury, may also result in pericardial tamponade. The fluid in the pericardium restricts the cardiac movement and thereby diminishes the cardiac throughput—fast diagnosis is thus essential.

! Patients with preexisting aortic aneurysms (see p. 85) or lipomatosis of the mediastinum (Fig. 14.**29g**) or infants with a well-developed thymus also demonstrate a wide mediastinum on the CXR.

Paul scrutinizes the CT with great care image by image. He diagnoses a pseudoaneurysm of the aortic arch. Later the finding is confirmed during aortography (Fig. 14.**30**).

Patient C

By now the third heavily traumatized patient (C, name unknown, female, about 45 years of age) is wheeled into the resuscitation room. She is conscious and is breathing spontaneously; several peripheral venous cannulas have been inserted and she wears a cervical collar. Joey is now in charge of the ultrasound machine.

Radiography of the chest and rib series: The CXR is felt to be within normal limits. A skin bruise on the left lateral thorax and pain in this area prompt a rib series (Fig. 14.**31a**). This shows a fracture of the 8th rib.

! A fracture of the lower bony thorax should alert you to potential severe trauma of underlying abdominal organs and must be correlated with an ultrasound or CT examination of the abdomen.

Patient B

a Radiograph of the chest

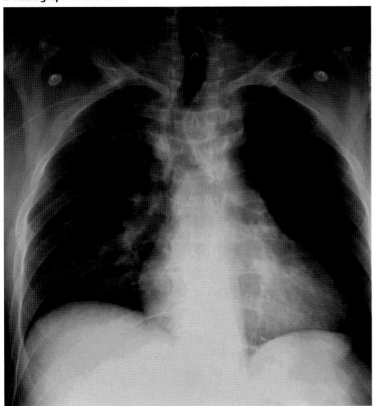

Fig. 14.**28 a**   This is the chest radiograph that led to the immediate transfer of the patient to the trauma center. The upper mediastinum appears widened. Are you sure the patient is well positioned?
b Go ahead and trace the aortic arch and its branches on the consecutive slices. Try to form a three-dimensional model of the arch in the back of your mind. Now try to rotate it.

b Chest CT

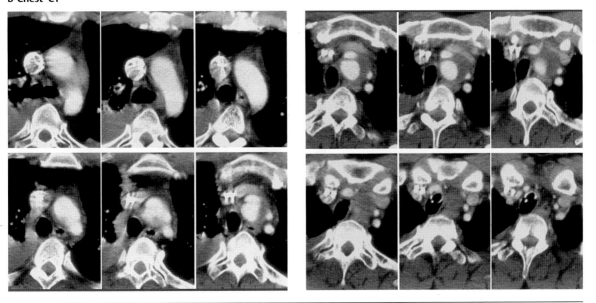

Causes of Mediastinal Widening

a Incomplete aortic rupture

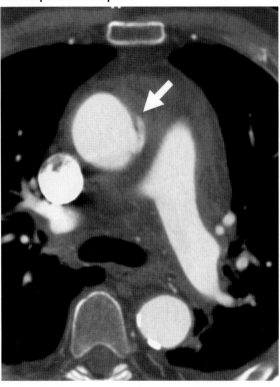

Fig. 14.**29 a**   This CT shows an incomplete rupture of the ascending aorta. The leakage of contrast into the defect of the intima and media is seen well (arrow). **b** In this patient a pseudoaneurysm has formed in the typical location close to the ligament of Bothalli (star). **c** The sagittal reconstruction of the aortic arch shows the aneurysm (star) in its relation to the spine to better advantage. **d** The sagittal reconstruction of the thoracic spine depicts the fracture of the adjoining vertebral body emphasizing the brutal force of the trauma.

b–d Traumatic pseudoaneurysm

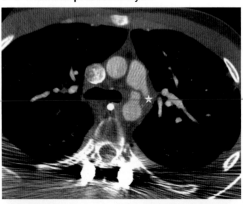 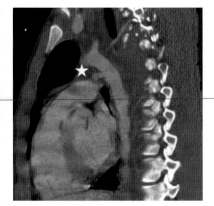

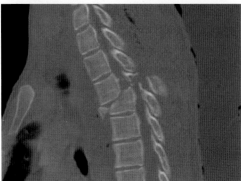

▶

Causes of Mediastinal Widening

e Aortic dissection

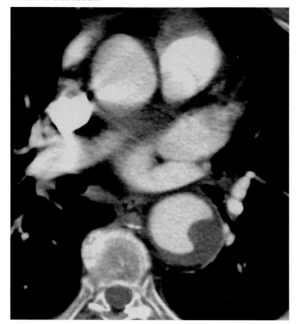

f Hematopericardium

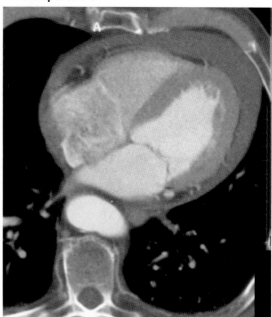

g Mediastinal lipomatosis

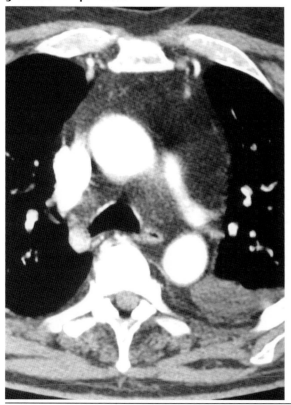

Fig. 14.**29 e** A hematoma of the wall of the descending aorta has been the sequel of a severe chest trauma in this patient. This is a precursor of a full-blown aortic dissection. **f** A heated exchange of arguments among friends climaxed in a knife stab directly into the heart. The pericardium is filled with blood—rapid surgical intervention is imperative. **g** The large vessels are surrounded by a wide fatty tissue cuff. Compare the density of the subcutaneous fat. Only CT can diagnose mediastinal lipomatosis with certainty in an emergency setting.

Patient B: Aortography

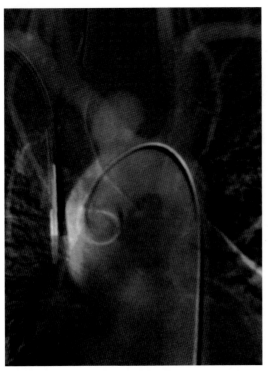

Fig.14.**30**   A catheter that has the shape of a pigtail is located in the aortic arch. This digital subtraction angiography image (the images acquired before and after contrast administration are subtracted from each other) shows the cranial bulge of the aortic lumen close to the origin of the brachiocephalic trunk. This is a false aneurysm. The diagnosis fits very well with the conventional chest radiograph findings (see Fig. 14.**28a**): The trachea has been displaced to the right by the aneurysm.

Ultrasound and CT of the abdomen: During the ultrasound examination, Joey takes a particularly good look at Morrison's pouch (Fig. 14.**31b**), where free fluid in the abdomen tends to accumulate first. Owing to its location and consistency, the spleen is the abdominal organ most at risk for blunt injury. Contusions, lacerations, and ruptures of spleen (Fig. 14.**32a**, **b**) and liver (Fig. 14.**32c**) as well as bleeds from larger vessels into the open abdomen (Fig. 14.**32b**) are readily appreciated on CT images.

> **!** Remember that the amount of hemorrhage may be decreased in severe shock. After circulatory stabilization, bleeds may intensify and manifest with some delay.

Free fluid in the abdomen in a trauma patient can also have other causes. Trauma may rupture the bowel or induce bursting of a full urinary bladder. Bleeds may also arise in the retroperitoneum, particularly in renal injuries, which often become symptomatic with hematuria (Fig. 14.**33**).

> **!** In a patient with polytrauma, the parenchymal organs of the upper abdomen and especially the retroperitoneum are not sufficiently examined by ultrasound. An abdominal CT is indicated in all cases of doubt and severe trauma. Ultrasound may be useful as a rapid screening tool to detect conditions that require immediate surgical attention even prior to a trip to the CT scanner, such as pericardial hematoma/tamponade, hemothorax, and large amounts of free fluid in the abdomen requiring immediate emergency laparotomy.

Joey immediately worries about splenic rupture, having seen the obvious fracture of the 8th rib on the left side. the ultrasound aspect of the space of Morrison reinforces

Patient C

a Radiograph of left hemithorax

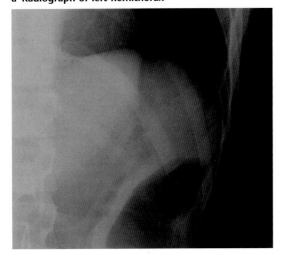

b Abdominal ultrasound

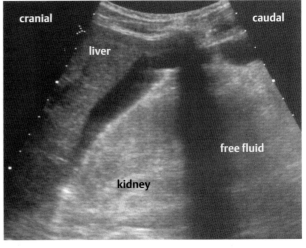

Fig. 14.**31**   Here you see the radiograph of the left lower hemithorax of patient C (**a**) as well as a parasagittal ultrasound section through the liver and the right kidney (**b**).

Causes of Free Fluid in the Abdomen

a Contained splenic rupture

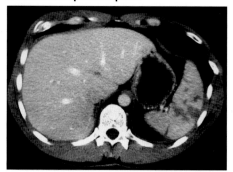

b Splenic rupture with active extravasation of blood

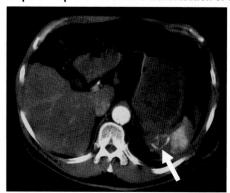

c Liver rupture

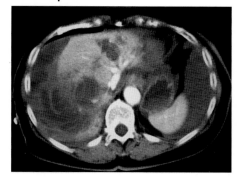

Fig. 14.**32 a** In this patient a splenic tear has occurred, which luckily has not led to a full-blown bleed into the into the peritoneum. This is an incomplete splenic rupture or splenic laceration. **b** This splenic rupture in another patient exhibits active extravasation of blood into the peritoneum. You recognize the active bleed by appreciating the contrast media-enhanced blood within the intra-abdominal hemorrhage (arrow). This young man was not the victim of an motor vehicle accident but—chained to his own bed—of rather unorthodox sexual habits of his latest boyfriend. In a sexual frenzy the friend attacked and stabbed him with a knife—26 times. Luckily the patient recovered to full health, but he became a little more fussy picking his sexual partners. In any case, the injuries kept the trauma surgeons entertained for quite a while. **c** This is a liver rupture (compare the normal liver in **a** and **b**) due to a blunt abdominal trauma. This lady was treated with thrombocyte aggregation inhibitors because of advanced coronary arteriosclerosis. She called the ambulance during a heart attack. When the ambulance team arrived, she could still open the door but then collapsed. The team resuscitated her successfully on the spot but noted signs of shock a little later. The liver rupture caused by the resuscitation was diagnosed rapidly with an abdominal CT and was later addressed surgically. The patient was lucky: the surgery was successful and she returned home a few weeks later. Hepatic and splenic ruptures and pericardiac injuries occur rarely during resuscitations—rib fractures are common.

Retroperitoneal Hemorrhage

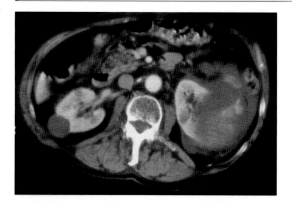

Fig. 14.**33** On this image you see documented a rupture of the left kidney associated with a retroperitoneal bleed. Fractures of the transverse spinous processes were also seen on that side. The patient had severe hematuria after a motor vehicle accident.

his suspicion: There is a considerable amount of fluid between the liver and the right kidney, indicative of visceral organ rupture—most likely of the spleen. The spleen itself is difficult to image in its entirety as it is partially obscured by the overlying lung. Abdominal CT is performed immediately and confirms the diagnosis (Fig. 14.**34a**).

Radiographs of the spine: Meanwhile, the radiographs of the spine are ready for Joey's analysis (Fig. 14.**34b**). He studies them with great care and quietly, despite the trauma surgeons' breathing down his neck.

First of all Joey looks at the configuration of the spinal column. Do all the auxiliary lines along the anterior and posterior edge of the vertebral bodies and along the spinous processes appear smooth and well defined? Are the individual vertebral bodies configured normally? Joey looks at every single body, trying to imagine a three-dimensional and complete model of it in the back of his mind.

Patient C

a Abdominal CT

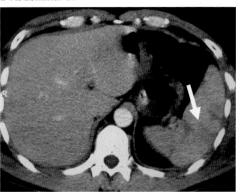

Fig. 14.**34 a**   The spleen is ruptured (arrow). **b** Note the radiograph of the patient's lumbar spine. Does anything strike you as abnormal? **c** The second and third right foraminal arches of the sacral bone are interrupted (arrow), which means that the right sacral ala is fractured.

b Radiographs of the spine

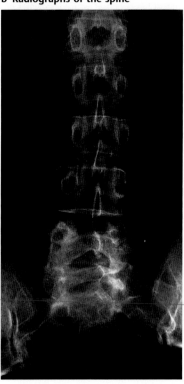
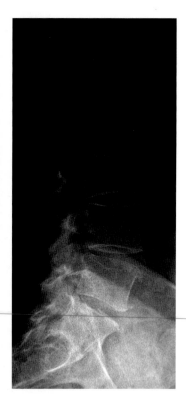

c Radiograph and CT of the pelvis

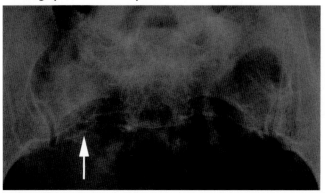
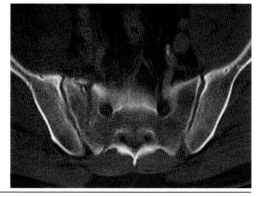

! One predominant question in the evaluation of a spinal column fracture is whether the spinal canal and/or the neural foramina are involved and how.

Does a fracture affect the posterior column of the vertebral body? This is always the case if the vertebral body is diminished in height dorsally. To determine this, measure the height of the vertebral body immediately underneath and immediately above—vertebral body height normally increases incrementally in the caudal direction. Does the spinal canal appear narrowed? This is of particular importance above the level of L3 because the spinal cord reaches down to that level. Is the dorsal vertebral arch involved? If that is the case, instability looms, which can seriously damage the spinal nerves along their course through the potentially narrowed neuroforamina.

Joey makes up his mind and calls a fracture of the anterior vertebral edge of L3. The keeper of the notes hardly suppresses a yawn because the staff surgeon had called this diagnosis minutes before when Joey was still busy doing the ultrasound.

Radiograph and CT of the pelvis: In the meantime, the radiograph of the pelvis has also been put up on the viewbox (Fig. 14.**34c**). The evaluation of the pelvis, particularly of the sacral bone, is frequently compromised by the superimposition of bowel content. Helpful structures are the sacral neuroforamina: analyze their outline carefully and in comparison to the contralateral side. Are they completely visible and smooth or are there defects, a step-off, or irregularities? Frequently a fracture of the sacral bone continues on cranially into the lumbar transversal processes. Are these truly intact? In the region of the iliac bone and the anterior pelvic ring, superimposition is less of a problem. But remember that posterior pelvic fractures often go along with another fracture of the anterior pelvic ring and vice versa. If no fractures are found, the width of the pubic symphysis and the iliosacral joints should be scrutinized. Somewhere the pelvic ring must have given way. By the way, the pubic symphysis is wider in women who have given birth than in those who have not.

Joey has not detected any fractures in a first quick glance over the pelvic radiograph. Gregory, who seems to be everywhere at the same time today, puts his finger on the film. The foraminal arch of S2 on the right is interrupted. CT confirms a sacral fracture (Fig. 14.**34c**).

14.2 Luxations and Fractures

The severe, acute, and life-threatening injuries of the polytraumatized patients from the highway collision have been taken care of radiologically by now. Our students return to the routine radiological examinations and procedures occurring in the Emergency Room of any vibrant city in this world. What is better to describe the numerous dislocations and "small" fractures than a good old fashioned movie style row? By the way: all fractures can be classified. Check your favorite trauma surgery book for the latest fashion in nomenclature.

Checklist: Luxations and Fractures

• Is the relevant region documented in two projections?
• Are the projections truly perpendicular to each other?

Eastside Story

There has been a brawl between two rival youth gangs on the outside staircase of the beer garden quite close to the hospital. One of the participants is well known to the emergency team head, Mr. Webber, and is welcomed with a warm handshake. Members of both groups are now sitting in the waiting zone, groaning with pain but still irreconcilable, and kept at a distance only by one robust policewoman. She knows just about enough about what has gone on during the confrontation: a certain "Ayeesha" and a lot of alcohol. The x-ray techs cross the injured off their worklist one by one. Fortunately, the hotheads become a little calmer in the x-ray room once their peers disappear from

Fractures of the Metacarpal Bones 4 and 5

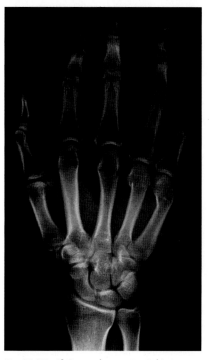

Fig. 14.**35** If Dung does not get his temper under control he will get this typical fistfighter injury more often. His 4th and 5th metacarpal bones are fractured and deviated to the palmar side. The respective radiograph of Sylvester Stallone or Bud Spencer would certainly be of interest for comparison.

sight. Joey calls Ajay and Paul as a reinforcement. Each grabs a couple of report forms and jots down the consequences of the brawl.

Dung apparently punched Ayeesha's brother Fuad with his fist when Fuad screamed at his sister and wanted to slap her in the face. Since then his hand hurts badly (Fig. 14.**35**). Fuad's jaw withstood the punch but while evading the attack he lost balance and fell a few steps down the stairs and on his hand (Fig. 14.**36a**). He dragged his drunk friend Eyad with him, who tried clumsily to stop his own fall with his left hand (Fig. 14.**36b**). The colossal Eyad got so mad he tore a wooden picket off the fence and assaulted Dung with it. Dung's friend Nam intervened and fended off the move forward (Fig. 14.**37**). Hoang jumped on Eyad's back, only to be shaken off and get his hand stuck between the pickets of the fence (Fig. 14.**38**). Faris, Fuad's first-degree cousin, lost his balance on the staircase while trying to draw himself up to full size and fell off the side of the stairs onto the concrete. Now his lower arm is swollen and hurts considerably (Fig. 14.**39**). Thanh had just a little hand in Faris's fall, which is why Faris's buddy Ghazi pushed him to the ground. His elbow joint is now immobile and painful (Fig. 14.**40**).

Oh yes, and Ayeesha took the opportunity to have a nice cappuccino with Dung's sister Hue in a close-by street café. From there the two girls called a bunch of ambulances to the site by mobile phone. They figure the boys are off their backs for the next few hours.

Meanwhile Joey, Ajay, and Paul are sick and tired of looking at radiographs of people who smash themselves up and they all leave for a cup of coffee. Hannah has dropped in a little too late to get the eastside action but she is definitely ready for some more.

Distal Radius Fracture

a Extension fracture (Colles type)

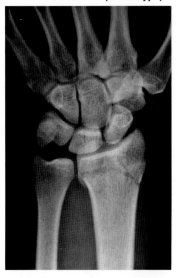
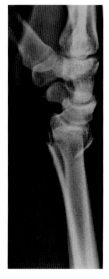

b Radius edge fracture (Smith type)

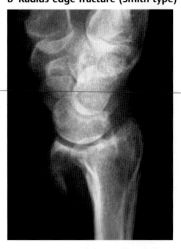

Fig. 14.**36 a** Fuad has suffered the most frequent fracture of the distal radius, the extension fracture of the Colles type. In this type of injury the distal fragment of the radius is displaced and angled dorsally, giving it the appearance of a fork (fourchette or bayonet configuration). Fuad is lucky—the articular surface is not involved and the ulna is positioned correctly. An ulnar protrusion would point to an injury of the triangular fibrocartilage and would have to be corrected in due time. **b** Eyad has landed on the back of his hand: he has a Smith-type flexion fracture in which the distal fragment is deviated to the palmar side. Unfortunately, Eyad's fracture involves the articular surface.

Ulnar Fracture

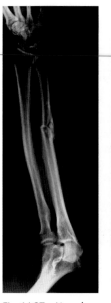
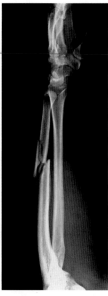

Fig. 14.**37** Nam has warded off the blow with his forearm, or parried it. An isolated wedge fracture of the ulna has resulted—also called the "parry fracture." The little notch at the radial head is a sequel of a previous injury.

Fracture of the Scaphoid Bone

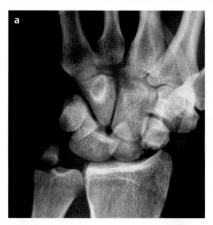

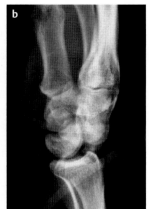

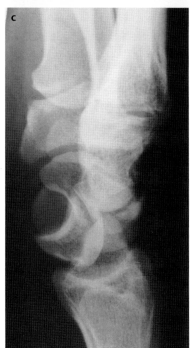

Fig. 14.**38 a–c** Hoang is out of luck. The bony avulsion of his ulnar epicondyle is his smallest problem (**a**). The scaphoid is fractured, with a couple of rather displaced fragments. The run of the mill scaphoid fracture is often so subtle it can be missed on standard projection. For that reason additional angled special projections are ordered if a scaphoid fracture is anticipated. Fractures may easily interrupt the blood supply to the scaphoid fragments, which is why the healing process may be impaired and a pseudoarthrosis may eventually develop. Hoang also has a perilunate carpal luxation: compare the configuration of the lunate and capitate bone on the lateral projection (**b**) with the correct situation seen in Fig. 14.**36a** (lateral projection). An isolated lunate luxation can also occur (**c**): compare the position of the radius with that of the lunate to determine whether they are aligned or not.

For all of you who haven't given up on German classes here is an anatomical helper:

> *Das Schiffchen (scaphoid) fährt im Mondenschein (lunate)*
> *im Dreieck (triquetrum) um das Erbsenbein (pisiform),*
> *Vieleck groß (trapezium) and Vieleck klein (trapezoid),*
> *der Kopf (capitate), der muss beim Hammer (hamate) sein.*

It is all about a **little ship** that sails in the **moonlight** in a **triangular** course around some **pea bone** and about a **large polygon** and a **small polygon** and the **head** having to be close to the **hammer** (the last of which we should all subscribe to).

Galeazzi Fracture

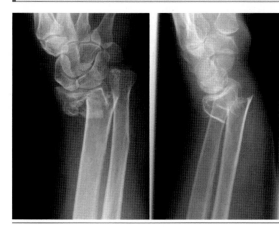

Fig. 14.**39** Faris has sustained a severe distal radial fracture and a dislocation of the distal ulna. This is a common fracture named after Galeazzi. If the ulna is fractured proximally and the capitulum of the radius is luxated, this is called a Monteggia fracture. The difference between the two can be remembered using the following if rather homespun and complicated memory hook:

Bella *ragazza* (Italian for "beautiful girl") – radius fracture (*Ra*) = Galeazzi (*gazza*).

Fracture of the Radial Head

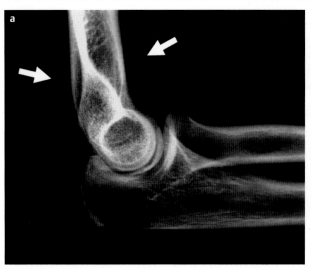

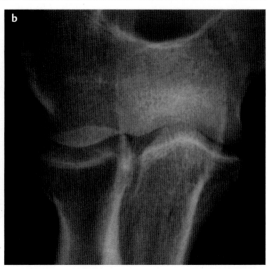

Fig. 14.**40 a** Thanh has an effusion in his elbow joint. The effusion lifts the fat pads normally located in the coronoid and olecranon fossa and adherent to the articular capsule out of hiding (arrows). When you see this positive fat-pad sign, the patient has an elbow fracture until proven otherwise, most likely of the radial head. **b** The anterior–posterior projection confirms the suspicion: There is a subtle step in the contour of the head on the ulnar side.

Shoulder Luxation

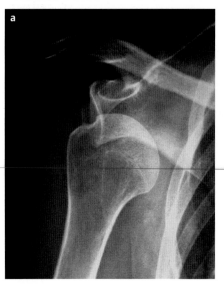

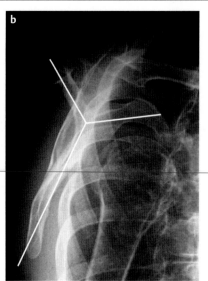

Fig. 14.**41 a** Mr. McClellan has an anterior shoulder dislocation, the most common type. **b** The tangential view of the scapula (also called Y- or "Mercedes star" view owing to the form of the scapula in this projection) shows the humeral head ventral and caudal to the glenoid, which is situated in the center of the Y. If the anterior instability is severe and recurrent, it often results in varying degrees of impression fracture of the dorsolateral circumference of the humeral head ("Hill–Sachs lesion," but subtle in Mr. McClellan's case). In addition, during dislocation, impact of the humerus on the bony anterior glenoid process of the scapula may occur ("Bankart lesion").

Medial Femoral Neck Fracture

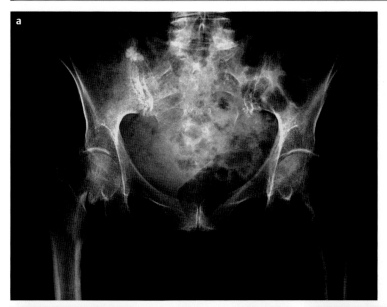

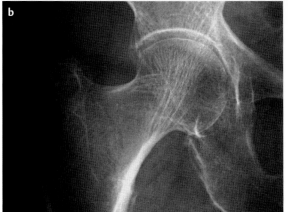

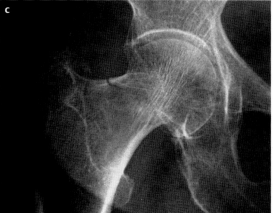

Fig. 14.**42 a** Nadine Rothman has suffered an injury quite typical for her age: a medial femoral neck fracture, which she is at risk for because of her osteoporosis. The fracture is classified according to its angle as Pauwels I–III (approx. 30°, 50°, and 70°). The more acute the angle of the fracture, the higher the degree of instability and the risk of avascular necrosis of the femoral head or pseudoarthrosis formation. What do you think of a Pauwels III in this case? A femoral neck fracture is not always so obvious. **b** In Mrs. Rothman's girlfriend, Anastasia, no fracture was found on the initial radiograph taken right after a fall and consecutive pain in the right hip. **c** A week later (the pain did not recede) the radiological diagnosis was clear. In such cases bone scintigraphy may also be helpful because it shows the increased bone turnover at a fracture site at an early stage when it might otherwise be invisible. MRI is more costly but would also show the bone bruise.

Unlucky Fellows

While on his daily walk through the Royal Botanic Garden this morning, retired stockbroker Rob McClellan lost his balance on slippery ground and fell on his shoulder. He has not been able to move his shoulder since (Fig. 14.**41**). His girlfriend Nadine Rothman tried to help him up but also fell on the slippery concrete. Now her right hip is painful and she cannot move her leg anymore (Fig. 14.**42a**). McClellan's grandson

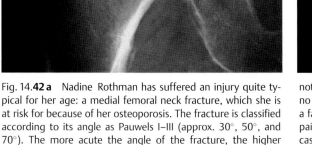

Philipp who had joined them for the walk, tried to come to their help on his inline-skaters at full speed and fell on his arm in the process of braking (Fig. 14.**43**). Hannah has a look at the radiographs of the pitiful bunch.

Greenstick Fracture

a   b

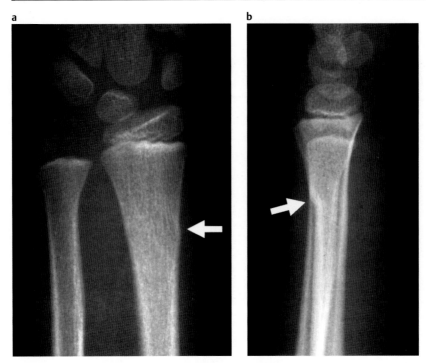

Fig. 14.**43**   In children the bone can break without seriously in-juring the periosteal cuff around it. This is called a greenstick fracture. Frequently the only sign is a little bulge of the cortex (arrow in **a** and **b**). Philipp has a greenstick fracture of the distal forearm, which will heal rapidly when sufficiently immobilized with a cast.

Femoral Shaft Fracture

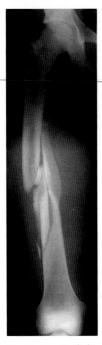

Surfing

The opportunities for avid surfers within the city are limited—but there are ways for the desperate and the airheaded. Hank and his friend Dude are a little bit of both, and to a dangerous degree. After partici-pating in the annual Mardi Gras parade, drunk as skunks, they surfed on the train coupling of the last suburban line to Bondi Junction and fell off at full speed. Fortunately, they were found quite quickly by some other nighthawks. Hank is lying apathetically on a vacuum mattress with his right thigh severely swollen (Fig. 14.**44**), Dude complains about pain in his right knee (Fig. 14.**45**) and left foot (Fig. 14.**46**). Han-nah reviews the films toward the end of her shift.

Fig. 14.**44**   Hank has suffered a comminuted fracture of the femoral shaft. The soft tissue shadow indicates a severe hema-toma and soft tissue injury.

Tibial Head Fracture

a

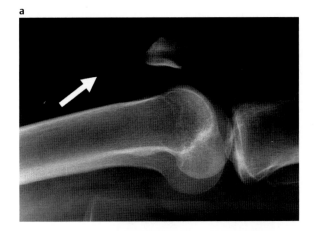

b   **c**

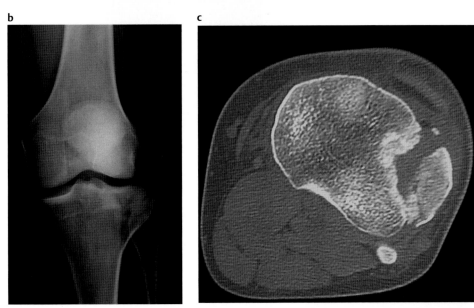

Fig. 14.**45 a**   The lateral radiograph already points to a fracture of the tibial head. The pronounced knee joint effusion in the suprapatellar bursa shows a fluid–fluid interface (arrow) indicating a suspended layer of fat, which proves the communication of the joint to the fatty bone marrow. (By the way, this image also helps to understand why life-threatening fat embolism can occur after fractures of large tubular bones.) Only CT could theoretically exclude a fracture in this setting with sufficient certainty. **b** The anterior–posterior radiograph clearly demonstrates the tibial fracture. **c** Before approaching this articular fracture, the surgeons often ask for a CT with 3D reconstructions to find out preoperatively which type of screws should be put in and where. The reconstruction of the articular surface is crucial for the treatment result.

Ankle Joint Fracture

a   b   c

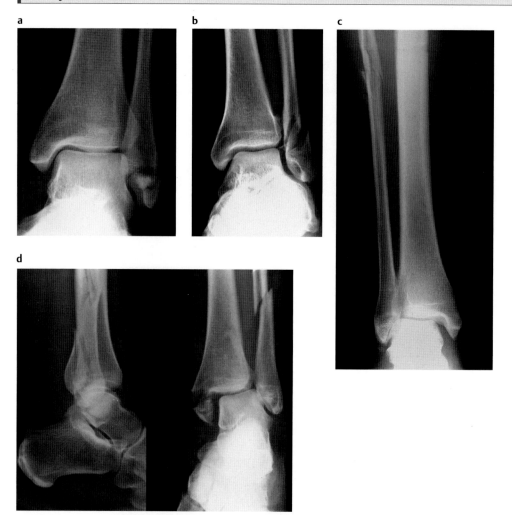

d

e

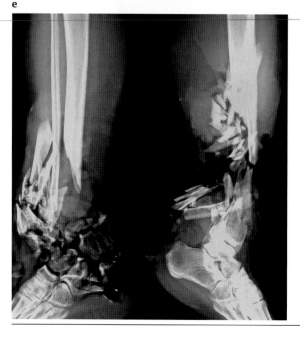

Fig. 14.**46**   Dude has suffered a fracture of his left lateral ankle. These fractures are classified according to Weber. The important issue is the involvement of the distal fibulotibial syndesmosis: If it is torn, the bony fork of the lateral and medial ankle that is tightly fitted around the talus becomes dysfunctional, giving the talus a lot more slack. **a** The fibular fracture of the Weber A type that Dude has suffered is located distal to the syndesmosis. The syndesmosis and the upper ankle joint are thus intact. **b** With a fibular fracture of the Weber B type, the syndesmosis is involved and loses its stability. **c** The fibular injury of the Weber C type is a fracture proximal to the syndesmosis, which is, however, also disrupted. If the Weber C-type fracture is located very high in the proximal fibula, that is, outside of the region normally imaged for an ankle joint problem, it is called a Maisonneuve fracture. The syndesmosis is also torn in this fracture type. Note the widened medial joint space of the upper ankle joint. **d** In addition, the medial ankle and the dorsal tibial edge ("Volkmann-triangle") can also be fractured. **e** How dangerous surfing metropolitan trains can be is documented by these radiographs of an equally careless but considerably less fortunate peer of Hank and Dude.

14.3 Hannah's Test

Hannah is just about to leave the trauma imaging unit as Greg turns the corner. "Where is everybody?" he asks Hannah in despair. "Giufeng, Joey, Ajay, Paul—they all seem to have left. Probably hitting the student pubs and gargling ale by now. Typical!" Greg complains. "No-one to play with, is that it, Gregory?" grins Hannah. "Actually I'm really on my way myself but you could do me a favor and run through these cases with me (Fig. 14.**47**), before I go to Giufeng's party." Gregory pales. "Now don't tell me you don't know of the party, Greg!" Gregory gives a deep sigh and collapses into the seat in front of the viewbox. "Good lord, Greg, this seems to be really serious. Have you been misbehaving?" Gregory waves his hand weakly. "Come on, Greg. Be tough. This is an academic department, remember? Let's do these cases and then you can simply come along with me." Hannah taps his shoulder.
Go ahead and help Gregory! He and Hannah really want to get going to this private beach party.

One Truly International Colleague Who Made a Dent in Trauma Survival

Geoffrey Jefferson was a Manchester-born neurosurgeon who worked in St. Petersburg during World War I, where he served in the Anglo-Russian Hospital, a gift of the British Empire to the Russian ally. Obviously he gained a lot of experience with severe trauma during that time. He became a skeptic witness of the 1917 communist October revolution. He earlier practiced in Canada where his wife came from; later in the war he worked in France. He described the typical fracture of the atlas in 1920. One of his wise sayings comes in handy to end this book:

"Material gains play a small role in life's equation. The great advantage is to be allowed to work with things you enjoy."

Test Cases

a This patient cannot move his arm after a fall.

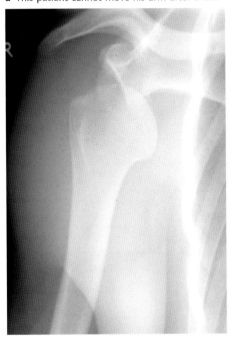

b This history is withheld, but we still want the complete diagnosis.

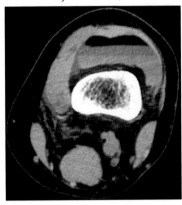

c This patient came straight off the highway and is in shock.

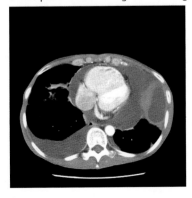

Fig. 14.**47** ▶

Test Cases

d This patient has just been brought in by helicopter.

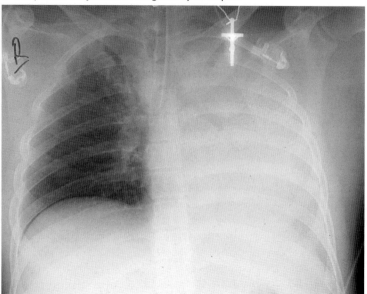

e Question: Cervical fracture?

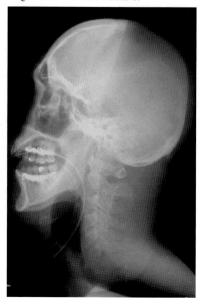

f This child was brought in comatose by the parents.

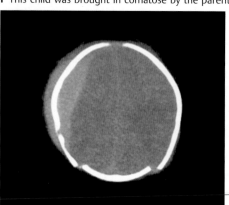

g This patient had a high-speed motor vehicle accident and the chest radiograph was abnormal.

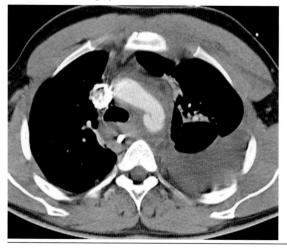

h Unspecific abdominal pain of two weeks' duration.

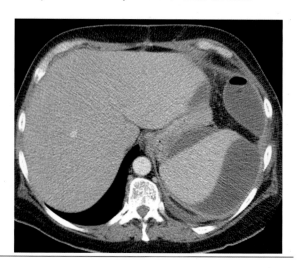

Test Cases

i–l This is the great wrapper-upper case of this book. Observe, analyze, reason, remember, discuss, and reach a comprehensive diagnosis! All images belong to one patient. Go one by one. Take your time. Write us an email (george.w.eastman@thieme.com) if you made it. Good luck!

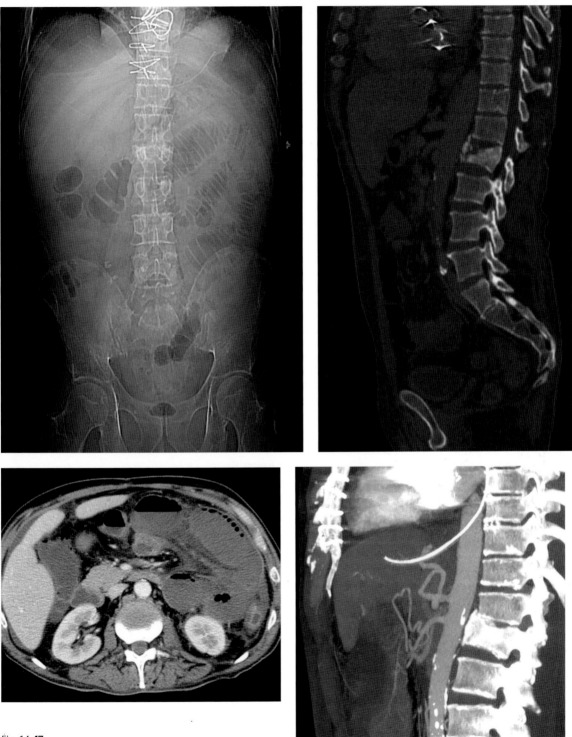

Fig. 14.**47**

Solutions to the Test Cases

Chapter 6

Fig. 6.**76** **a** This is a type B aortic dissection—the dissection is limited to the descending aorta. The false lumen can be distinguished from the true lumen by residual fiber strands connecting the intimal flap to the media. The true lumen is the smaller lumen—which shows more contrast enhancement in this case. **b** There is a large tumor in the anterior mediastinum. The trachea is narrowed down to a "saber sheath" configuration. In an acute setting, such as in this case with upper venous congestion, a lymphoma is the most likely cause. A large retrosternal goiter could produce a similar appearance. **c** This CT image shows massively dilated bronchi over all lung fields. This is severe bronchiectasis in cystic fibrosis. **d** The redistribution, the Kerley lines, an accentuated horizontal fissure, unsharp vascular markings, "bronchial cuffing," and an enlarged heart prove a cardiogenic pulmonary edema. **e** The thick-walled cavern in the right lung apex occurred in an HIV-positive patient—this is tuberculosis until proven otherwise. Tuberculosis it turned out to be. What would you do next if you saw this patient? Of course, for starters you would make sure the patient had a face mask. **f** The radiograph depicts a pneumonia of the right upper lobe and some of the middle lobe. The bronchi are well seen against the background of the pus-filled alveoli. **g** The severely increased interstitial markings in the periphery (Kerley lines) and centrally (reticular or netlike pattern) suggest an interstitial process. The HRCT (**right**) confirms the thickened interlobular septa in a patient with carcinomatosis of the pulmonary interstitium. **h** The left lung is overly transparent, hypovascular, and volume-reduced in this patient. He suffered from recurring pulmonary infections in early childhood until the age of 12. Right—this is Swyer–James syndrome.

Chapter 7

Where and when should the informed consent of the patient be achieved? This should best be done the day before the study, either in the office or on the ward but never where and when the study is performed. Which parameters should be watched? Prothrombin time should be >50%, partial thromboplastin time <35 seconds, and thrombocyte count >50 000/μl. Acetylsalicylic acid (ASA/aspirin) should be discontinued a week before deep-body interventions are performed.

Here is the great case: Figure 7.**18a** shows a close up view of the ribs. The infracostal margins are very irregular—they are being remodeled by the enlarged and varicose intercostal arteries in aortic coarctation. Compare this to the normal ribs of Fig. 6.**5a**. As the aorta is stenosed in this entity (see the sagittal T1-weighted MR; **b**), the descending aorta is filled via intercostal collaterals and via arteries in the abdominal wall (see the MR angiography; **c**). After the insertion of a stent (see the conventional angiography; **d**), the stenosis is reduced to a moderate level without the risks of open chest surgery (see the sagittally reconstructed CT; **e**).

Chapter 8

Fig. 8.**83** **a** There is malalignment at the C4/C5 level much like the degenerative spondylolisthesis seen in the lumbar spine. Ventral osteophytes and disk space narrowing in the lower cervical spine support the notion of a degenerative cause. **b** The C2 vertebral body in this man has turned sclerotic: this is an osteoblastic metastasis of a prostate carcinoma. **c** The hand appears demineralized in comparison to the radial metaphysis. The soft tissues appear to be swollen. This was Sudeck disease. Remember: The clinical symptoms must fit! **d** The width of the radiocarpal joint space is diminished radially. The bordering bone is sclerosed. The scaphoid shows a little osteophyte, the lunate seems a little out of line. This is a posttraumatic osteoarthritis and lunate malalignment. **e** This is a patient with ankylosing spondylitis: both iliosacral joints appear to be fused, more so on the right. **f** They do not come more pathognomonic than this: a gigantic chondrosarcoma engulfs the right half of the pelvis. **g** This is a typical nonossifying fibroma—no further measures are needed. **h** Right. This is an osteoid osteoma of the talus. **i** It is a severe inherited osteosclerosis of the Camurati–Engelmann type. **j** The patient suffers from multiple myeloma. **k** The os lunatum shows a dense inhomogeneous structure. You are looking at an osteonecrosis of the lunatum, also termed Kienboeck disease. It is a little sister of the femoral head necrosis. If you diagnosed this by yourself, either you are a genius or you have leafed through one of those fat books on skeletal radiology. In either case—congratulations! **l** This patient suffers from low back pain. Paget's disease of the sacral bone is the diagnosis.

Chapter 9

Fig. 9.**70** **a** This is a carcinoma of the hypopharynx that originates from the piriform recess. **b** Sentinel loops in the small intestine with air–fluid levels at different heights point to a mechanical (obstructive) ileus. **c** This is a diverticulosis of the descending colon. **d** A scrotal hernia is present bilaterally. **e** Did you diagnose the splenic cyst alright? **f** This is the radiograph of a neonate without any air in the stomach and small intestine. This is a definite sign of esophageal atresia. **g** This is what a tapeworm looks like in a barium study. **h** This patient suffers from chronic pancreatitis. **i** Have you recognized the liver metastases and the ascites? **j** Did you notice that most air is in the small bowel but none in the distant colon and rectum? Did you also see the dilated air-filled loops of the proximal colon? This a cecal volvulus! Some contrast media rests in the bowel are also appreciated. **k** This is a cecal volvulus. **l** This patient was referred from a mental institution because he had ingested something. What material might it be? (It was mercury taken from an old thermometer.) **m** No excuses if you did not get this one: It is a severe gangrene of small and large bowel due to mesenteral infarction. **n** Now this one was for the real eggheads: Contrast is in the vena cava and the liver veins, but not in the aorta. Two theoretical possibilities that one can think of: (a) This is remote: the contrast is given via a vein of the lower extremities—that would never give you that solid filling of the ves-

the venous return of the kidneys would mix in. (b) This is the solution: The patient has severe right heart insufficiency so the contrast flows through the superior vena cava past the heart right into the inferior cava and the liver veins. Of course, the contrast is given via the veins of the arm, as almost always. And, by the way, some people call this the "playboy bunny" sign. **o** This patient felt uneasy after a long flight as a "body packer." The sealed drug packages were swallowed before the flight. A leakage of the containers, of course, means serious health trouble for the poor fellow.

Chapter 10

Fig. 10.**21   a** This is a pelvic kidney with a renal cell carcinoma. **b** Here you see a posttraumatic priapism. The pubic symphysis is torn, the left iliosacral joint is opened: The configuration is also called an "open book" injury. The genitals are enlarged owing to hemorrhage, thrombosis, or edema. **c** This is what a calcified transplant kidney looks like. **d** There is a tumor thrombus that has grown through the vena cava into the right atrium. This patient had a renal carcinoma. **e** Did you diagnose the renal hematoma alright? **f** Did you detect the concrement in the left kidney? This is nephrolithiasis. **g** The lesion in the kidney is a manifestation of lymphoma. If you appreciated the tumor in the mesentery ventral to the aorta you probably got it right. If you overlooked that tumor, remember the "satisfaction of search" effect (Chapter 3).

Chapter 11

Fig. 11.**57   a** There is a C7 diskal prolapse on the left that significantly compresses the spinal nerve. **b** This coronal MR image of the lumbar spine at the level of the kidneys shows an extra-axial, intrathecal tumor—a typical meningioma. The tumor has expanded the spinal canal **c** This spinal canal is extremely narrow owing to a congenital stenosis. **d** A right foraminal prolapse is seen on this CT. **e** If you have not detected it yet, take a step back! The left basal ganglia are hypodense—an early infarction may not become more obvious. CT perfusion would make the diagnosis a lot easier to reach. But there is no hemorrhage: thrombolytic treatment could start. **f** This dense media sign is pretty obvious: this is an early infarction of the right hemisphere. **g** This CT shows a frontal intracranial hemorrhage in combination with extreme edema.

Chapter 12

Fig. 12.**29   a** What you are seeing is a typical plasma cell mastitis. **b** The breast carcinoma (left image, large arrows) shows pronounced acoustic shadowing (right image small arrows).

Chapter 13

Fig. 13.**30**   The 48 is an impacted wisdom tooth; the 28 tooth has come through. A granuloma is visible at the root of the 45 tooth. The bridge between 25 and 27 is intact; the bridge anchored on tooth 14 reaches out into nothing. The crown of tooth 16 is broken and ground down. There are root fillings in tooth 16 and 35. Superimposed over 42–44 a sialolith is visualized sitting in the main duct of the submandibular gland.

Chapter 14

Fig. 14.**47   a** You are seeing a typical caudal shoulder luxation. You should now worry about impression fractures or avulsions of the glenoid. **b** Now this should have been so easy. If you did not diagnose this tibial head fracture by its indirect signs, go back and check Fig. 4.**4b**. This is the Dutch flag sign—this time in CT. **c** Extensive pericardial and pleural hemorrhage in a traumatized patient: an immediate chest intervention is necessary. **d** The tip of the tracheal tube sits in the right main bronchus. A complete atelectasis of the left lung has resulted. Thank god you were the one to analyze the image—you did get this one right, didn't you? **e** This is a cephalad malposition of the tube. Severe injury to the glottis will result. **f** A scalp hematoma and a subdural hematoma with severe edema was diagnosed in this young child. In not so clear trauma in children, always exclude battered child. **g** This is a posttraumatic aortic dissection (see the flap?) with left-sided hemothorax. **h** Two weeks after abdominal trauma this patient presented with pain—a delayed spleen rupture is present. **i, j, k, l** This was your chance to prove you've understood it all, you know how to reason, and you are just a little lucky. The scout view of the abdominal CT **(i)** displays an air-filled dilated loop of small bowel in the mid-abdomen. Note: A vertical beam is used in normal scout views, so air–fluid levels would not show. There is a definite problem of bowel peristalsis. The axial CT image **(j)** confirms the dilated small bowel and finds little air bubbles in the intestinal wall—the "string of pearls" sign. A necrosis of the bowel wall is most likely present. The sagittal reconstruction of the trauma spiral CT **(k)** tells you why the patient came to the hospital in the first place. The L2 vertebral body has been crushed in a deceleration trauma. What else might have happened in the process? The last CT reconstruction **(l)** wraps it all up: The trauma impact caused the L2 fracture and a dissection of the superior mesenteric artery, which led to the bowel necrosis, which was at the base of the developing ileus. Now go through the timewarp back to the first image **(i)** and search for the "string of pearls" and the fracture in that image—it was all our forefathers had for diagnosis.

Post Scriptum

Our group of students has meanwhile left us, of course, and others are now in their shoes. We have, however, not forgotten this bright bunch and have kept an eye on their fate inside the global village with curiosity.

For starters, there is Paul—our born "mother's-milk" radiologist. He has actually started ENT training in Melbourne. In addition, he runs an internet shop specialized in French lingerie together with his brother. The shop's illustrated homepage and special sale event e-mails keep the department amused. We are not really worried about his future.

Giufeng has moved to Stockholm, of all places, where she is getting ready to move into neuroradiology at the Karolinska Institute. Her last postcard from the subpolar city of Hammerfest also bore the signature of a certain Ingmar, igniting fantasies in some members of the CT team. People remember her for her pleasant, easygoing personality.

Ajay is still looking around in the United States for a good residency program. He has also toured Canada and Europe and might consider the Charité in Berlin. But then again his wife has not decided yet.

Some knew it all along but chose to keep it to themselves. First a postcard from Joey arrives in the angio section. It is from Boston, where Joey has paused during a sightseeing trip through New England at the end of which he plans to visit his grandparents on Martha's Vineyard. The French croissants at Harvard Square really are something, he writes. Is that special research slot in angiography is still open? Chief Waginaw promises to check.

A week later another postcard showing a stunning sundown at Niagara Falls reaches the bone section. Hello to everyone and she is feeling terrific, writes Hannah. Both pieces of information find their way to the department's coffee counter, where little imagination is needed to get the whole picture: Those two who would have thought? Hannah has, of course, already gotten herself a job with the trauma surgeons. How she did it nobody knows, but the surgeons sure got themselves a great young colleague.

OK, what else? Well, let's not forget about Greg, who also gets what he deserves: The chairman has asked him to apply for an assistant professorship. Life is tough on some, Gregory!

Index

Note: page numbers in *italics* refer to figures and tables